Health
and
Health
Care
in
Developing
Countries

Temple University Press

Philadelphia

Health
and
Health
Care
in
Developing
Countries

Sociological Perspectives

EDITED BY

Peter Conrad
and
Eugene B. Gallagher

Temple University Press, Philadelphia 19122
Copyright © 1993 by Temple University. All rights reserved
Published 1993
Printed in the United States of America

The paper used in this publication meets the minimum
requirements of American National Standard for Information
Sciences—Permanence of Paper for Printed Library Materials,
ANSI Z39.48–1984   ∞

Library of Congress Cataloging-in-Publication Data

Health and health care in developing countries : sociological
perspectives / edited by Peter Conrad and Eugene B.
Gallagher.
    p.   cm.
    Includes bibliographical references and index.
    ISBN 1–56639–027–3 (cl. : alk. paper)
 1. Social medicine—Developing countries.   I. Conrad, Peter,
1945–   . II. Gallagher, Eugene B.
    [DNLM: 1. Developing Countries.   2. Health Services.
3. Sociology.   WA 395 H4324]
RA418.3.D48H43   1993
362.1′09172′4—dc20
DNLM/DLC
for Library of Congress   92-49629

Contents

Introduction

PETER CONRAD *and*
EUGENE B. GALLAGHER

Disease and infirmity are universal problems, and all societies have developed means by which to attempt to control or influence the health and illness of their members. Most societies have developed some type of indigenous "health system," and many have designated healing specialists.

During the era of colonization, European medicine—usually in the person of medical missionaries—was exported to the colonies in an effort to spread European culture and religion and to pacify the natives (Comaroff 1992). Because the colonials' economic and political interests far outweighed their medical ones, Western medicine had a limited impact. Although the specifics varied by society, when the former colonies emerged as independent nations in the post–World War II period, they were often left with some amalgam of very limited Western medicine alongside traditional forms of indigenous healing. In the past three decades, however, the influence of Western medicine has penetrated these developing societies, often with the help of governments and international donor organizations. In most developing societies now we find complex health systems (Kleinman 1980), often manifesting dilemmas between the Western and traditional health care sectors (Zeichner 1988).

The health problems in these Third World or developing countries are enormous. Enhanced sanitation and public health measures, especially vaccination, have improved health in some developing societies in recent years; yet disease remains endemic and devastating in many others. Amplified by a lack of safe water and inadequate nutrition, infectious disease rates in many countries are very high. This is especially evident in the high infant mortality from such diseases as diarrheal disease, measles, neonatal tetanus, whooping cough, and malaria (UNICEF

1990, 17). Infant mortality rates range from 147 per 1,000 births in Malawi, 116 in Bangladesh, 51 in Ecuador, to 44 in Egypt, compared with 7 to 12 in most Western developed countries. The life expectancy in developing countries ranges from the mid-forties in many African countries to the mid-sixties in most Latin American countries; this is compared with the mid-seventies for most developed countries (USAID 1990).

Western medicine is making an impact on the developing world, especially in terms of public health and the training of tens of thousands of doctors. In' countries like Mexico and Pakistan, however, thousands of physicians are unemployed in the cities, largely because many do not want to work in rural areas and the urban medical system cannot economically absorb them. Many countries still relegate the majority of their medical resources to urban areas, even though the highest rates of disease occur among rural peoples. While doctor-centered Western curative medicine is often exported to developing countries, limited health dollars may be better spent training community primary health workers than doctors.

Although it is sometimes useful to lump societies together as "developing," there is a huge range in the development of these countries. On the more developed end are the newly industrialized countries, such as Korea, Taiwan, and Singapore, with per capita gross national products (GNPs) of about $8,000; on the other end are some of the poorest countries in the world, such as Ethiopia, Chad, and Bangladesh, with per capita GNPs of $150. There is also great variety in terms of size (e.g., China and Haiti), history of colonialism (e.g., India and Nepal), and type of government (e.g., Cuba, Saudi Arabia, and Costa Rica), as well as location, religion, population, age structure, and so forth. For the most part, what these developing countries have in common is that they tend to be non-Western (except for Latin American countries) and in the early 1960s had very little industry and were generally economically poor. As these countries have developed in different directions and at different rates, the range of development among them is now much greater than in 1960. But the vast majority of these countries remain poor; in 1987 over sixty of these countries still had a per capita GNP of less than one thousand dollars (World Bank 1989).

It is not clear that Western development strategies, including modern biomedicine, are always appropriate in Third World situations. Contemporary industrial societies historically shifted from agricultural to industrial production and from rural to urban settlement before modern medicine and public health had substantially reduced the burden of infectious disease and lengthened life expectancy. Illness and early death were dreaded but expected and accepted. The developing nations now face a more demanding set of conditions, expectations, and challenges. Many wrestle with poverty, overpopulation, and disrupted patterns of community life. In the face of numerous obstacles, they must modernize in health care even as they shift to factory production, expand educational opportunity, and provide services for the burgeoning urban populations. In addition to rising expectations for longevity and general health, there are rising expectations for recovery from chronic diseases and disabilities. Health care, however, like other "modern" projects such as mass communication and highway construction, cannot be introduced in isolation, apart from a so-called infrastructure that includes administrative know-how, cultural resources (e.g., literacy), and a supportive physical environment—all of which are scarce. Many Third World countries are also distracted by ethnic and religious factionalism, which retards health care's progress along with much else.

Because the administrative structures of health care are still being laid down in the developing world, the influence of rational planning on health policy—bureaucratic initiatives implemented from the center outward, such the World Health Organization's "Health for All by the Year 2000" (HFA/2000)—is critically important. Yet in sharp contrast to the ultramodern spirit of biomedical health planning, traditional medicine—its theories of illness, practitioners, and remedies—remains as much more than a vestigial element in Third World health care. The range and complexity of health phenomena in the developing world are great; but it seems clear, in countries that can afford it, that Western medicine is becoming the ideal and standard of medical care.

Drift toward Medical Dominance in Third World Health Care

Recent trends of thought in the Third World have considered the history of health care development in the industrialized world with ambivalence. Developing countries want to emulate the health care accomplishments of the West, yet they are also determined not to repeat mistakes made there. This new thinking has called into question both the centrality of the physician's role and the relevance that clinical medicine oriented to the individual patient has for alleviating the major health problems faced by these societies: inadequate sanitation, infectious disease, high infant–child mortality, and a lack of family planning.

Similar questions can be raised about the place of clinical medicine in developed societies. Although life expectancy is higher and the burden of chronic disease heavier in developed societies, many of their health problems cannot be addressed by clinical medicine. For example, widespread respiratory disease attributable to tobacco use is more a challenge to health educators and public health authorities than to doctors. Other so-called life-style diseases or conditions, such as obesity and hypertension, are apt targets for preventive rather than clinical medicine (Levine and Lilienfeld 1987). But clinical medicine is so strongly entrenched and such an essential feature of modern society that searching questions about its relevance and limits are largely confined to a small band of "critics of medicine" (which includes, incidentally, a number of medical sociologists).

Medical dominance is not yet an established fact in Third World societies. The health care system is still in a formative flux. For example, many health planners, including social scientists and public health physicians, wish to curtail the production of physicians in favor of other professionals—nurse-midwives and community health workers, for example—who are trained to meet the needs of the populace with preventive resources, rather than concentrate on the curative needs of the national upper class. The goal is to democratize the health care provider labor structure, as well as to widen the distribution of health care. This is seen as a way of avoiding the mistakes of the developed societies, which allowed the medical profession to assume an inordinately important role in carrying out health care.

The foregoing health care ideology has been important in the programmatic thinking of many developing countries (Bryant 1969). It has not, however, dissuaded most of them from investing in medical care, organization, and education modeled closely on the West's. Given the limited resources of most developing societies, the investment has often been substantial.

The health policy debate discussed here can be phrased as a question of whether a health system should emphasize the role of clinical medicine and individual physicians or community and preventive medical resources—or what kind of balance to strike between the two. There are great opportunities here for social scientists to make significant contributions to understanding and even shaping health care in the developing world.

Medical Sociology and the Developing World

Social science research has already contributed significantly to our understanding of health and health care in the developing world. A perusal of the literature, however, reveals that it is overwhelmingly anthropologists, epidemiologists, international health planners, and physicians who are researching and writing on these issues. Indeed, anthropologists have been working in the "international health" arena for decades (Foster 1982). Specific medical sociological work in this area can rarely be found.

Over the past three decades, medical sociologists have developed a base of concepts and research tools for looking at health and health care phenomena in industrialized societies. This base includes studies of illness behavior; the sick role; doctor–patient relationships; health professional socialization; the organization of health services; medicalization; the social production of disease; the experience of illness; the relation of stress and social support to health; the effects of race, class, and gender on health and disease; the impact of medical technology; and the health care system as part of total societies. Sociological research depends upon many sources and methods: interviews, ethnographic observation, patient biographies and diaries, official documents, survey questionnaires, health care utilization statistics, health care personnel inventories, economic reports, and clinical studies.

With very few exceptions, however, medical sociologists have neglected the study of developing societies. This is not unique to medical sociology; as Alejandro Portes notes, "A major gap . . . exists between theoretical perspectives chosen by modern sociology and the recurrent dilemmas and restrictions faced by the non-industrialized world" (1976, 51). Western sociology often demonstrates parochialism and ethnocentrism, with sociologists assuming that concepts derived in a Western context can be universally applied (Smith 1990). In some instances, Western sociological concepts may not be appropriate for examining developing societies (e.g., the sick role or compliance may be Western constructs); by contrast, research on developing societies would likely enrich and broaden many of our Western-based sociological conceptualizations. This would force us to reexamine our knowledge in a global sense, while simultaneously shedding a fresh light on health dilemmas in the Third World.

Over the years a few articles by sociologists on health and development have appeared in journals such as *Social Science and Medicine* and *International Journal of Health Services* or in special monographs (e.g., Zeichner 1988), but these have remained on the periphery of medical sociology. A few medical sociologists, such as Ray Elling and Howard Waitzkin, have consistently examined health problems in a Third World context, but they are obvious exceptions. In the last few years, however, there have been signs that this may be changing. The fourth edition of the *Handbook of Medical Sociology* contained a chapter on "Health Care in Developing Countries" (Najman 1989), and in 1989 a special issue of *Journal of Health and Social Behavior* was dedicated to "Sociological Studies of Third World Health and Health Care."

Two of the goals of this book are to draw attention to the significance of medical sociology for understanding Third World health problems and to show how examining developing societies may necessitate reframing or modifying some of our standard sociological notions. We believe that sociological perspectives can be useful in understanding health and health care in the developing world. It seems likely that unless medical sociologists become serious about examining health issues in comparative or Third World contexts, much of our accumulated knowledge will prove irrelevant for most of the world. It would be regrettable if medical sociology were to become an artifact limited to American or Western societies; after forty years of disciplinary development, medical sociology would seem to have a great deal to offer and productive interchange to gain.

Overview of the Book

Our selections for this book were slanted toward papers we saw as conceptual, empirical, and sociological. Most of the contributors are sociologists; and although a couple of papers were contributed by anthropologists, the issues they addressed or perspectives they used are broadly sociological.

The Social Production of Disease

Evidence from Western societies has suggested that social factors may have had a greater impact than medical factors historically on the reduction of infectious disease (McKinlay and McKinlay 1977). Therefore it is not surprising that social factors may be fundamentally involved with the production of disease.

The two chapters in Part I examine the social production of disease in diverse Third World contexts. In the context of the worldwide epidemic of acquired immunodeficiency syndrome (AIDS), Charles W. Hunt examines the development and spread of AIDS in Africa. He challenges the commonly held notion that AIDS originated in Africa and, more importantly, presents a persuasive analysis of the emergence of a particular pattern of AIDS in Africa. While in the United States the epidemiological pattern of the disease has involved predominantly men and homosexuals, in Africa it consists equally of male and female heterosexuals. The variance in risk pattern suggests that different social forces may be abetting the transmission of the human immunodeficiency virus (HIV). By examining the geographic patterns of the disease, Hunt locates the transmission of HIV specifically in the migratory labor system found in Africa. He contends this system creates long absences from home and family breakdown, promoting prostitution and sexually transmitted diseases. Although the virus may be the same in the West and the Third World, the social production of disease in developing countries is different and devastating.

Rita S. Gallin's chapter focuses on Taiwan, a more developed Third World society. Like Hunt, she shows how the social organization of the economy can affect health and illness, but her lens focuses specifically on a community. Using ethnographic methods, Gallin studied a rural village where married women with children were central to the labor force. Despite long work hours and conflicts between responsibilities at work and home, which under some conditions would make women more susceptible to disease, she found the women to be markedly healthy. Because this contradicts to a degree the predictions of stress theories, Gallin examines the social production of good health. She finds that in the context of traditional family values and the developing Taiwanese economy, the meaning work has in the local culture seems to have engendered a type of social resistance to disease among these women.

Seeking Medical Care

The social context has an important effect on if, when, and how people seek medical care (and, as noted in the Part III, what type of care they seek). Medical sociologists have examined illness behavior, help-seeking, and utilization to try better to understand the process of seeking medical aid. These issues are also significant in a Third World context, although the parameters may be quite different. The two chapters in Part II examine specific ways the social context affects seeking medical help.

Peter Conrad presents an analysis from a study of the use of emergency medical services in urban Indonesia. In the first place, the very notion of "emergency" regarding a health situation is a Western concept. Many non-Western societies do not necessarily conceptualize events of illness or injury as emergencies that need immediate attention. In the second place, as Conrad shows, only about 7 percent of cases coming to the four emergency departments his group studied could be classified as medical emergencies. Thus, in a manner similar to Western countries, the emergency department is used frequently for primary and nonurgent care. One of the most interesting findings in this study was a transportation issue: only a tiny fraction of trauma patients arrived by ambulance, yet three-fourths of the "emergency" patients arrived within an hour. How is it that most patients arrive so quickly, and what does that mean in terms of investing in "modernizing" the system with spiffy ambulances and an emergency medical services (EMS) system? Conrad concludes his chapter with a reflection on some of the dilemmas of conducting sociomedical research in a Third World context.

In Chapter 4, Stella R. Quah examines the link between ethnicity and health behavior in Singapore. Singapore is a multiethnic island republic that has Chinese, Indian, and Malay populations. Like Taiwan, Singapore has developed rapidly in the past two decades, although there has been uneven development among ethnic groups. Focusing on behavioral and life-style risk factors for heart disease and cancer and using data collected in a stratified random interview study, Quah discusses how ethnic factors especially affect preventive attitudes and behavior. The Malays showed a stronger inclination toward prevention than the Chinese or Indians; Quah shows how religious and cultural values underlie this preventive orientation (although this is not without interesting contradictions; for instance, Malay men are known to have the highest percentage of smokers). The preventive orientation has a payoff: the Malays have lower mortality rates from cancer and heart disease. As Quah notes, even in the context of rapid modernization, ethnic factors still have a significant impact on life and death.

Traditional and Modern Medicines

In virtually all developing societies, before the introduction of Western medicine indigenous or traditional medicine flourished. In some cases, such as India or China, traditional medicine was highly developed and systematized; in others, local groups had healers who gained their knowledge from other healers. Although traditional medicines varied in their ability to affect health and disease, they were intertwined with culture and usually offered explanations and comfort, even when they were unable to reshape the course of disease.

When Western medicine was first introduced into these cultures, some expected that the apparent technical superiority of modern medical interventions would cause traditional medicine eventually to wither away. But this has not been the case: traditional medicine still thrives and, in some situations, competes favorably with modern medicine.

The two chapters in Part III reflect the relationship between traditional and modern medicine. Janardan Subedi and Sree Subedi examine the case of Nepal, where the introduction of modern medicine was relatively recent. They describe a medical system that includes folk, traditional, and modern medicines; as the authors note, despite international assistance and government support, modern medicine has not achieved universal acceptance. It remains a "foreign" medicine, more expensive than and culturally distant from traditional medicine. Thus the medical system remains "incompletely differentiated" and pluralistic, with three legitimate and competing medical systems providing services. As in other studies, Subedi and Subedi find that patients use traditional and modern medicine at different points in an illness career and for different problems.

In Chapter 6, Collins O. Airhihenbuwa and Ira E. Harrison argue that it is commonly believed that traditional medical practitioners can (and should) learn from modern medicine and become more effective healers. Using the example of Nigeria, they suggest that this knowledge flow— from modern to traditional—needs to be more of an interchange, creating a reciprocity between traditional and allopathic concepts. They show the utility of some of the long-established traditional medical treatment concepts, which could be adopted by modern medicine. Because consumers already use both services, the authors contend that medical providers need to offer some integration, particularly in terms of causality concepts and the context of local culture. This two-way technical and cultural interchange would enhance both medicines and, more importantly, the health services available to people in developing societies.

Modern Medicine in Developing Societies

The three chapters in Part IV, by Eugene B. Gallagher, Joseph W. Schneider, and Mary-Jo DelVechhio Good and associates, look at the ways in which supposedly standard features of modern medicine are modified when they are taken into developing societies. The three features considered here are medical education, the hospital care of patients, and doctors' communication with patients about disease. The developing societies are, respectively, the United Arab Emirates, China, and Mexico (although the chapter by Good and her colleagues also deals with the United States and Japan).

The reader will note that we qualify these features as *supposedly* standard. The issue behind that qualification is whether the given feature of modern medicine under inspection is indeed standard. It is not difficult to assert that a Gambro hemodialyzer or the bacterium *Vibrio cholerae* is the same whether found in North America or Kenya. But can we say as much for medical education, hospital care of patients, and doctors' communication with patients? The latter features of modern medicine do vary from one place to another. The variations might be thought of as empirical variations around a central, ideal type—perhaps random variations, or perhaps variations induced by cultural or environmental forces. Another way to think about such variations, however, setting aside the notion of an ideal type, is to say that when a feature of biomedicine moves from a place or society of origin to another place or society of destination, it may be changed—modified, transformed, skewed, deformed, improved—by its introduction into a different social environment.

Although these are abstract, partly semantic questions of concern to sociologists who wish to observe accurately and conceptualize clearly, they also capture issues that are important to real social actors in social situations, not only to sociologists. The reader may wish to keep these questions in mind as a critical viewpoint in reading these chapters. We use this viewpoint in summarizing them.

Gallagher's chapter deals with curriculum planning for a medical school in the United Arab Emirates and with the conceptions that the medical students there hold toward "being a doctor." The curriculum issue revolves around the question of whether the curriculum should take into account the health needs of the society, or whether it should strive for standards of scientific and clinical excellence embodied in Western medical education. According to Gallagher's observations of the particular school, the planners eventually decided to create a copy of Western medical education. The idea of a model or ideal was very much on their minds. They wanted to turn out students trained in this model, whose knowledge and skill would be acceptable anywhere in the world. This way of creating a new medical school diverges markedly from the priorities held by many educators and planners elsewhere in the Third World.

Educators as a rule believe that there are right and wrong ways to go about educating students. They will on occasion adhere strenuously to a model, resisting random or structured departures from the model, for the sake of their educational ideals. But what about the hospital care of patients, as Schneider describes it in China? Everyone agrees that patients everywhere should be made to feel as comfortable as possible during their stay; but does it matter whether it is a hospital orderly or the patient's relative who mops the floor around his or her bed and who carries a urine sample from the patient to a hospital lab?

Although there are dominant overall similarities between the purposes and functioning of American and Chinese hospitals, the role of relatives is far more circumscribed in American hospitals. Schneider's insightful study helps us to believe that the stronger Chinese role may derive from traditional Chinese values about the duties of family members toward one another, perhaps with the additional contemporary socialist blessing for proletarian everyday labor performed in a spirit of service.

Schneider's Chinese hospital carries out sophisticated, modern medical interventions, such as peritoneal dialysis, that are performed according to a universal standard (e.g., avoiding peritonitis by sterile procedure). But one can scarcely argue that the Chinese way of hospital care of patients is better or worse than the American way, or that either way is a closer approximation to *the* modern way of caring for patients.

In dealing with doctor–patient communications, Good, Linda Hunt, Tsunetsugu Munakata, and Yasuki Kobayashi examine another feature of modern medicine that displays great variation from one society to another. The specific question they deal with has no ideal solution: How does the physician inform the patient that he or she has cancer? They find that American physicians tend to be forthright, trying to encourage the patient's faith in the anticancer treatment regimens. The Japanese doctors tend to shield the patient from the bad news, yet they increasingly feel that they must tell the patient enough to promote the patient's interest in and compliance with treatment. The Mexican doctors tend toward assertive frankness. The authors tie the behavior of the Mexican physicians to the fact that, given Mexican underdevelopment, many of their patients are poor and uneducated; the physicians believe they must be blunt to get across to the patient.

The authors note that American medicine is a recognized world leader in anticancer technology. By extension, there is considerable interest outside the United States in American oncological practice, including communication with patients. This does not mean, however, that physicians elsewhere agree with American oncological approaches or that there is a universal standard for communication about the diagnosis.

The Sociopolitics of Health Care

In all countries—developed and developing—governments at national, provincial, and local levels can play an important part in regulating financing for and directly providing health care and in using state powers to maintain a healthful environment. In relation to this general paradigm, however, the actual pattern and content of governmental activity vary enormously from one nation to another.

Public expectations for health care have surged over recent decades because of greater recognition of the effectiveness of medicine, both preventive and curative. Third World governments have attempted to meet these expectations, but their performance often falls short of the intention and the promise. In Chapter 11, S. Ogoh Alubo shows the difficulties of establishing effective health care at local levels in Nigeria; Kenyon Rainier Stebbins presents a similar picture of Mexico in Chapter 10. The similarity is remarkable given the economic and social differences between the two countries.

In comparing the situations in Nigeria and Mexico, one gets the impression that Mexico is somewhat closer to the goal than Nigeria. Mexico's national independence and autonomy date back to some five decades before Nigeria's, and Mexico has closer integration (though still problematic) between medical education and health care delivery than does Nigeria.

Alubo and Stebbins also show the relevance of WHO's HFA/2000 as a broad strategy for health progress in developing countries. Their studies reveal, by ethnography and by the analysis of official documents, how the translation of health care strategy into health care reality becomes attenuated and sometimes corrupted. Both studies also suggest that the sociopolitical process is so ramified that even feeble or failed attempts to provide health care can become impervious to evaluation in terms of the worth of actual services provided.

Applying Sociological Knowledge in Health Settings

Readers familiar with the history of sociology will recall that many founders of sociology—pioneers such as Robert Park and Emile Durkheim—earnestly wanted it to contribute to the improvement of society. They believed that sociological investigations would bring the social evils of their era into a corrective illumination, leading to reform and human progress. Seventy years later, applied sociology is one of the American Sociological Association's most active interest areas. Many sociologists who have strong research interests in medical sociology are also concerned with the practical uses of knowledge about disease, health, and health care. Understandably, however, their concerns are directed toward health conditions in the United States. The thrust of this book takes us outside the United States while still maintaining the concern with application. Therefore the three chapters in Part VI take up the question of the relevance and application of sociology in Third World settings.

Chapter 12, by Carol J. Pierce Colfer and Eugene B. Gallagher, is set in Oman and compares birthing at home with lay midwife support and birthing in a regional hospital with professional services. The impetus to this study came from the observation that many Omani women, ignoring official encouragement, were reluctant to go the hospital for delivery. What could be done to increase hospital deliveries? By interviewing the midwives, Colfer learned much about home birth and came to see that it contrasted considerably with hospital birth, both in technique and in spirit. This research started out with a practical problem, formulated a practical approach to gather relevant information, and then ameliorated the problem by bringing the information to a relevant audience of professionals. The final phase of this application loop took the form of showing hospital staff that their unrelaxed, schedule-oriented approach to birth grated on the sensibilities of the Omani women.

Sally E. Findley's chapter analyzes the general research application paradigm, within which the Colfer–Gallagher research falls. Applied researchers will recognize the basic features of Findley's paradigm: an initial health problem, deficiency, or crisis that generates a felt need for social knowledge; the gathering of knowledge according to a feasible research strategy; and then a report, often with accompanying recommendations, to those caught up in the initial problem. But this description is a great oversimplification of the complex communication structure with which Findley deals precisely. She argues that, to increase their effectiveness, social scientists must leave behind the technical language of research and speak in the idiom of the professional or layperson, for whom their research results are intended. Even before that, the social scientist must have a clear conception of whom the recipient is; and, above all, the social scientist must not assume that research results will simply apply themselves in the field of action. Findley's chapter is a sustained exposition of the art and craft of applied research that many readers will, we believe, find to be a penetrating statement of a familiar subject, uncovering aspects about which they were not yet cognizant.

Medical sociologists often bewail what they see as a lack of conceptual bridging from general sociology into their specialty; they feel stranded on an island that is well stocked with solid empirical generalizations about the social causes of illness and the distribution of health resources, but poorly stocked with basic concepts. Gallagher's chapter, the last in the book, applies and tests the value of sociological concepts, especially those in modernization theory, for understanding health developments in the Third World. It looks at health care as a carrier of modernity and, on that basis, is able to account for phenomena such as the overconcentration of resources in the metropolitan areas—phenomena that may seem puzzling, if not perverse, according to a rational assessment of the needs of Third World societies.

REFERENCES

Bryant, Jack. 1969. *Health and the Developing World*. Ithaca, N.Y.: Cornell University Press.

Comaroff, Jean. 1992. "The Diseased Heart of Africa: Medicine, Colonialism and the Black Body." In *Ethnography and the Historical Imagination*, ed. John Comaroff and Jean Comaroff. Boulder, Colo.: Westview.

Foster, George M. 1982. "Applied Anthropology and International Health." *Human Organization* 41:189–97.

Gallagher, Eugene B., ed. 1989. Sociological Studies of Third World Health and Health Care (special single-topic issue). *Journal of Health and Social Behavior* 30 (4).

Kleinman, Arthur. 1980. *Patients and Healers in the Context of Culture*. Berkeley: University of California Press.

Levine, Sol, and Abraham Lilienfeld, eds. 1987. *Epidemiology and Health Policy*. New York: Tavistock.

McKinlay, John B., and Sonja McKinlay. 1977. "The Questionable Contribution of Medical Measures to the Decline of Mortality in the United States in the Twentieth Century." *Milbank Memorial Fund Quarterly* 55:405–28.

Najman, Jakob M. 1989. "Health Care in Developing Countries." In *Handbook of Medical Sociology*, 4th ed., ed. H. E. Freeman and Sol Levine, 1332–46. Englewood Cliffs, N.J.: Prentice-Hall.

Portes, Alejandro. 1976. "On the Sociology of National Development: Theories and Issues." *American Journal of Sociology* 82:55–85.

Smith, Harold E. 1990. "Sociology and the Study of Non-Western Societies." *American Sociologist* 21:150–63.

UNICEF. 1990. *The State of the World's Children*. New York: Oxford University Press (published for United Nations Children's Fund).

USAID. 1990. *Child Survival: A Fifth Report to Congress on the USAID Program*. Washington, D.C.: U.S. Agency for International Development.

World Bank. 1989. *World Bank Development Report 1989*. New York: Oxford University Press (published for the World Bank).

Zeichner, Christiane I., ed. 1988. *Modern and Traditional Health Care in Developing Societies: Conflict and Co-Operation*. Lanham, Md.: University Press of America.

Part I

The

Social

Production

of

Disease

Chapter 1

The Social Epidemiology of

AIDS in Africa:

Migrant Labor and

Sexually Transmitted Disease

CHARLES W. HUNT

Acquired Immune Deficiency Syndrome:
History and Explanations

Acquired immune deficiency syndrome (AIDS) was first discovered in the spring of 1981, after the detection of a series of unusual infections in previously healthy young men in the Los Angeles area. Most of these illnesses were not usually seen in healthy adults but were generally found in individuals who were either very young or very old and who had compromised immune systems. Some of the diseases were endemic to the United States but usually of such mild symptoms as to pass almost unnoticed in the population. Such diseases as Kaposi's sarcoma (a type of skin cancer), toxoplasmosis (a usually harmless parasitic disease, often spread by cats and chickens), pneumocystis carinii pneumonia, thrush, and herpes began to appear in patients, along with severe weight loss and fevers of unknown origin. The young men who had these infections died as a result.

The infections were termed "opportunistic" because they took the opportunity provided by the compromised immune system to strike. The patients were twenty to forty years old, supposedly the time of greatest health and vigor; as the spring turned to fall, the Centers for Disease Control (CDC) in Atlanta began to see more of these cases, concentrated in Los Angeles, New York, and San Francisco. Because all the early victims were homosexuals, this cluster came to be referred to as Gay Related Immune Deficiency, or GRID (Altman 1986, 33). This was never the official designation, however. Almost a decade later, in the 1990's, the designation has long disappeared and has been replaced by the internationally accepted designation of AIDS. In the public mind, however, this mysterious immune deficiency is still strongly associated with homosexuality.

Early theories concerning AIDS pursued this correlation. Therefore, in keeping with the prevailing explanations for such diseases as heart and blood vessel disease, high blood pressure, and cancer, AIDS was seen as a likely result of life-style factors in the gay community. "Poppers," amyl nitrate inhalants, were investigated and correlated—spuriously, it was later determined—with the syndrome (Vandenbroucke and Pardoel 1989). Other life-style factors were investigated and discussed as possible causes of AIDS; all of this work assumed that the syndrome would continue only in the male gay community.

The likelihood of AIDS being caused by a life-style factor was greatly diminished when, in mid-1982, it was discovered that the syndrome was not confined to the gay community. Intravenous (IV) drug users in a number of cities began to evidence the syndrome. AIDS began to appear among females and also among Haitian males. Hemophiliacs began to evidence the disease syndrome, and by December 1982 the first cases of AIDS linked to blood transfusions were noted, as well as the first appearance of AIDS in female sexual partners of those in high risk groups. By 1984, the communicable retrovirus that caused AIDS was discovered and identified, thereby finally eliminating explanations for the syndrome that relied exclusively on life-style. Although these discoveries decisively refuted the association of AIDS with the gay community, the early media blitz that created that association left a permanent impression in the public mind worldwide (Curran 1985, 7–9).

Noticed, but relatively little discussed at first, AIDS began to appear in the Third World. AIDS was first discovered in Africa when it was diagnosed in upper-class Africans traveling to and seeking treatment in European hospitals. The first African cases were diagnosed in Europe shortly after the first diagnosis of AIDS occurred in the United States (Quinn et al. 1986). Some confusion occurred initially because the opportunistic disease that accompanied the immune compromise were not always the same as those that appeared in the United States (Quinn et al. 1986). Whereas Kaposi's sarcoma, toxoplasmosis, herpes, and pneumocystis pneumonia were the common opportunistic diseases in North America, diseases of the digestive system and severe wasting were the common characteristics of the African immune compromise. However, these were often also accompanied by evidence of lung disease. The syndrome became known as "slim disease" in Uganda (Serwadda et al. 1985).

One characteristic of the epidemiological pattern was quite striking in the AIDS cases in Africa, right from the point of discovery. The sex ratio of AIDS cases in Africa was equal consistently one-to-one, with an equal number of women suffering from the immune compromise as men (Biggar 1986, 1987; Brunet and Ancelle 1985; Carael et al. 1988; Clumeck et al. 1985; Curran et al. 1985; Mann and Chin 1988; Mann, Chin, et al. 1988; Mann, Francis, Quinn, et al. 1986; Mann, Francis, Davachi, et al. 1986; Piot et al. 1988; Quinn 1987; Quinn et al. 1986). This was in marked contrast to the sex ratio in North America and other developed areas, where initially in the epidemic the ratio had been heavily weighed toward men. In fact, the early sex ratio in the United States was sixteen-to-one, reflecting the prevalence of the syndrome among male homosexuals, IV drug users, and hemophiliacs (Quinn et al. 1986). Why was the appearance of the disease epidemiologically distinctive, remarkably different, in the developed world from its appearance in the Third World? Formulating and answering this question is the major thrust of this paper.

The initial Western reaction to the equality of sex ratios in Third World cases of AIDS involved a complex combination of sexism and racism, expressed through a popular prism of hysteria. It was asserted that the human immunodeficiency virus (HIV-1), which caused the syndrome, had originated in Africa; specifically, it was theorized that the virus had originated in the Lake Victoria area of eastern and central Africa. It was known that a syndrome somewhat similar to AIDS existed in monkey populations from those regions currently held in captivity in the United States, and it was assumed that a crossover had occurred at some time in the past, the monkey virus transferring its infectivity from animal to human (Gallo 1987). Certainly, previous viruses had followed this pattern; Jenner's vaccine against smallpox, in fact, was derived from cowpox precisely because of the evolution of smallpox from that parent form. An animal origin was even advanced in the African equatorial green monkey; it was based on the use of this monkey for food, in supposed shamanistic rituals, and so forth, which, Western authorities hypothesized, had provided the opportunity for the crossover to occur (*The Economist* 1986). Therefore, in this approach, which was a sort of natural history view of the syndrome, AIDS had begun in a small community or perhaps in the gay population in Africa. This was considered to be the earliest stage of the syndrome. Then, over considerable time, it progressed into the heterosexual community. This explained the differing sex ratios in the two areas of the developed world and the Third World. We were simply seeing the natural history, the natural development, of the syndrome and its progression.

The natural history explanation caught on in the West with a fury. It caused considerable fear in the developed world, because it meant that the heterosexual community could no longer ignore AIDS and its consequences. Its members would suffer the syndrome also. This was part of the cause for a shift in the amount of attention the AIDS epidemic began to receive. By the mid-1980s, AIDS had become a constant topic in the media.

Research began to be directed at the syndrome, and money began to flow into research organizations directed toward controlling and, eventually, conquering the epidemic. Although the epidemic might have been ignored if it only struck homosexuals and IV drug users, if it was a threat to all, particularly heterosexuals, it needed considerable attention. The concept of the African origins of HIV-1 and the AIDS epidemic entered the public consciousness with the same indelible strength as the original association of homosexuality and AIDS.

The natural history explanation had a number of assumptions attached to it that were testable and could assist in confirming the theory. First, the green monkey virus must be, of necessity, a close genetic relative of HIV-1; the former would be the ancestral form of the latter, and genetic research should be capable of confirming this relationship. It might even be possible, on the Jenner model, to use the ancestral form to develop a vaccine to combat the epidemic. Second, the theory assumed that the epidemic of AIDS had been present on the African continent for considerably longer than it had been present in the developed world and North America. In some cases it was asserted that the virus had been dormant for decades or centuries in rural Africa, only to be spread suddenly, exploding into an epidemic due to modernization or the disturbance of "traditional" ways of life. Third, as a frequently advanced corollary it was assumed that the syndrome progressed from the gay community into the heterosexual community over time. There are many other testable assumptions of the African origins theory, but these three at least can be examined closely.

By the summer of 1988, genetic experiments and comparisons had been done between the green monkey viruses of the equatorial region of Africa and HIV-1 of AIDS. They were not closely related. The former was decisively not the ancestral form of the latter (Mulder 1988). Perhaps the most significant prop of the African origins theory had collapsed.

However, this was not the only support for the theory that disappeared in the latter half of the 1980s. It became clear that AIDS was a quite recent syndrome to the African continent as a whole and, particularly, to the areas hardest hit in eastern and central Africa, countries such as Uganda, Burundi, Rwanda, Tanzania, Kenya, Zaire, Zambia, and the Congo Republic. Physicians who had spent their lives studying and treating infectious diseases in the area were absolutely certain that this syndrome had not appeared prior to its appearance in North America (Carswell 1987; Carswell et al. 1986; Serwadda et al. 1985). The counter-assertion was that the detection system in Africa was simply inadequate to screen and detect cases. This deficiency has been denied by physicians in Uganda (particularly Carswell et al. 1986).

Furthermore, early AIDS cases began to be discovered in the United States (Garry et al. 1988). It was soon discovered that the earliest case of confirmed HIV-1 infection and AIDS had occurred in the United States in 1953. Subsequent cases of confirmed AIDS occurred in Europe and Israel in a scattering of incidents throughout the 1950s, 1960s, and early 1970s. The first case of confirmed AIDS in Africa occurred in Uganda in 1973, according to careful retrospective study and analysis of medical reports (Huminer et al. 1987). This was almost twenty years after the first case detected in the United States. It seems highly unlikely that AIDS occurred on the African continent first, as the African origins theory would require. Further, the syndrome was rapidly fatal in the African context; it hardly acted as though it had been endemic to the southern, eastern, and central African peoples. Endemic infectious diseases—that is, those long associated with a population—usually do not have a high case fatality rate during an epidemic. The host and infectious agent have usually had time to adjust to each other and become less virulent. In the case of HIV-1 in Africa, the case fatality rate approaches 100 percent. It also takes less time for fatalities to result from HIV-1 infection and diagnosis with AIDS in Africa than in the United States, although this may be an artifact of later diagnosis in Africa.

Much of the support for an African origins theory came from early blood analysis done to test for the presence of HIV-1 in the blood of various African populations. Thus, it was claimed, testing done for HIV-1 on stored blood from such countries as Zaire had established the presence of HIV-1 in Africa in the late 1950s. Further, very high rates of HIV-1 positive blood were found in many African populations in Uganda, Kenya, Zaire, and Congo. This, many argued, showed how many were infected and how widely prevalent the syndrome was and argued for a longer term over which it must have been spreading. Low levels of HIV-1 positive blood in rural areas argued for a low level of endemic disease in these areas.

The difficulty with this evidence was twofold. First, the particular blood test—the Enzyme Linked Immunosorbent Assay (ELISA) test—used to search for HIV-1 in Africa was not reliable when used on stored blood. It produced a high level of false positive when so used, due to the increased "stickiness" of such blood. Second, when the HIV-1 test employed in the early 1980s was used on blood that had various blood-borne diseases present, particularly malaria, the test and the manner of its interpretation produced very high numbers of false positives. These false positives meant that high numbers of blood samples were being interpreted as having HIV-1 infection when, in fact, they did not. We can conclude that the blood tests performed to detect HIV-1 in African populations throughout the first half of the 1980s were totally unreliable. The tests and the data are false (Biggar et al. 1985; Norman 1985).

All of this argued that HIV-1 and AIDS were new to Africa and the African population. Further, the idea that there was some isolated population in remote, rural Africa that could have harbored the virus for decades, or perhaps centuries, and released it upon some calamity or through modernization belies the development of Africa for the past hundred years. Such events were possible within a few years of conquest in the late 1800s and, in fact, did occur. They seem highly unlikely today. There simply are no such areas left of any consequence that could harbor such a pathogen.

If it was determined that the virus was not genetically related to an African original virus and the retrovirus itself was only recently introduced to the African continent, then it was also established that the syndrome had never been associated with homosexuality in Africa. Despite constant and repeated attempts by researchers to establish this link between homosexuality and AIDS in Africa in the early research of the 1980s, it was clear that HIV-1 in Africa was transmitted heterosexually and always had been (Biggar 1986, 1987; Brunet and Ancelle 1985; Quinn 1987; Quinn et al. 1986; Melbye et al. 1986). This may be because of differing sexual roles, definitions, and practices in the African cultural context (Moodie 1988). At any rate, the natural history argument, that one only needed to put the AIDS epidemics in Africa and North America side by side to see the natural progression of the syndrome, fell apart. There was a corresponding decrease in interest in the AIDS epidemic as it was realized that, if the natural history theories were incorrect, the AIDS epidemic and HIV-1 were not necessarily going to strike the heterosexual community in North America and the developed world. Attention to AIDS flagged in the political and social arenas of the United States.

The natural history theories concerning AIDS collapsed by 1988. One prop of the theory, however, the African origins of the AIDS epidemic and HIV-1, although standing on no scientific basis or support whatsoever, still continues in the public mind. Ask anyone in the United States where the AIDS virus comes from and that person will almost inevitably reply that it originated in Africa. There may be many reasons for this persistence; two reasons can be given specifically. First, the combination of sexuality, disease, and death is so explosive that North Americans—and humans generally—do not want to take responsibility for initiating such a disaster. Therefore they blame someone else for the origins of the problem. This occurs even when the disease is not as emotionally charged as AIDS. For instance, we do not have cases of the Washington flu in the United States; we have cases of the Hong Kong flu. When picking whom to blame, making international victims the culprits seems to be the order of the day where AIDS and HIV-1 are concerned (Hunt 1988).

The second reason for the persistence of the unsupported theory of

African origins for AIDS and HIV-1 is pure and simple racism. The steaming jungles and strange shamanistic rituals of black Africans are cited, and frequently have been cited, as the origins of the crossover of HIV-1 from the green monkey. Some of this material has written a shameful chapter in the history of anthropological research in the 1980s. The acceptance of some of this material is ludicrous; its widescale adoption into the AIDS discussion can only be seen as racism (Hunt 1988).

If the natural history of the syndrome does not explain the epidemiological differences between African and North American AIDS cases, what does? The biological cause of the syndrome, HIV-1 is the same in both places. There are not variants of HIV-1 in eastern, central, and southern Africa that are significantly different genetically from HIV-1 in North America. Surely the biological cause cannot explain the epidemiological differences between AIDS in the Third World and AIDS in the developed world.

The next attempt to explain the differences between the AIDS epidemic in the two areas was still based upon biology. If HIV-1 was the same in both places and could not be the cause of different epidemics, perhaps the human beings in North America were different in some significant biological way from those in eastern, central, and southern Africa. Sociobiologists asserted that they were significantly different.

Two sociobiological researchers asserted that Africans have a genetically determined pattern of sexuality that is quite different from the genetically determined sexuality or reproductive strategy of Caucasians. Using long discredited research data and materials concerning intercranial capacities, intelligence quotient (IQ) ratings, rates of criminal activity, and other data, these researchers have attempted to establish that Africans have a reproductive strategy that maximizes numbers of offspring while minimizing offspring care (Rushton and Bogaert 1989). This is opposed to supposed Caucasian reproductive strategies, which produce small numbers of offspring with maximum care for the offspring. These differing strategies for reproduction supposedly make African populations susceptible to sexually transmitted diseases (STDs) and AIDS (Rushton and Bogaert 1989). Needless to say, not only has the evidence used by these two researchers been invalidated, but the link between family size (termed "litter size" in the article), care of children, criminal records (particularly for sexual crimes), and other factors used as evidence in their work is tenuous at best. Many would assert, as this author does, that the link is so obviously heavily affected by social environmental factors as to make the sociobiologists' assertion of a genetic link untenable. The sociobiological explanation of differences in the AIDS epidemic in Africa and the United States, in sum, rests on refuted evidence and unproven and highly untenable assumptions concerning the origin of social behavior. It is racist in the classical and extreme sense.

If, however, we are to dismiss the sociobiological explanation for the epidemiological differences in the AIDS epidemic between Africa and the United States—and I believe that we must dismiss this work from both a scientific and a political standpoint—then we are faced with a dilemma. There is no longer any way to explain these differences from a biological point of view. If there are no differences in the biology of hosts and infectious agents between the AIDS epidemics in Africa and the United States, why do the epidemics appear quite different and distinctive? Perhaps the explanation must be pursed in the realm of social organization, rather than in that of biological relationships. We take up this task in the remainder of this discussion.

African Social Organization

Having essentially rejected as unsupported, unhelpful, and inappropriate the biological explanations for the epidemiological patterns of African AIDS, we must look to social explanations. What is it about African social organization, as opposed to social organization in North America, that might explain the patterns of AIDS?

The most obvious differences in social organization concern the position of eastern, central, and southern Africa in the world system, as opposed to the position of the United States and the other developed countries. In the case of Africa, and particularly the regions of Africa with which we are concerned, the countries' position in the world system is on the periphery, as opposed to the core position of the United States, Western Europe, and the developed world (Wallerstein 1984; Stavrianos 1981). In a remarkable way, the two basic patterns of the AIDS epidemic mirror the difference between these two areas of the world. The AIDS epidemic with a distinctively imbalanced sex ratio—the epidemic of the developed world, what is termed by world-system theorists as the "core"—is often called Pattern One AIDS. The epidemic with a balanced sex ratio of one-to-one—the epidemic of the Third World, what is termed by world-system theorists as the "periphery"—is often called Pattern Two AIDS.

What is distinctive in these two areas? Of what significance is the core–periphery dichotomy for the social organization of these areas and the AIDS epidemic? It is clear that the organization of the labor market, the characteristics of the proletarianization of workers, the separation of the labor force from the land, the terms of employment, and the resulting household formation (and sexual and reproductive relations) in the periphery diverge markedly from the corresponding features in the core (Martin 1984; Stavrianos 1981; Wallerstein 1984; Wallerstein and Martin 1979). It is these differences, arising out of the particular manner of insertion into the world system of the periphery, that I contend socially create a population susceptible to STDs. This population has shown evidence of this susceptibility in the past, due to these same social or organizational factors. Further, the previous epidemics of STDs, which the features listed above have helped cause, also assist in shaping the AIDS epidemic in Africa, because previously untreated STDs increase the susceptibility to HIV-1 infection and resulting AIDS (Simonsen 1988). The position of Africa as a peripheral area, which I contend shapes this population for susceptibility to STD, arises from the relationship Africa has had historically with European imperialism and expansionism. To understand this connection, we must look closely at the colonial period in the histories of eastern, central, and southern Africa.

The African Migrant Labor System and Sexually Transmitted Disease

African conquest by the European imperial powers came relatively late in the development of the world system (Stavrianos 1981). The conquest of the African continent, following the slave trade, began in earnest only after the Berlin African Conference of 1884–85. As L.S. Stavrianos relates in the monumental text *Global Rift: The Third World Comes of Age* (1981):

> The Berlin African Conference was held in 1884–5 to set down the ground rules for future acquisitions of African lands. It was agreed that notice of intent should be given, that claims had to be legitimized by effective occupation and that disputes were to be settled by arbitration. This treaty cleared the way for the greatest land grab in history. In 1879 the only colonies in Africa were those of France in Algeria and Senegal, of Britain along the Gold Coast and at the Cape, and of Portugal in Angola and Mozambique. By 1914 the entire continent had been partitioned, except for Ethiopia and Liberia. (281–82)

European colonialism's conquest of Africa took approximately thirty years and was completed well before the First World War. Plans for the development of the continent met with a considerable obstacle, however: How would the European powers create a labor force on the African continent? The residents of the continent were made up of many different social formations, or social organizational types, which ranged from sophisticated states to hunter–gatherer groups (Rodney 1982). The vast majority of the peoples of Africa, no matter what their social organizational type, were not integrated into any sort of a wage employment system; a money economy was foreign to most of the continent. One could offer a wage, but an employer so doing would not find any workers. The various African social formations were adequately providing for their members without the added input of resources that a wage system represented. It was this problem that the Europeans faced in the early 1900s and that they determined, by various means, to solve. How Europeans solved this problem is well known and well documented.

To force Africans to enter wage labor, the conquering Europeans for a time used forced labor. In other words, they simply placed a gun and bayonet at the back of the African worker and ordered that worker to labor on pain of death. This was, however, an inefficient method of obtaining labor and had largely disappeared by the turn of the century. A much more effective method of obtaining wage labor was the use of economic force; various taxes—head taxes, poll taxes, and hut taxes—were imposed upon the African household and community members. These taxes were to be paid in cash, not in kind or by barter. The necessity of cash meant that the African must either sell possessions, such as herd animals or crops, or go to work for a cash wage. When herd animals were sold, it was only a matter of time before poverty set in and wage labor commenced anyway, unless taxes were set low enough that the reproduction rate of the herd could keep up—a consideration the imperial power was not likely to extend. In the case of the sale of crops, the farmer needed to have enough of a crop left over to feed a family. Again, if the tax was higher than to allow this, poverty and destitution resulted with wage labor following soon after (Stavrianos 1981, 302–4).

Another way in which wage labor was created, one in which the alternative of selling herd animals or crops was avoided, was for the imperial power intentionally to underdevelop areas that were not integrated into the larger economy (Mamdani 1976). Areas were intentionally created by the governing imperial power that had no infrastructure to transport crops and cattle to markets, thereby preventing their sale. Often these areas were actually prevented from producing crops or livestock of a type that could be sold on the market. Further, the areas so designated were often the poorest in terms of land productivity and fertility.

With this policy, areas in eastern, southern, and central Africa were intentionally underdeveloped so that their major—in fact, their only—export crop would be human labor and human beings. In sum, the Europeans attempted, through the imposition of taxes and the intentional underdevelopment of geographical areas, to break the ability of Africans to live and reproduce themselves and their society. Once the money economy was introduced and put in place and the ability to reproduce society was broken, the African would labor simply to obtain the necessities of life. Africans would no longer have to be forced at gunpoint to work; they would be forced by a desire to survive—no external coercion would be necessary.

This system was effective in producing the wage labor to meet the colonial requirements. The result of the system was the emergence of

large geographical regions in the countryside that were systematically underdeveloped and impoverished (Mamdani 1976; Rodney 1982). Over-
crowding led to land overuse and fertility decline, which further led to an
inability to support a family in these regions. The regions became known
as "labor reserves." The system of labor that resulted had as its pillar the
migration of labor from these reserves into enclaves of employment some
considerable distance away (Crush 1984; Davidson 1983; Doyal 1981, 11–
119; Freund 1984, 1988; Gugler 1968; Gutkind and Wallerstein 1976; Karugire 1980; C. Leys 1975; R. Leys 1974; Mamdani 1976; Parpart 1983;
Roberts 1979; Sathyamurthy 1986; Stichter 1985; Turshen 1977, 1984;
Wallerstein and Martin 1979). The latter employment areas became the
developed enclaves in the rural–urban dialectic of colonial Africa. Thus
mining, railroad work, plantation work, and primary production facilities
absorbed capital investment and became enclaves of development in an
immense, underdeveloped continent. Just as these industries absorbed
capital, they absorbed large quantities of labor from the rural areas, con-
centrating large numbers of predominant, male workers. The effect on
these men and on their families is described well by Lesley Doyal in *The
Political Economy of Health* (1981):

> The migrant labor system affected Africans' lives in many funda-
> mental ways. Whatever the miseries of industrialization in Brit-
> ain, it was usually possible for workers to keep their families
> together, but this has not been the case in third world countries.
> In Tanganyika, for example, male workers were typically re-
> cruited from designated labour supply areas great distances from
> the centres of economic activity. This entailed prolonged family
> separation which had serious physical and psychological reper-
> cussions for all concerned. The populations of African towns "re-
> cruited by migration" were characterized by a heavy prepon-
> derance of men living in intolerably insecure and depressing
> conditions and lacking the benefits of family life or other cus-
> tomary supports. (114)

In many areas of Africa, women established land tenure. It is the
woman's residence upon the land in the labor reserve that establishes the
right to that land and safeguards a tenuous social security in land for the
family. Therefore there is considerable pressure for a wife to remain
home, do the farming, and raise the children on the labor reserve, while
the male member of the family migrates to contractual labor for periods
of one or two years at a time. Unfortunately, this system has led to serious difficulties in food production and in family care. Women labored
alone, without male help, and frequently failed to clear new land, overus-
ing the old. Due to the declining fertility of the land, crops such as millet
became less productive. Cassava was substituted because of its higher

productivity; however, cassava is a high carbohydrate food and millet is a high protein food. Protein deficiencies in children resulted from the substitution of cassava for millet. Calorie deficiencies resulted when even the cassava failed to produce adequately (Murray 1981; McCance and Rutishauser 1975; Stichter 1985).

Women busy with the farming had difficulty taking time to care for children adequately. Some studies show that simply the increased labor demand on women, with the accompanying reduction in time to attend to their children's nutritional concerns, led to declines in children's nutritional status whether or not cropping patterns and crops have changed (Vaughn and Moore 1988). One solution to these problems was to increase the number of laborers at both the tasks of child care and farming. Large families resulted, because children at an early age could do farming work. At a later age they could tend other, younger children. The large family made larger demands upon the meager resources of the labor reserve and the cycle continued.

The situation of the migrant laborer in the developed enclave did not reduce the difficulties on the labor reserve. Male laborers were paid a bachelor wage, just enough money to feed themselves and house themselves from day to day. The wage reproduced the laborer for a day; it did not provide for long-term reproduction of the working class. The latter task was left to the overtaxed resources of the labor reserve and women back home (Stichter 1985). A consistently declining agriculture, poor child care, and increasingly poor nutrition resulted.

In addition, and particularly in recent decades, many unmarried rural women saw no means of adequate support for a family on the labor reserve and so emigrated to the city at a young age. Family conflict and separation also have caused many young women to migrate to the cities and to concentrations of male laborers (Murray 1977, 1980, 1981; Stichter 1985). Unfortunately, very few women have found wage labor or work of any kind in the primary labor sectors in eastern, southern, and central Africa. There is little wage employment for women in the developing African economy in these regions (Doyal 1981; 116; Stichter 1985, 144–78). Some—perhaps many—of these women become prostitutes and beer brewers, entering the marginal or secondary labor markets in the areas surrounding the large concentrations of men and development (Doyal 1981; Stichter 1985).

The combination of the migrant labor system with a heavy preponderance of male laboring jobs and long familial separations has caused a breakdown in family and sexual patterns in central, eastern, and southern Africa (Murray 1977, 1980, 1981; Wren 1990). An explosion of both prostitution and STDs in these populations occurred well before the AIDS virus made an appearance (Bennett 1962, 1964, 1975; Brown et al. 1985;

Rampen 1978; Sajiwandani and Baboo 1987; Sathyamurthy 1986; Wren 1990). As Doyal (1981) states:

> Venereal disease became—and still remains—a major health problem in many parts of the third world where it was previously unknown. It is hardly surprising that the disruption of the economy and personal foundations of family life led to the disintegration of long-established marital and sexual patterns. In this context, the growth of prostitution represented one form of adaptation to the intolerable strains faced by men and women alike. In the case of male migrants, the absence of their wives was compounded by the fact that their new environment was almost exclusively masculine. This unequal sex ratio made it difficult for men to establish stable sexual liaisons with women, and encouraged prostitution. For the women involved, prostitution was usually a matter of sheer economic necessity. . . . The structure of the colonial economy made it virtually impossible for women to sell their labor . . . most were compelled to live off the low wages of male workers. Often this involved either formal or informal prostitution. (115–16)

The development of the migrant labor system led to serious health consequences, particularly to an epidemic of STDs in central, eastern, and southern Africa. This pattern is clear even in 1981, when Doyal wrote the passage above (Osoba 1981).

In addition to the "pull" effect of industrialization and the migrant labor markets, and the "push" effect of declining agriculture with reduced labor inputs on the labor reserve, a "push" effect was produced by capital's takeover of African agriculture (Loewenson 1988; Sanders and Davies 1988). As in many Third World countries, the best and most fertile lands are taken over by capital to produce agricultural products for export. Local food production is marginalized onto poor land; rural labor needs become seasonal; and as a result of large-scale monoculture and mechanization, rural "overpopulation" is pushed into urban slum areas. In these areas poor health, disease, and malnutrition abound. Employment is difficult, especially for women; family life may also become difficult (Stichter 1985). The result, as with the pull effect of large capital developments, is the social creation of a population especially vulnerable to STDs and, particularly, to AIDS (Epstein and Packard 1987, 10–17).

As a consequence of the migrant labor pattern and the capitalist takeover of rural African agriculture, therefore, AIDS had a ready population that suffered from an unusually high level of STDs. As recent research has indicated, the higher incidence of previous venereal disease, especially if untreated, increases the likelihood of contracting AIDS, due to the presence of remaining lesions and injury (Quinn et al. 1986, 957–58; Stamm et al. 1988).

The manner in which labor is handled in migrant labor situations worsens epidemics. Such a labor system, with recruitment of migrant workers from rural areas surrounding industrial and extractive developments, does not require that care be taken concerning the health or safety of the working population. As long as labor power is in surplus in the rural areas (due to the expansion of capitalist agriculture and the resulting rural overpopulation, along with the continued high birth rate in the labor reserves), injured or incapacitated workers may be replaced easily by further migrants. Workers who can no longer continue to work under such conditions simply return to their villages for care (Doyal 1981, 119). Further, the ability of workers to combat poor working conditions and to demand health care and benefits from employment is severely compromised, because migrant workers are historically difficult to unionize or organize for resistance to employers (Stichter 1985).

Following the same pattern as migrant laborers, urban slum dwellers, lacking any medical care due to their unemployment, also regularly return home when ill, carrying urban disease back to rural villages (Doyal 1981). Thus a women who is a prostitute and becomes ill is very likely to return to her home village to be cared for by relatives.

In the case of STDs and many other diseases, the return home with illness has a tragic consequence. Like tuberculosis in the past, STDs today are carried back to the village, infecting areas where these diseases were not seen before and populations that lack resistance or previous exposure to these illnesses. "Whether or not these migrants survived their diseases, the diseases invariably survived them, often spreading rapidly among an increasingly susceptible population" (Doyal 1981, 119).

There is little question, therefore, that AIDS strikes a population not only made susceptible to STDs but also socially structured to hasten the transmission of HIV-1. This social structuring of a population that makes it vulnerable to STDs is an integral part of the peripheral status of eastern, central, and southern Africa. The social structuring of the family unit and labor migrancy is, as is argued above, closely related to partial proletarianization and incomplete separation from the land, characteristics of a peripheral labor force (Wallerstein 1984; Friedman 1984; J. Smith 1984; Martin 1984; Wallerstein and Martin 1979).

Past data on the prevalence of STDs has clearly indicated that the pattern of STD spread detailed above has occurred. For instance, in studies completed in the 1960s and early 1970s, the primary risk factor for gonorrhea in eastern Africa was male labor migrancy, with a pool of infection in the female prostitute population (Verhagen and Gemert 1972; Bennett 1962). The pattern of spread from urban and labor concentrations to rural areas was also confirmed for gonorrhea (Bennett 1964).

Prevalence data also establishes that there are higher rates of STDs in general around labor concentrations.

Thus the pattern of the eastern, southern, and central African labor market—a migrant labor system based on labor reserves, surpluses of laborers, and a laboring population only partially separated from the land—may account for a great many of the differences between the AIDS epidemic in the United States and AIDS as it appears in the African population. AIDS required in each case, in Africa as in North America, a population that was vulnerable to STDs. In each case, this is where the virus first made its inroads. In Africa, a population socially structured by capitalist agriculture, early imperialism, and later dependency development patterns—that is, by its peripheral position in the world system—gave AIDS the foothold that it required. The prevalence of malnutrition, malaria, measles, and other diseases that have resulted from the collapse of local food production and the dependency-development pattern of Africa has resulted in a population whose health is continually compromised. Large numbers of persons have immune systems weakened not only from disease but also from malnutrition, a condition that also may set the stage for AIDS infection (Epstein and Packard 1987; Hall and Langlands 1975; McCance and Rutishauser 1975). In North America, a gay population that for at least a decade had an STD problem was the foothold for HIV-1 (Altman 1986; Shilts 1987). In each case, the initial stages of the epidemic have been determined by the population in which the virus was able to begin its infection. In both cases, it appears that these beginnings, while affecting profoundly the perceptions of AIDS, will not be the limits to which HIV-1 confines itself. These were simply the populations that were most vulnerable at the outset.

This model for the spread of the AIDS epidemic in Africa relies not only upon the scientific understanding of HIV-1 and its methods of transmission but also upon the historical patterns of development in eastern, central, and southern Africa. The peripheral status of eastern, central, and southern Africa in the world system must be understood to make sense of the epidemiology of the AIDS epidemic.

Testing a Theory

If the model that has been presented above is valid for the AIDS epidemic in eastern, central, and southern Africa, then the pattern in which the epidemic appears should show some evidence of the modes of transmission that this exposition of the epidemic would expect. In other words, if the epidemic occurs geographically in areas with high concentrations of male migrant laborers and particularly with men and women who have high levels of heterosexual activity, then high prevalence or incidence rates should appear first geographically in those areas where labor is concentrated. Further, two populations groups in these areas should be affected, the male migrant laborers themselves and their partners, usually female prostitutes living near the enclave of development. Therefore a high rate of infection in these two groups would fit the model advanced.

If the spread of HIV-1 occurs through the return, due to illness, of male migrant laborers and female prostitutes to their villages, then the second geographic area that should begin to show high rates of infection are those areas in eastern, central, and southern Africa known as labor reserves. Assuming that the rural areas are infected with HIV-1 after the infection of the labor-concentration areas, these rural areas should show prevalence rates that are lower than the labor-concentration areas. The rural labor reserves, however, should show higher rates of infection than surrounding rural areas that do not provide migrant labor. Thus the areas from which migrant workers are drawn (in contract form, to provide the workers necessary for production) in prevalence should lag somewhat behind the areas where these workers labor. This model assumes that these workers return home carrying HIV-1, they will pass this infection on to their partners and others by their return.

The prostitutes from these areas of male migrant labor concentration also tend to return home when illness prevents them from continuing to work. This trend may be less definite, because prostitutes are not formally dismissed by someone else from work. They may continue prostitution activities and delay returning home, even though quite ill. That is, despite their illness, they may be able to continue to work and generate some income, although their capacity to work and produce income may be reduced considerably.

The brief discussion in this chapter concerning the historical, social, and economic development of eastern, central, and southern Africa points in a number of directions for further research and study. As a start, however, available data concerning HIV-1 seropositivity and AIDS prevalence can be used to test the pattern of the epidemic. Does the available data on seropositivity and AIDS prevalence fit the pattern that would result from the description presented above? We can generate the following hypotheses based upon the above argument:

1. Geographically, areas of migrant labor concentration should show high prevalence rates of HIV-1 infection. This includes mining areas, commercial plantation areas, and some large cities.
2. Also geographically, areas from which migrant laborers are drawn (labor reserves) should show high rates of prevalence for HIV-1 infection.
3. The prevalence of HIV-1 infection in labor reserves should be

higher than in other rural areas that do not form labor reserves.

4. Geographic areas from which young women migrate to become prostitutes should show high prevalence levels of HIV-1 infection. These rates also should be higher than for other rural areas of stable peasant commodity production.

5. HIV-1 seropositivity should appear earlier in the rural labor reserves, than in surrounding rural areas or areas of stable peasant commodity production, due to earliest transmission by migrant labor to the former areas.

6. The HIV-1 infection prevalence rates for areas where migrant labor is concentrated should be somewhat higher than the areas from which migrant labor is drawn.

7. Temporally, HIV-1 seropositivity should appear earliest in the areas where migrant labor is concentrated, such as mining areas, plantations, and cities.

8. Migrant laborers should show higher rates of HIV-1 infection than other men within the population.

9. There may be a correlation between an increase in the rate of HIV-1 seropositivity among male migrant workers and the length of their labor contracts or time spent away from their families.

10. There should be a lower rate of HIV-1 infection prevalence among permanent migrant laborers, those who are allowed to take their families with them to the job site.

11. Prostitutes concentrated in areas where male migrant labor is located should show higher rates of HIV-1 infection than other women in the population. Further, prostitutes located in areas of migrant labor concentration should show higher levels of HIV-1 seropositivity and AIDS than prostitutes in areas where migrant labor does not concentrate. These rates should bias the age and marital status data concerning women who are infected with HIV-1. Therefore, women infected should be younger and more often single than men who are infected.

12. Higher prevalence and earlier occurrences of HIV-1 infection should appear among those who have previously suffered STDs. This is the population that is socially and biologically constructed to transmit these diseases.

13. There should be lower prevalence of HIV-1 infection among those persons on the rural labor reserves who have not migrated for laboring contracts and among their families.

14. HIV-1 seropositivity should evidence a complex pattern of spread. The epidemic will not be from rural areas to the city, as would be posited by a disease that has been endemic for

long periods of time in rural areas and, that due to social disruption, breaks out into the larger population. Such a pattern would show earlier and higher prevalence in rural areas. Rather, HIV-1 seropositivity should evidence a movement from areas of labor concentration to rural labor reserves and outward from the latter focuses of infection to the general rural community. The degree of movement of HIV-1 seropositivity and AIDS into a labor reserve should depend upon the quantity of migrant labor employed from that reserve, the length of time of contracts or absences, the age of migrant laborers leaving, the type of employment to which migrants are moving, the number of women leaving for the city and the work they obtain, and the rate of return of ill women and migrant laborers. The direction of movement should depend upon where the major quantity of migrant labor originates, where recruiting occurs, and from what home areas women are leaving.

In other words, numerous factors that influence the sexual and migratory patterns in eastern, central, and southern Africa will affect the spread and transmission of HIV-1 seropositivity and AIDS. The principal organizing factor, however, is the system of labor migration and the labor reserve. From this central understanding, one can begin to investigate the variations and complex movement of the epidemic.

Data and Prevalence Surveys

Does the available data support the fourteen hypotheses that have been presented? Are the actual AIDS prevalence and seropositivity studies done in eastern, central, and southern Africa in conformity with these hypotheses? Caution should first be advised, because data is, in some cases, unreliable and fragmentary. It may be reiterated that the ELISA test for HIV-1 immune response may also be much less reliable in African than elsewhere (Biggar et al. 1985). Of course, the use of the World Health Organization (WHO) case definition in Uganda (Berkley, Okware, and Naamara 1989), which does not rely on laboratory work, makes this unreliability less of a problem. (The WHO case definition has been shown to be quite reliable in the Ugandan context.)

Further, the process of transmission of HIV-1, which has been outlined above, is dynamic. Much of the data is prevalence data, which can be examined spatially or geographically. There is relatively little incidence data. Prevalence data is inherently static, not dynamic. Therefore we can only infer the dynamic process from the static data.

Specific areas that are labor concentrations and labor reserves in

Uganda can be determined. Upon request, I will provide the reader with a map highlighting the labor-concentration areas and the labor-reserve areas in Uganda (see Figure 1.1). This map is derived from historical accounts of Uganda development, as well as migration data derived from the Ugandan census (Kabera 1982; Mamdani 1976; Gimui 1982).

HYPOTHESES 1 THROUGH 7. These hypotheses concern the geographical and temporal distributional evidence for the pattern of HIV-1 transmission outlined. Geographical distribution is capable of eliciting transmission patterns in some diseases (Hall and Langlands 1975; Meade 1980; McGlashan 1972; Hunter 1974; Prothero 1977, 1983; Pyle 1979).

It is clear that AIDS cases and HIV infection have generally been most serious in cities in Uganda and much of eastern Africa (Mugerwa, Widy-Wirski, and Okwake 1987; *The Economist* 1987; Harden 1986, 1987; Mugerwa and Giraldo 1987; Georges et al. 1987; Van de Perre 1984; Biggar 1986; Mann, Francis, Quinn, et al. 1986; Berkley, Okware, and Naamara 1989). These are areas of labor concentration. This is also confirmed by cumulative prevalence data from Uganda (Figure 1.2), which establishes that the highest prevalence rate of AIDS in Uganda is contained in the half-moon area along the shore of Lake Victoria, particularly in the Masaka and Kampala–Entebbe areas (Berkley, Okware, and Naamara 1989, 83).

The problem with this data is that it reflects not only the possible reality of the epidemic but also the availability of medical facilities in these regions of Africa. Medical facilities capable of recognizing and diagnosing AIDS in central, eastern, and southern Africa are almost exclusively concentrated in cities (Hall and Langlands 1975; Navarro 1974). Therefore these areas will show a predominant number of diagnosed cases. Individuals from rural areas may not even be able to travel to the cities for diagnosis and may be either misdiagnosed or not treated at all. This tendency has been counteracted somewhat in the case of Uganda, however, because of the widespread nature of the surveillance system in that country and because of the training provided by the government to all health workers in the rural and urban areas of the country (Berkley, Okware, and Naamara 1989). We would expect, therefore, that this difficulty would be minimized in the Ugandan context, compared to the rest of eastern, southern, and central Africa.

It has frequently been commented that AIDS patients in eastern Africa are more well-to-do than the average population (Georges et al. 1987; Harden 1987; Van de Perre 1984). This may also reflect the comparative ease with which these classes can access the medical system, as opposed to poorer or rural individuals.

In Uganda, however, it has been claimed that the prevalence of HIV-1 seropositivity does not seem as high in Kampala as elsewhere (*The Economist* 1987). It has been claimed that the southwestern areas of the coun-

FIGURE 1-1. Map of Labor Concentrations and Labor Reserves in Uganda

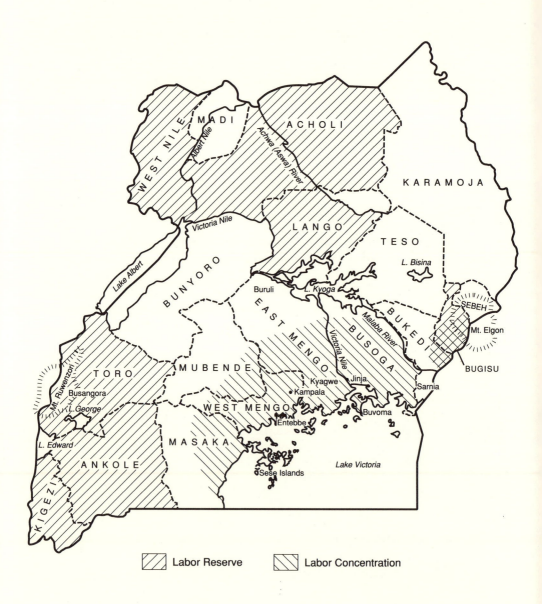

FIGURE 1-2. AIDS Cumulative Prevalence by District in Uganda.

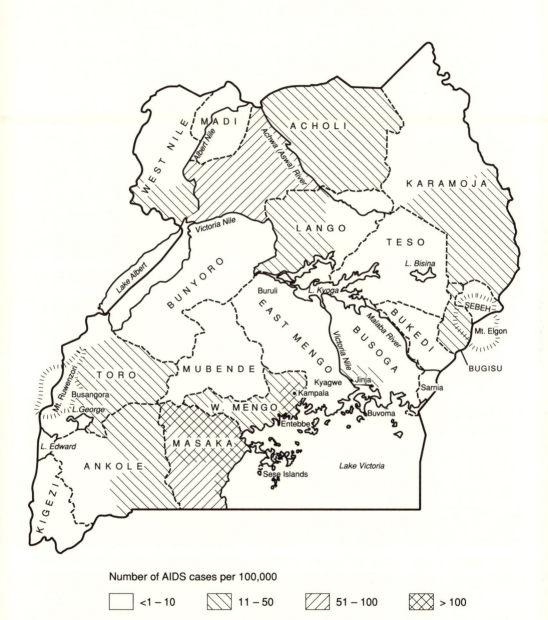

Number of AIDS cases per 100,000

<1 – 10   11 – 50   51 – 100   > 100

Source: From Berkeley, Okware, and Naamara 1989.

try have higher HIV-1 prevalence rates. This conclusion seems to be refuted by recent and more comprehensive studies and cumulative prevalence data (Carswell 1987; Berkley, Okware, and Naamara 1989; also see Figure 1.2). In general, rural residents, particularly in the peasant-farming areas of central Uganda, seem to have a low rate of HIV-1 seropositivity and AIDS (Carswell 1987; Van de Perre 1984; Harden 1987; Berkley, Okware, and Naamara 1989). In Rwanda and Zaire, the infection rate in the country is very small, compared to a very high rate in the cities (Specter 1986). We can say, however, that rural southwestern Uganda appears to have high prevalence of AIDS cases and HIV-1 infection (Serwadda et al. 1985; *The Economist* 1987; Berkley, Okware, and Naamara 1989). It has been estimated that one-third of the members of the population in this area are infected with HIV-1 (*The Economist* 1987). It is clear from the cumulative prevalence data of AIDS cases that the southwestern areas of Uganda, particularly Anchole and Toro, have quite high rates of AIDS cases, ranging from the 11 to 50 per every 100,000 persons. These two areas are labor reserves, having high rates of circulating migration, to and from the core developed areas in Uganda.

In studies of prostitutes in the town of Rakai, south of Kampala, some 86 percent were found to be HIV-1 positive (WHO 1988). Barmaids were 80 percent seropositive in this same area of major labor concentration. The area south of Kampala has one of the highest rates of AIDS in Uganda, comparable to the Kampala–Entebbe area.

In the countries of Burundi and Rwanda, there has not been established an AIDS surveillance system like the one in place in Uganda. There are, however, some cumulative figures for AIDS cases from the WHO. These figures were accumulated until 31 December 1988, and they establish that Burundi has a prevalence rate of AIDS cases of 13 per 100,000 persons, with a total of 1,408 cases of AIDS (WHO 1989, 113). This rate is comparable to the high rate found in such labor reserves in Uganda as the West Nile, Lango, Ancoli, Bugisu, Toro, and eastern Ancholi. Further, it establishes Burundi as having the second highest national cumulative prevalence rate of AIDS cases in Africa. Burundi's prevalence rate is even higher than the overall rate for Uganda (WHO 1989, 113).

According to these figures, however, Rwanda has a cumulative AIDS case rate of only 2.8 per 100,000 persons. This would place its rate much lower than that of other labor reserves. In like manner, the labor reserve in the extreme southwest of Uganda, Kigezi, has a low case rate in the range of 1 to 10 per 100,000 persons. In the latter case may be reflected a diminished rate of circulating migrant labor, with increases in permanent settlement outside Kigezi (Kabera 1982). This is only speculation, however, as we have no really accurate figures for the trends in migratory labor from this district in the 1970s and 1980s.

The low figures for both Rwanda and the Kigezi district may reflect underreporting, although this is most likely for the Rwanda figures. Underreporting seems likely in the Rwandan case because the infection rate in Kigali, Rwanda, has been estimated at 25 percent (Van de Perre 1984). The infection rate in rural areas of Rwanda has been estimated to be very low (Van de Perre 1984; Harden 1987), so it is also possible that the combination of these two rates produces the somewhat lower rate. Prostitutes in Rwanda have had the highest infection rates reported in the world for this subgroup overall, with 80 percent reported as infected in 1983–84 (Mann, Francis, Quinn, et al. 1986; Padian 1988, 414). This level of infection was not reached by any other prostitute population studied until 1987, when 535 incarcerated women were studied in Nairobi, Kenya. They had an 85 percent infection rate (Padian 1988, 414). It is possible that the early (1983–84) figure for Rwandan prostitutes reflected ELISA tests that were not properly interpreted due to malaria contamination. This seems unlikely, however, given Rwanda's high altitude and relatively low level of malaria infection.

It seems likely that the reported rate of HIV-1 infection in the WHO figures underestimates the actual infection rate in Rwanda. However, Rwanda has not necessarily joined in the openness that other eastern African nations have begun to evidence with regard to AIDS. In the Kigezi case, underreporting seems less likely, especially because the area was served (at least in the 1960s) by two government hospitals, two mission hospitals, two health centers, and a number of dispensaries and maternity units (Hall and Langlands 1975, viii). This might be an area for further research. The surveillance system in Uganda is passive, not legally required, and thus cases may be underreported (Berkley, Okware, and Naamara 1989, 82). The Kigezi district, however, would have to have a systematic underreporting bias to explain the lower rate of AIDS cases than is found in other labor reserves. At present such a systematic bias is unknown, and therefore the low rate may be seen as unsupportive of the hypotheses put forward on geographical distribution.

In the West Nile district in the north of Uganda, cumulative AIDS case prevalence figures establish that the rate is also in the 11 to 50 per 100,000 person range in the southern areas of the district. In the northern areas, the case rate is lower, 1 to 10 per 100,000 persons. This is despite the fact that a low rate of infection has been claimed for the entire area of the West Nile (Carswell 1987). Why does this variation exist, and why is there a relatively low rate in the northern section of the West Nile?

There is some indication that the Tanzanian invasion and subsequent civil war, starting in 1978 and continuing until 1985, impeded the movement of commerce and migrant labor from the West Nile district to the Kampala area, thus delaying the spread of HIV-1 (Avirgan and Honey 1982; Carswell 1987; Mamdani 1988). Further, the Nile River itself often forms a "formidable barrier to communication" and interchange (Cars-well 1987). Unlike many previous wars and conflicts, the fighting in Uganda, by slowing the flow of migrant laborers from the West Nile area into Kampala, may have slowed down the spread of disease in the opposite direction. Certainly, the present prevalence of AIDS in the West Nile area is lower than in the Kampala area. There is some indication that the army, in its movements into the northwest to suppress the recent rebellion in this area of Uganda, may be spreading HIV-1 (*The Economist* 1987). The generally high rate of AIDS cases in the southern section of the West Nile, combined with the difficulties in commerce in the seventies and eighties, may be seen as supportive of the hypotheses that we have advanced for the AIDS epidemic, temporally and spatially.

In the central northern area of Acholi, which many cite as the leading area of migratory labor (Kabera 1982; Mamdani 1976), the cumulative rate of AIDS cases is second only to the labor concentrations around Kampala–Entebbe and Masaka, with a 51 to 100 per 100,000 person rate of cases in the western sections of Acholi. The western section of Lango and the eastern section of Acholi also contain unusually high cumulative rates of AIDS, at 11 to 50 cases per 100,000 persons. Both of these findings support the hypotheses on spatial and temporal distribution of AIDS.

In eastern sections of Uganda, a high cumulative AIDS-case prevalence rate occurs in the Bugisu area, also a major labor reserve and a source of migrant labor, although this rate of 11 to 50 cases per 100,000 persons extends northward into the Karamoja district. The latter development is unexplained by the labor-reserve theory advanced. It is possible that the extension into the Karamoja district reflects a labor migration from this area into Kenya, and a resulting spread of AIDS as a consequence of that migration and subsequent returns to the district of ill laborers. Internal census data and most historical data for the region deal not with interstate migration but with internal migration. Therefore it may be hypothesized that the extension of AIDS northward into the Karamoja district is a result of migration into the nearby labor concentrations of Kenya. In general, these results are supportive of hypotheses 1 through 7.

It is difficult to determine if the syndrome occurred earlier in the cities—that is, the areas of labor concentration—than in the labor reserves, but one can argue that the higher cumulative prevalence rates in the Kampala–Entebbe and Masaka areas are consistent with an earlier appearance there. Certainly, it can be argued that AIDS seems to have had a longer time in which to reach high epidemic levels in these areas.

When considering countries other than Uganda, Burundi, and Rwanda, the evidence is consistent with a higher rate of spread of HIV-1 in areas of labor concentration such as the copper mines of Zambia and Zaire (Harden 1987). In Lusaka, the capital of Zambia, the HIV-1 infection rate for blood donors was 15 percent in 1986. In the northern copper-belt areas, the rate of HIV-1 seropositivity among blood donors was 13 percent (Harden 1987; Melbye et al. 1986). Zambia has always had a clearer pattern of labor concentrations and labor reserves than Uganda, because the copper belt has dominated the economic development of the country (Mamdani 1976; Parpart 1983; Kay 1967; Roberts 1979). There is, unfortunately, little data from labor-reserve areas in Zambia to compare with the data from the northern copper belt.

In Zaire, it is clear that the rural prevalence of HIV-1 is low (Nzilambi et al. 1988) and that urban prevalence, at least in Kinshasa, is quite high (Mann, Francis, Davachi, et al. 1986). There is little data on the labor-reserve areas in Zaire, however, with which to compare these results.

HYPOTHESES 8 THROUGH 10. Migrant laborers should show higher rates of HIV-1 infection than other men in the population, and this data should correlate with family factors and length of contracts. There is a paucity of data on this point. Only two studies concentrate upon laborers who are migrant workers in the eastern, southern, and central Africa, and we may also use some national data to draw some conclusions concerning this group.

Seventy-four truck drivers for a large freight company in the Kampala region of Uganda were tested in 1986 for HIV-1. Some 55.9 percent were seropositive. (*The Economist* 1987; Carswell 1987). The overall HIV-1 infection rate for Kampala was estimated in 1986 to be approximately 10 percent (Harden 1986). Therefore we can say that, in Uganda, truck drivers have a much higher rate of infection than others in the population. These truck drivers and their mates, known as "turnboys," were either Ugandan or Kenyan nationals and had high numbers of sexual partners, particularly prostitutes (Carswell 1987).

In South Africa, the country with the most "developed" system of migrant labor, we might expect more clarity with regard to HIV-1 seropositivity. South Africa has a very systematic labor-reserve policy, termed a "homelands" policy, and workers are usually banned from living with their families close to where they contract to work. Thus familial separation is more clearly enforced in South Africa. This is particularly true in the mining regions of that country.

In 1987, South Africa reported an overall infection rate of 0.1 percent, with only forty-six cases of full-blown AIDS. By 1990 this had grown to five hundred cases of full-blown AIDS in a population of thirty-seven million, five million of whom are white (Wren 1990). Since 1987, the South African government has been testing migrant laborers from other countries for HIV-1 infection and refusing to admit infected laborers (the Malawi government has refused to allow its migrant laborers to be so tested, and so no Malawian workers have been admitted to South Africa). Migrant laborers already working in the mines who are infected with HIV-1 are not sent home, however, as long as they can work. It is estimated that, by 1990, approximately 1 percent of the black adult population in South Africa was infected with HIV-1, and "the number is rising fast" (Wren 1990). It would appear, therefore, that the AIDS epidemic will be concentrated in the migrant labor population in South Africa. The mechanisms outlined above for the spread of the epidemic will function also in South Africa. This is recognized by South African medical authorities studying the situation in that country (Ijsselmuiden et al. 1988; Sher 1986; Schoub et al. 1988; Wren 1990).

Finally, with regard to migrant laborers, the countries of Rwanda and Burundi, as mentioned earlier, seem to have a serious problem with AIDS infection (Harden 1987; Mann and Chin 1988; Mann et al. 1988; Brunet and Ancelle 1985; Biggar 1987; Quinn et al. 1986; WHO 1989). It is noteworthy that these two countries send massive numbers of migrant laborers to the labor-concentration areas of Uganda. In fact, these two mountainous countries comprise labor reserves for Uganda and, in the past, there have been some 380,000 Rwandans and 140,000 Rundi living in Uganda. These people come to Uganda as migrant laborers and usually are only temporary residents. A heavy proportion of the migrant laborers in the areas around Kampala come from Rwanda and Burundi (Hall and Langlands 1975, 7–8). The high cumulative prevalence rate of AIDS cases in Burundi, and the likelihood of a high prevalence in Rwanda, would argue strongly for the hypothesis that AIDS prevalence will be high among migrant laborers.

It is impossible from this data to determine if the earliest cases of AIDS in South Africa or in central or eastern Africa occurred among migrant laborers. Assuming, however, that in many of these areas the epidemic of AIDS is new to the region (see Carswell et al. 1986), we may say that the prevalence data gives an indication of where the epidemic really got its start. Thus, although there may be cases that show up earlier among isolated groups in South Africa, the prevalence among migrant laborers argues for an early appearance in this group. Unfortunately, there is little data on other migrant laborers and their family and sexual patterns; nor is this data correlated with length of contract, working conditions, and so forth. The lack of data mitigates against truly definitive conclusions.

HYPOTHESIS 11. One of the best documented facts concerning the epidemic of AIDS in Africa is the syndrome's incredibly high prevalence rates among prostitutes in all countries. Prostitutes are at high risk for HIV-1 infection (Mann et al. 1988), and the prostitute as a transmitter of HIV-1 infection has been recognized as a worldwide problem (Day 1988; Padian 1988; Carael et al. 1988; Hudson et al. 1988). The practice of prostitution varies in different areas of the world, from a professionalization associated with "marked distance between their working and private lives" (Day 1988, 421) in the United States to the much more informal types of prostitution practiced in sub-Saharan Africa, where prostitution is difficult to define (Day 1988, 424).

"Rates of infection among some prostitute groups range from 27 percent in Kinshasa, Zaire, to 66 percent in Nairobi, Kenya, and 88 percent in Butare, Rwanda" (Mann, Francis, Davachi, et al. 1986). Kigali, Rwanda, has an infection rate among prostitutes of approximately 25 percent, although rural infection rates are almost 0 percent (Van de Peere 1984; Harden 1987). In the Central African Republic, in a survey of 327 prostitutes concluded in 1986, 19 percent were HIV-1 seropositive. This is compared to a 4 percent overall infection rate in the republic (Specter 1986). In Tanzania, a study of 225 prostitutes in 1986 established a 29 percent HIV-1 seropositivity rate (Padian 1988, 414).

In a study in Kenya, it is also easy to see the growth in the HIV-1 infection incidence rate among prostitutes (Kreiss 1986). There was apparently a 4 percent rate of HIV-1 infection among prostitutes in Nairobi in 1980. In 1987, there was an infection prevalence rate among 115 prostitutes in Nairobi of 65 percent. All of these women had been uninfected by HIV-1 only one year before. Over half of the new cases were attributed to the presence of genital ulcers and to the use of birth control pills, which, it was claimed, increased the probability of HIV-1 infection (Specter 1986).

The overall HIV-1 infection rate for women is consistently much lower than for prostitutes, as would be expected. The overall infection rate for sexually active persons of both sexes is approximately 20 percent (Mann et al. 1988, 85). In fact, in Kampala, Uganda, women of childbearing age evidenced an infection rate of approximately 10 to 15 percent in 1986 (Harden 1987). In one hospital in Kampala, of one thousand pregnant women in 1986, 13 percent were found to be HIV-1 seropositive. The same hospital showed a seropositivity rate of 24 percent one year later in the testing of 170 pregnant women (Carswell 1987; Harden 1987).

In all of the countries of central, eastern, and southern Africa, the mean age of men with HIV-1 seropositivity was greater than the mean age of women who were infected (Quinn 1987; Quinn et al. 1986; Mann, Francis, Quinn, et al. 1986). Women have accounted for a majority of the AIDS cases in the twenty to twenty-nine age group in Kinshasa, Zaire, but the majority of cases are male in the forty to forty-nine and fifty to fifty-nine age groups, although both of these groups are generally smaller cohorts of AIDS cases than the twenty to twenty-nine age group (Mann, Francis, Quinn, et al. 1986). Among those suffering from AIDS, women were more likely to be unmarried than men (Quinn 1987; Quinn et al. 1986; Mann, Francis, Quinn, et al. 1986).

All of this evidence points to an STD in which the number of partners increases the risk of exposure to the infection (Carswell 1987; Clumeck et al. 1985; Kreiss 1986; Van de Perre 1984; Serwadda et al. 1985). Prostitutes, who have large numbers of partners, are particularly at risk. But the pattern also fits the larger social model that has been advanced. Young women, migrating to concentrations of male migrant labor, become prostitutes to earn a living in an environment in which women are rarely employed in wage labor or other "legitimate" sector jobs.

HYPOTHESIS 12. There is little question that those who were previously infected by STDs are at higher risk for HIV-1 infection (Pepin et al. 1989). This is due to the continued high number of sexual partners for those in this group and may be evidence of a life situation, such as migrant laboring, that structures an unstable sexual life. Further, this group increases risk if STDs are untreated or if lesions and ulceration are present, thereby allowing easier infection.

HYPOTHESIS 13. Unfortunately, it is not possible to compare migrant workers with those from the same labor-reserve area who do not migrate, because there seems to be little data that tests migrant workers themselves. Thus at present there is little ability to compare prevalence rates for the two groups.

HYPOTHESIS 14. There is little question of the complex nature of the AIDS epidemic in central, eastern, and southern Africa (Biggar 1987; Carswell 1987). The complex advance of this epidemic is capable of blinding observers to the patterns still present, just as a lack of geographical, historical, and economic information makes the map of cumulative prevalence of AIDS virtually unintelligible.

What is quite clear from much of the data dealing with urban and rural prevalence of HIV-1 seropositivity and AIDS cases is that a rural-to-urban spread pattern is not present. Urban infection rates are considerably higher than rural ones (Wender et al. 1986; Recene et al. 1987; Nzilambi et al. 1988; Van de Perre 1984; Peterson et al. 1987; Clumeck et al. 1985; Carswell 1987; Carswell et al. 1986; Berkley, Okware, and Naamara 1989). This data is refutation of the argument that HIV-1 was somehow endemic in rural Africa, then broke out into the broader community because of war and social disruption. Such an argument would not evidence the prevalence patterns we have seen. Much more logical is the spread of AIDS according to the complex patterns of migratory labor in the eastern, central, and southern African economy. This would explain the complex pattern of cumulative AIDS prevalence that is seen in Uganda. The effects of this system of labor on sexual practices and on the stability of the African family help to set up the pattern of AIDS epidemic, which we can see in outline form from the evidence available.

There seems to be substantial evidence, particularly in geographical cumulative prevalence data and also in HIV-1 seropositivity prevalence data for some specific population groups and geographical areas, to support the model that we presented for the AIDS epidemic in eastern, central, and southern Africa. In rather a striking manner, the evidence supports the theory that HIV-1 and resulting AIDS first struck the labor concentrations in Uganda and then moved outward to the labor reserves, carried by migrant laborers and prostitutes as they returned to their birthplaces for care and assistance with illnesses consequent to infection by this virus.

Conclusions

The evidence of the data and prevalence surveys supports the dynamics of the AIDS epidemic that we presented earlier in this exposition. A migrant labor system, founded in pre-World War I European imperialism, continues today in eastern, central, and southern Africa. The African continent—particularly the eastern, southern, and central regions—exists in a peripheral relationship with the core capitalist countries in the capitalist world system.

The migrant labor system has profound effects on the health of the population in these areas. This essay has argued that one of the consequences of peripheral status and such a labor market is the social structuring of a population for susceptibility to STDs. This social structuring and its consequences in STD patterns in eastern, southern, and central Africa determine the nature of the AIDS epidemic in these regions. It is this structuring that fixes the epidemiological patterns that are so distinctive from those of North America. A number of implications arise from this conclusion.

It would seem clear that prevention of HIV-1 infection should target those groups who enter the migrant labor pool. Educational, preventative, and general health resources need to be directed toward these groups. It is precisely these groups who frequently have the fewest health resources available to them. This needs to be reversed.

There are a number of other areas in the world in which Pattern Two AIDS occurs. These areas are also peripheral in the world system. An investigation should proceed to determine if a link between migrant labor and AIDS is present in such areas. This investigation would include such countries as Haiti. We know, for instance, that there is considerable migratory labor between Haiti and the Dominican Republic. Is migrant labor spreading AIDS in these areas? Are the dynamics the same as or different from the African dynamics? What about other areas of the Third World, which may be a patchwork quilt of Pattern One and Pattern Two AIDS—does migratory labor contribute to the different patterns in these areas? South America has been presented by some research as such a patchwork area of Pattern One and Pattern Two AIDS.

The implications for such countries as South Africa, which clearly has a very developed and rigidified migratory labor system—a system encased in legal *apartheid*—would seem particularly precarious (Becker 1986; Sher 1986; Schoub et al. 1988). Recent developments do indicate that the connection between migratory labor and AIDS may create a very difficult and explosive expansion of the AIDS epidemic in this area. Heterosexual cases of AIDS in South Africa among blacks in the labor reserves and squatter camps are growing in number at an alarming rate. "It is estimated that 1 percent of the country's black population is carrying the AIDS virus and that this number is rising fast. Two Johannesburg researchers have forecast that as many as 446,000 adult South Africans, almost all of them black, could be infected by the end of next year" (Wren 1990).

Much as occurred in northwestern Uganda because of the civil war, South Africa's isolation due the antiapartheid movement appears to have spared the country from AIDS for some time. As Christopher Wren (1990) states:

> Although the country's relative isolation because of its apartheid may have helped protect its people from contact with AIDS, truck drivers and guest workers from countries to the north are believed to have introduced the disease into the black population. . . . The spread has been accelerated by the country's internal migrant labor system, which forced blacks to leave their families in rural areas and seek work in mines and factories around the white cities. This has caused a breakdown of the traditional family and an increase in prostitution and other promiscuity.
>   "The pillar of the educational program is one sexual partner. . . . But with the migrant labor system, it's condoned for a man to have a sexual partner where he's working."

The implications for South Africa's future may be quite serious, to say the least. It is estimated that a 10 percent incidence of AIDS in South Africa could devastate the nation's economy (Wren 1990). Incidence rates of this magnitude have easily been reached in other areas of Africa, which have the combination of an AIDS and HIV-1 epidemic and migrant labor systems. It is ironic that the isolation of South Africa because of its apartheid system has apparently also limited the information it has received concerning AIDS and AIDS-control strategies, thereby limiting its ability to organize a defense against the disease (Ijsselmuiden et al. 1988; Wren 1990).

In a somewhat more theoretical vein, there seems little, if any, evidence at present to support the theory of an African origin for the AIDS epidemic or HIV-1. Insofar as the epidemiological pattern of the AIDS epidemic in Africa can be traced to the syndrome's rapid spread by the migratory labor system, the African origins theories would seem to be further undermined. It is not necessary to argue a long stay on the African continent for HIV-1 to reach high levels of prevalence; at least, it is not necessary when there is such a mechanism for transmission as the migratory labor system.

As a further theoretical note, it would also seem unnecessary to make extreme assumptions, as have certain sociobiologists, concerning racial differences in reproductive strategies to explain the nature of the AIDS epidemic in Africa. Despite the tendency for North Americans to use science to explain events, biology is not necessarily definitive in explaining the epidemiology of AIDS in Africa. The AIDS epidemic in Africa is rooted in the social, historical, and economic fabric of the continent. As a medical sociologist stated well over a decade ago, epidemics are social events (Stark 1977).

REFERENCES

Altman, Dennis. 1986. *AIDS in the Mind of America*. Garden City, N.Y.: Anchor/ Doubleday.
Amin, Samir. 1976. *Unequal Development: An Essay on the Social Formations of Peripheral Capitalism*. New York: Monthly Review.
Anderson, R. M., R. M. May, and A. R. McLean. 1988. "Possible Demographic Consequences of AIDS in Developing Countries." *Nature* 332(6161):228.
Avirgan, Tony, and Martha Honey. 1982. *War in Uganda: The Legacy of Idi Amin*. Westport, Conn.: Lawrence Hill.
Becker, W. B. 1986. "HTLV-III Infection in the RSA." *South African Medical Journal* supplement 70(8):26–27.
Bennett, F. J. 1962. "The Social Determinants of Gonorrhoea in an East African Town." *East African Medicine* 39(6) :332–42.
———. 1964. "Gonorrhoea: A Rural Pattern of Transmission." *East African Medical Journal* 41(4):163–67.
———. 1975. "Venereal Disease and Other Spirochaetal Diseases." In *Uganda Atlas of Disease Distribution*, 64–65. *See* Hall and Langlands, eds., 1975.
Berkley, Seth, Samuel Okware, and Warren Naamara. 1989. "Surveillance for AIDS in Uganda." *AIDS* 3(2):79–85.
Biggar, Robert J. 1986. "The AIDS Problem in Africa." *Lancet* 1(8472):79–83.
———. 1987. "AIDS in Subsaharan Africa." *Cancer Detection and Prevention* supplement 1:487–91.
Biggar, Robert J., Mads Melbye, Prem S. Sarin, Paul Demedts, Charles Delacollette, Wim J. Stevens, Paul L. Gigase, Luc Kestens, Anne J. Bodner, Leopold Paluku, and William A. Blattner. 1985. "ELISA HTLV Retrovirus Antibody Reactivity Associated with Malaria and Immune Complexes in Healthy Africans." *Lancet* 2(8454): 520–23.
Brandt, Allan M. 1985. *No Magic Bullet: A Social History of Venereal Disease in the United States since 1880*. New York: Oxford University Press.
Brown, Stuart T., Fernando R. K. Zacarias, and Sevgi O. Aral. 1985. "STD Control in Less Developed Countries: The Time Is Now." *International Journal of Epidemiology* 14(4):505–9.
Brunet, J. B., and R. A. Ancelle. 1985. "The International Occurrence of the Acquired Immunodeficiency Syndrome." *Annals of Internal Medicine* 103(5):670–74.

Carael, Michel, Philippe H. Van de Perre, Philippe H. Lepage, Susan Allen, Francois Nsenquimuremyi, Christian Van Goethem, Melanie Ntahorutaba, Didace Nzaramba, and Nathan Clumeck. 1988. "Human Immunodeficiency Virus Transmission among Heterosexual Couples in Central Africa." *AIDS* 2(3):201–5.

Carswell, J. Wilson. 1987. "HIV Infection in Healthy Persons in Uganda." *AIDS* 1(4):223–27.

Carswell, J. Wilson, N. Sewankambo, G. Lloyd, and R. G. Downing. 1986. "How Long Has the AIDS Virus Been in Uganda?" *Lancet* 1(8491):1217.

Chavkin, Wendy, ed. 1984. *Double Exposure: Women's Health Hazards on the Job and at Home.* New York: Monthly Review.

Clumeck, Nathan, Marjorie Robert-Guroff, Philippe Van de Perre, Andrea Jennings, Jean Sibomana, Patrick Demol, Sophie Cran, and Robert C. Gallo. 1985. "Seroepidemiological Studies of HTLV-III Antibody Prevalence among Selected Groups of Heterosexual Africans." *Journal of the American Medical Association* 254(18):2599–2602.

Crush, Jonathan. 1984. "Uneven Labour Migration in Southern Africa: Conceptions and Misconceptions." *South African Geographical Journal* 66(2):115–32.

Curran, James W. 1985. "The Epidemiology and Prevention of the Acquired Immunodeficiency Syndrome." *Annals of Internal Medicine* 103(5):657–62.

Curran, James W., Meade Morgan, A. M. Hardy, H. W. Jaffe, W. M. Darrow, and W. R. Dowdle. 1985. "The Epidemiology of AIDS: Current Status and Future Prospects." *Science* 229:1352–57.

Davidson, Basil. 1983. *Modern Africa.* New York: Longman.

Day, Sophie. 1988. "Prostitute Women and AIDS: Anthropology." *AIDS* 2(4):421–28.

DeLancey, Mark W. 1978. "Health and Disease on the Plantations of Cameroon, 1884–1939." In *Disease in African History: An Introductory Survey and Case Studies,* ed. Gerald W. Hartwig and K. David Patterson, 151–79. Durham,: N.C. Duke University Press.

Doyal, Lesley (with Immogen Pennell). 1981. *The Political Economy of Health.* Boston: South End.

The Economist. 1987. "In the Heart of the Plague." March 21–27:45.

Epstein, Paul, and Randall Packard. 1987. "Ecology and Immunity." *Science for the People* (January–February):10–17+.

Epstein, Samuel S. 1976. "The Political and Economic Basis of Cancer." *Technology Review* 78:1–7.

———. 1978. *The Politics of Cancer.* San Francisco: Sierra Club.

Eyer, Joseph. 1975. "Hypertension as a Disease of Modern Society." *International Journal of Health Services* 5(4):539–58.

———. 1977. "Prosperity as a Cause of Death." *International Journal of Health Services* 7(1):125–50.

Eyer, Joseph, and Peter Sterling. 1977. "Stress-Related Mortality and Social Organization." *Review of Radical Political Economy* 8(1):1–44.

Foster, John Bellamy. 1986. *The Theory of Monopoly Capitalism: An Elaboration of Marxian Political Economy.* New York: Monthly Review.

Frank, Andre G. 1967. *Capitalism and Underdevelopment in Latin America.* New York: Monthly Review.

Freund, Bill. 1988. *The African Worker.* New York: Cambridge University Press.

Freund, William. 1984. *The Making of Contemporary Africa: The Development of African Society since 1800.* Bloomington: University of Indiana Press.

Friedman, Kathie. 1984. "Households as Income-Pooling Units." In *Households and the World Economy,* ed. Joan Smith, Immanuel Wallerstein, and Hans-Dieter Evers, 37–55. Beverly Hills: Sage.

Gallo, Robert C. 1987. "The AIDS Virus." *Scientific American* 256(1):46–56.

Garry, Robert F., Marlys H. Witte, A. Arthur Gottlieb, Memory Elvin-Lewis, Marise S. Gottlieb, Charles L. Witte, Steve S. Alexander, William R. Cole, and William L. Drake. 1988. "Documentation of an AIDS Virus Infection in the United States in 1968." *Journal of the American Medical Association* 260(14):2085–87.

Georges, Alain J., Paul M. V. Martin, Jean-Paul Gonzalez, Daniele Salaun, Christian C. Mathiot, Gerard Grezenguet, and Marie-Claude Georges-Courbot. 1987. "HIV-1 Seroprevalence and AIDS Diagnostic Criteria in Central African Republic." Letter in *Lancet* 2(8571):1332.

Gimui, Kiboma. 1982. "Spatial Inequalities and Population Redistribution with Reference to Uganda." In *Redistribution of Population in Africa*, ed. John I. Clarke and Laszek A. Kosinski, 146–49 London: Heinemann.

Gugler, Josef. 1968. "The Impact of Labor Migration on Society and Economy in Sub-Saharan Africa: Empirical Findings and Theoretical Considerations." *African Social Research* (December 6):463–86.

Gutkind, Peter C. W., and Immanuel Wallerstein. 1976. *The Political Economy of Contemporary Africa.* Beverly Hills: Sage.

Hall, S. A., and B. W. Langlands, eds. 1975. *Uganda Atlas of Disease Distribution.* Nairobi: East African.

Harden, Blaine. 1986. "Uganda Battles AIDS Epidemic." *Washington Post* (June 2):A1, A18.

———. 1987. "AIDS Seen as Threat to Africa's Future." *Washington Post* (May 31):A1, A18.

Hilts, Philip J. 1987. "AIDS Takes Heavy Toll of African Children." *Washington Post* (October 10):A6.

Hooper, Ed. 1987. "AIDS in Uganda." *African Affairs* 86(345):469–77.

Hooper, K., and Sally Guttmacher. 1979. "Rethinking Suicide: Notes toward a Critical Epidemiology." *International Journal of Health Services* 9:417–38.

Hudson, Christopher P., Anselm J. M. Hennis, Peter Kataaha, Graham Lloyd, A. Timothy Moore, Gordon M. Sutehall, Rod Whetstone, Tim Wreghitt, and Abraham Karpas. 1988. "Risk Factors for the Spread of AIDS in Rural Africa: Evidence from a Comparative Seroepidemiological Survey of AIDS, Hepatitis B and Syphilis in Southwestern Uganda." *AIDS* 2(4):255–60.

Huminer, David, Joseph B. Rosenfeld, and Silvio D. Pitlik. 1987. "AIDS in the Pre-AIDS Era." *Review of Infectious Diseases* 9(6):1102–8.

Hunt, Charles W. 1988. "Africa and AIDS: Dependent Development, Sexism and Racism." *Monthly Review* 39(9):10–22.

Hunter, John M., ed. 1974. *The Geography of Health and Disease.* Chapel Hill: University of North Carolina Department of Geography.

Ijsselmuiden, C. B., M. H. Steinberg, G. N. Padayachee, B. D. Schoub, S. A. Strauss, E. Buch, J. C. A. Davies, C. DeBeer, J. S. S. Gear, and H. S. Hurwitz. 1988. "AIDS and South Africa—Towards a Comprehensive Strategy." *South African Medical Journal* 73(8):461–64.

Kabera, John B. 1982. "Rural Population Redistribution in Uganda since 1900." In *Redistribution of Population in Africa*, 192–201. *See* Gimui 1982.

Karugire, S. R. 1980. *A Political History of Uganda.* Nairobi: Heinemann.

Kay, George. 1967. *A Social Geography of Zambia.* London: University of London Press.

Kibukamusoke, J. W. 1975. "Diseases of the Genito-Urinary System." In *Uganda Atlas of Disease Distribution*, 121–24. *See* Hall and Langlands, eds., 1975.

Konotey-Ahulu, Felix I. D. 1987. "AIDS in Africa: Misinformation and Disinformation." *Lancet* 2(8252):206–7.

Kreiss, Joan K. 1986. "AIDS Virus Infection in Nairobi Prostitutes: Spread of the Epidemic to East Africa." *New England Journal of Medicine* 314(7):414–18.

Langlands, B. W. 1975. "Introduction: The Geographic Basis to the Pattern of Disease in Uganda." In *Uganda Atlas of Disease Distribution*, 1–10. *See* Hall and Langlands, eds., 1975.

Leys, Colin. 1975. *Underdevelopment in Kenya: The Political Economy of Neo-Colonialism*. Los Angeles: University of California Press.

Leys, R. 1974. "South African Gold Mining in 1974: 'The Gold of Migrant Labour.'" *African Affairs* 74(295):196–208.

Loewenson, Rene. 1988. "Labour Insecurity and Health: An Epidemiological Study in Zimbabwe." *Social Science and Medicine* 27(7):733–41.

McCance, R. A., and I. H. E. Rutishauser. 1975. "Childhood Malnutrition." In *Uganda Atlas of Disease Distribution*, 89–92. *See* Hall and Langlands, eds., 1975.

McGlashan, N. D., ed. 1972. *Medical Geography: Techniques and Field Studies*. New York: Harper & Row.

Mamdani, Mahmood. 1976. *Politics and Class Formation in Uganda*. New York: Monthly Review.

———. 1988. "Uganda in Transition: Two Years of the NRA/NRM." *Third World Quarterly* 10(3):1155–81.

Mann, Jonathan, and James Chin. 1988. "AIDS: A Global Perspective." *New England Journal of Medicine*. 319(5):302–3.

Mann, Jonathan M., James Chin, Peter Piot, and Thomas Quinn. 1988. "The International Epidemiology of AIDS." *Scientific American* 259(4):82–89.

Mann, Jonathan M., Henry Francis, Thomas Quinn, Pangu Kaza Asila, Ngaly Bosenge, Nzila Nzilambi, Kapita Bila, Muyembe Tamfum, Kalisa Ruti, Peter Piot, Joseph McCormick, and James W. Curran. 1986. "Surveillance for AIDS in a Central African City." *Journal of the American Medical Association* 255(23):3255–59.

Mann, Jonathan M., Henry Francis, Farzin Davachi, Paola Baudoux, Thomas C. Quinn, Nzila Nzilambi, Ngaly Bosenge, Robert L. Colebunders, Peter Piot, Ndoko Kabote, Pangu Kaza Asila, Miatudila Malonga, and James W. Curran. 1986. "Risk Factors for Human Immunodeficiency Virus Seropositivity among Children 1–24 Months Old in Kinshasa, Zaire." *Lancet* 2(8508):654–56.

Martin, William G. 1984. "Beyond the Peasant and Proletarian Debate: African Household Formation in South Africa." In *Households and the World Economy*, 151–67. *See* Friedman 1984.

Mayer, Jonathan D. 1988. "Migrant Studies and Medical Geography: Conceptual Problems and Methodological Issues." In *Conceptual and Methodological Issues in Medical Geography*, 136–54. *See* Meade, ed., 1988.

Meade, Melinda S., ed. 1988. *Conceptual and Methodological Issues in Medical Geography*. New York: Guilford.

Melbye, Mads, Anne Bayley, J. K. Manuwele, Susan A. Clayden, William A. Blattner, Richard Tedder, E. K. Njelesani, K. Mukelabai, F. J. Bowa, Arthur Levin, Robin A. Weiss, and Robert J. Biggar. 1986. "Evidence for Heterosexual Transmission and Clinical Manifestations of Human Immunodeficiency Virus Infection and Related Conditions in Lusaka, Zambia." *Lancet* 2(8516):1113–15.

Moodie, T. Dunbar. 1988. "Migrancy and Male Sexuality on the South African Gold Mines." *Journal of Southern African Studies* 14(2):228–56.

Mugerwa, R., and G. Giraldo. 1987. "Some Clinical Aspects of AIDS in Uganda." *Second International Symposium on AIDS and Associated Cancers in Africa*. Abstract S.3.2. Naples, Italy (October 7–9).

Mugerwa, R., R. Widy-Wirski, and S. Okwake. 1987. "Assessment of a Provisional WHO Clinical Case-Definition of HIV Related Illness in the Referral Hospital of Uganda." *Second International Symposium on AIDS and Associated Cancers in Africa*. Abstract TH–89. Naples, Italy (October 7–9).

Mulder, Carel. 1988. "Human AIDS Virus Not from Monkeys." *Nature* 333 (6172):396.

Murray, Colin. 1977. "High Bridewealth, Migrant Labour and the Position of Women in Lesotho." *Journal of African Law* 21(1):79–96.

———. 1980. "Migrant Labour and the Changing Family Structure in Rural Periphery of South Africa." *Journal of Southern African Studies* 6(2):139–56.

———. 1981. *Families Divided: The Impact of Migrant Labour in Lesotho*. Cambridge: Cambridge University Press.

Navarro, Vicente. 1974. "The Underdevelopment of Health or the Health of Underdevelopment." *Politics and Society* (Winter):267–93.

———. 1982. "The Labor Process and Health: A Historical Materialist Interpretation." *International Journal of Health Services* 12(1):5–29.

Navarro, Vicente, and Daniel M. Berman, eds. 1983. *Health and Work under Capitalism: An International Perspective*. Farmingdale, N.Y. Baywood.

Norman, Colin. 1985. "Politics and Science Clash on African AIDS." *Science* 230 (4730):1140–42.

Nzilambi, Nzila, Kevin M. DeCock, Donald N. Forthal, Henry Francis, Robert W. Ryder, Ismey Malebe, Jane Getchell, Marie Laga, Peter Piot, and Joseph B. McCormick. 1988. "The Prevalence of Infection with Human Immunodeficiency Virus over a 10-Year Period in Rural Zaire." *New England Journal of Medicine* 318 (5):276–79.

Osoba, A. O. 1981. "Sexually Transmitted Diseases in Tropical Africa." *British Journal of Venereal Disease* 57:89–94.

Padian, Nancy S. 1988. "Prostitute Women and AIDS: Epidemiology." *AIDS* 2(6):414–19.

Parker, Richard. "Acquired Immunodeficiency Syndrome in Urban Brazil." *Medical Anthropology Quarterly* 1(2):155–75.

Parpart, Jane L. 1983. *Labor and Capital on the African Copperbelt*. Philadelphia: Temple University Press.

Pepin, Jacques, Francis A. Plummer, Robert C. Brunham, Peter Piot, D. William Cameron, and Allan R. Ronald. 1989. "The Interaction of HIV Infection and Other Sexually Transmitted Diseases: An Opportunity for Intervention." *AIDS* 3(1):3–9.

Peterson, Hans D., Bjarne O. Lindhardt, Peter M. Nyarango, Tula R. Bowry, Alex K. Chemtal, Kim Krogsgaard, and Albert Bunyasi. 1987. "A Prevalence Study of HIV Antibodies in Rural Kenya." *Scandinavian Journal of Infectious Diseases* 19:395–401.

Piot, Peter, Francis A. Plummer, Fred S. Mhalu, Jean-Louis Lamboray, James Chin, and Jonathan Mann. 1988. "AIDS: An International Perspective." *Science* 239 (February 5):573–79.

Prothero, R. Mansell. 1977. "Disease and Mobility: A Neglected Factor in Epidemiology." *International Journal of Epidemiology* 3(6):259–67.

———. 1983. "Medical Geography of Tropical Africa." In *Geographical Aspects of Health*, ed. N. D. McGlashan and J. R. Blunden, 137–53. San Francisco: Academic.

Pyle, Gerald F. 1979. *Applied Medical Geography*. New York: John Wiley & Sons.

Quinn, Thomas C. 1987. "AIDS in Africa: Evidence for Heterosexual Transmission of the Human Immunodeficiency Virus." *New York State Journal of Medicine* 87 (5):286–89.

Quinn, Thomas C., Jonathan M. Mann, James W. Curran, and Peter Piot. 1986. "AIDS in Africa: An Epidemiological Paradigm." *Science* 234 (November 21):955–63.

Rampen, F. 1978. "Venereal Syphilis in Tropical Africa." *British Journal of Venereal Disease* 54:364–68.

Ratnam, Attili V., Shahida N. Din, Subhash K. Hira, Ganapati J. Bhat, D.S.O. Wacha, A. Rukmini, and Raphael C. Mulenga. 1982. "Syphilis in Pregnant Women in Zambia." *British Journal of Venereal Disease* 58:355–58.

Recene, U., S. Orach, and A. Petti. 1987. "HTLV III–TB Association in Northern

Uganda (Gulu District)." *Second International Conference on AIDS and Associated Cancers in Africa*. Abstract TH–80. ts. Naples, Italy (October 7–9).

Roberts, A. 1979. *A History of Zambia*. New York: Africana.

Rodney, Walter. 1982. *How Europe Underdeveloped Africa*. Washington, D. C.: Howard University Press.

Sajiwandani, Jonathan, and K. S. Baboo. "Sexually Transmitted Diseases in Zambia." 1987. *Journal of the Royal Society of Health* 5:183–86.

Sanders, David, and Rob Davies. 1988. "The Economy, the Health Sector and Child Health in Zimbabwe since Independence." *Social Science and Medicine* 27(7): 723–31.

Sathyamurthy, T. V. 1986. *The Political Development of Uganda: 1900–1986*. Brookfield, Vt.: Gower.

Saul, John S., and Giovanni Arrighi. 1973. *Essays on the Political Economy of Africa*. New York: Monthly Review.

Schall, Peter L., and Rochelle Kern. 1986. "Hypertension in American Society: An Introduction to Historical Materialist Epidemiology." In *The Society of Health and Illness: Critical Perspectives*, 2d ed., ed. Peter Conrad and Rochelle Kern, 73–89. New York: St. Martin's.

Schoub, B. D., A. N. Smith, S. F. Lyons, S. Johnson, D. J. Martin, G. McGillivray, G. N. Padayachee, S. Naidoo, E. L. Fisher, and H. S. Hurwitz. 1988. "Epidemiological Considerations of the Present Status and Future Growth of the Acquired Immunodeficiency Syndrome Epidemic in South Africa." *South African Medical Journal* 74 (August 20):153–157.

Serwadda, D., N. K. Sewankambo, J. W. Carswell, A. C. Bayley, R. S. Tedder, R. A. Weiss, R. D. Mugerwa, A. Lwegaba, G. B. Kirya, R. G. Downing, S. A. Clayden, and A. G. Dalgleish. 1985. "Slim Disease: A New Disease in Uganda and Its Association with HTLV-III Infection." *Lancet* 2(8460):849–52.

Sher, R. 1986. "Acquired Immune Deficiency Syndrome (AIDS) in the RSA." *South African Medical Journal* supplement 70(8):23–26.

Shilts, Randy. 1987. *And the Band Played On: Politics, People, and the AIDS Epidemic*. New York: Penguin.

Simonsen, J. Neil. 1988. "Human Immunodeficiency Virus Infection among Men with Sexually Transmitted Diseases: Experience from a Center in Africa." *New England Journal of Medicine* 319(5):1274–78.

Smith, Barbara E. 1981. "Black Lung: The Social Production of Disease." *International Journal of Health Services* 11(3):343–59.

Smith, Joan. 1984. "Nonwage Labor and Subsistence." In *Households in the World Economy*, 64–89. See Friedman 1984.

Sontag, Susan. 1978. *Illness as Metaphor*. New York: Farrar, Straus, & Giroux.

———. 1989. *AIDS and Its Metaphors*. New York: Farrar, Straus, & Giroux.

Specter, Michael. 1986. "AIDS Infection and Birth Control Pills." *Washington Post* (May 31):A18.

Stamm, Walter E., H. Hunter Handsfield, Anne M. Rompalo, Rhoda L. Ashley, Pacita L. Roberts, and Lawrence Corey. 1988. "The Association between Genital Ulcer Disease and Acquisition of HIV Infection in Homosexual Men." *Journal of the American Medical Association* 260(10):1429–33.

Stark, Evan. 1977. "The Epidemic as a Social Event." *International Journal of Health Services* 7(4):681–705.

Stichter, Sharon. 1985. *Migrant Laborers*. New York: Cambridge University Press.

Turshen, Meredeth. 1977. "The Impact of Colonialism on Health and Health Services in Tanzania." *International Journal of Health Services* 7(1):7–35.

———. 1984. *The Political Ecology of Disease in Tanzania*. New Brunswick, N.J.: Rutgers University Press.

Van de Perre, Philippe. 1984. "Acquired Immunodeficiency Syndrome in Rwanda." *Lancet* 2(8394):62–69.

Vaughn, Megan, and Henrietta Moore. 1988. "Health, Nutrition and Agricultural Development in Northern Zambia." *Social Science and Medicine* 27(7):743–45.

Verhagen, A. R., and W. Gemert. 1972. "Social and Epidemiological Determinants of Gonorrhoea in an East African Country." *British Review of Venereal Disease* 277(48):277–86.

Waitzkin, Howard. 1978. "A Marxist View of Medical Care." *Annals of Internal Medicine* 89(2):264–78.

———. 1983. *The Second Sickness: Contradictions of Capitalist Health Care.* New York: Free Press.

Waldron, Ingrid. 1986. "Why Do Women Live Longer than Men?" In *The Sociology of Health and Illness*, 34–44. *See* Schall and Kern.

Waldron, Ingrid, and J. Eryer. 1975. "Socioeconomic Causes of the Recent Rise in Death Rates for 15–24 Year Olds." *Social Science and Medicine* no. 9:383–96.

Wallerstein, Immanuel, 1984. "Household Structures and Labor-Force Formation in the Capitalist World-Economy." In *Households and the World Economy*, 17–22. *See* Friedman 1984.

Wallerstein, Immanuel, and William G. Martin. 1979. "Peripheralization of Southern Africa: Changes in Household Structure and Labor-Force Formation." *Review* 3(2):325–71.

Wender, I., J. Schneider, B. Gras, A. F. Fleming, G. Hunsmann, and H. Schmitz. 1986. "Seroepidemiology of Human Immunodeficiency Virus in Africa." *British Medical Journal* 293 (September 27):782–85.

White, Richard. 1978. *Africa: Geographic Studies.* London: Heinemann.

World Health Organization (WHO). 1988. "A Global Response to AIDS." *Africa Report* (November–December):13–16.

———. 1989. "Statistics from the World Health Organization and the Centers for Disease Control." *AIDS* 3(2):113–17.

Wren, Christopher. 1990. "AIDS Rising Fast among Black South Africans." *New York Times* (September 27):A12.

Chapter 2

Women and Work in Rural Taiwan:
Building a Contextual Model Linking
Employment and Health

RITA S. GALLIN

During the past two decades, Taiwan's economy has ranked among the
fastest growing in the developing world. As its economy has grown and
the demand for labor has increased, women have entered the wage labor
force in large numbers. Between 1956 and 1973, the proportion of female
workers in Taiwan increased from 20 to 40 percent (Greenhalgh 1985,
273); in 1986, women accounted for 45 percent of the labor force (DGBAS
1987, 6). Mature, married women make up a large part of this increase. In
1986, for example, over half (52 percent) of Taiwan's female employees
were thirty years of age and older (DGBAS 1987, 13); two-fifths (42 percent) were married (DGBAS 1982, 102–3).

To understand the meaning of work to women such as these, I lived
in the Taiwanese rural village of Hsin Hsing for four weeks during the
summer of 1982. The village and is people were already well known to
me; I had conducted seventeen months of field research there in the late
1950s, visited often in the 1960s while studying the migration of Hsin
Hsing residents to the capital city of Taipei, and lived and studied there
twice in the 1970s.[1]

During these thirty years of study, the economy of Hsin Hsing
changed dramatically from a system based almost purely on agriculture
to a system founded predominantly on off-farm employment. By 1979,
four-fifths of the village men were engaged in nonagricultural activities.

Reprinted from *Journal of Health and Social Behavior* 30 (Dec. 1985):374–85.

Village women had been drawn into the local off-farm labor force in large numbers to meet the great demand for workers by labor-intensive industries.

Most of these employed women held jobs that entailed physical hazards. Those who handled cotton fibers were exposed to cotton dust and the risk of respiratory disease. Others routinely came into contact with chemicals known to cause skin and eye irritations, as well as a variety of more serious conditions faced by workers in the textile, apparel, and electronics industries. Most worked at jobs that involved lifting, bending, carrying, and standing, all of which are likely to have adverse effects on health. A majority held jobs conducive to stress; in their dual roles as workers and as housewives, they also were exposed to repeated stressors. Thus the social aspects of their work, like the physical aspects, exposed these women to many health hazards.

I did not collect detailed or systematic data on the women's health. Yet in interviews about their work and its meaning to them, the women invariably discussed their health status and behaviors. They readily attributed a number of acute symptoms and illnesses to the physical aspects of their work. Without longitudinal data, however, it is impossible to evaluate the overall effects of these hazards on their future health (Waldron 1980, 443) or to assess the long-term health consequences of the social aspects of their work (House et al. 1986). Thus to understand what these consequences might be, I turned to the literature about women, work, and health in the United States.

In the literature I found two interpretations, or polar views, of the relationship between women's well-being and the social aspects of their work. These I labeled (1) the rewards model and (2) the stress–strain model. Both were based on the assumption that women's cognitive responses to employment mediated between health outcomes and individual situations (see, e.g., Haw 1982; Lewin and Olesen 1985; Stellman 1977, 40–80). One interpretation emphasized the perceived rewards of working and hence the positive effects of employment on health; the other stressed the perceived tensions of working and accordingly the negative consequences of employment on health.

Neither model, however, explained adequately the response of Hsin Hsing women to their work and life situations. My attempt to understand why this was so raised a number of questions: Why do women assign a variety of meanings to their situations? What do these meanings reflect about the political, economic, and social contexts in which they are situated? How is women's health or illness shaped by the dynamics of this larger system? The answers to these questions led me to develop an exploratory model linking employment and health. This model outlines the relationship between microphenomena, such as meanings attributed to work and health states, and macrophenomena, such as national political–economic processes and the world capitalist system. The purpose of this chapter is to describe women's work and its meaning in Hsin Hsing and to discuss the contextual model developed.

The chapter begins with a brief review of the two models that have been offered to explain the consequences of work for women's health. Next I discuss the development of Taiwan and the traditional Chinese family to establish the political, economic, and cultural context in which the women of Hsin Hsing live. After this discussion I present descriptive data about Hsin Hsing and explore the meaning of work to its women. In the final section I discuss the contextual model linking employment and health and consider briefly its applicability to Taiwan and the United States.

The Rewards Model and the Stress–Strain Model of Employment and Women's Health

Researchers who adopt the rewards model to explain the effects of employment on women's health[2] tend to focus on the positive aspects of the worker role in contrast to the negative aspects of the housewife role (Haw 1982; Kessler and McRae 1982; Nathanson 1980; Ross and Huber 1985; Thoits 1983). According to this view, working offers a challenge and opportunities for self-direction not found in housework and leads to favorable conceptions of self. Further, it provides relief from the isolation of housework by making social contacts and support available to women and by alleviating the boredom and the sense of meaninglessness considered endemic among housewives. Wages and salaries earned through work also are viewed as rewards; they are believed to give women a sense of independence, thereby mitigating the feeling—assumed to be common among housewives—of inability to change and control their lives. Earnings also are thought to improve women's position within the family; in recognition of their contribution to the household budget, their authority in decision-making increases.

Proponents of the rewards model, then, believe that the increased self-esteem, social interaction, autonomy, sense of meaningfulness, and status that accompany women's employment decrease women's susceptibility to illness and disease. In their view, working is positive for women's health. They often fail to recognize, however, that self-actualization is possible only under conditions of economic security. Many women enter the labor market not to fulfill themselves but to supplement the family's income or to guarantee its survival. For such women, the rewards of working may be outweighed by the stress and strain associated with it.

Although it is difficult to define stress, much evidence suggests that situations perceived as threats to a person's well-being can produce physiological changes (Selye 1976) and that repeated or prolonged stress can increase susceptibility to health problems (Cassell 1976; Makosky 1982). Four stress–strain models that explain this relationship have been developed.

Some researchers suggest that *role overload* is associated with an increase in symptoms of ill health (Barnett and Baruch 1985; Gove and Geerken 1977; Kandel, Davies, and Raveis 1985; Verbrugge 1984; Woods and Hulka 1979). Employed women who carry dual responsibilities for home and for job become debilitated by the effort needed to fulfill both sets of role requirements (Haw 1982; Haynes and Feinleib 1980; Miller et al. 1979). The pressures created by the two roles thus increase these women's susceptibility to disease.

Others believe that the demands of multiple roles on married women compete to create *role conflict* and result in vulnerability to ill health (Arber, Gilbert, and Dale 1985; Barnett and Baruch 1985; Gove and Geerken 1977; Powell and Reznikoff 1976). According to this view, when the wife's and the husband's expectations are incompatible, a woman experiences feelings of frustration, of being pulled in opposite directions in the performance of her different roles. In addition, when married women enter the labor force out of economic necessity, their inner conflict increases if their husbands resent their working because they hold traditional gender-role orientations. Thus women's exposure to pressures created by conflicting expectations and by active or passive resentment increases their risk of physiological and psychological problems.

A third explanation offered by proponents of the stress–strain model is the theory of *discrepancy* (Weissman and Klerman 1977). According to this view, "access to new opportunities, and efforts to redress the social inequalities of women in the United States are discrepant"; this discrepancy may be a contributory factor in the recent increase in depression among American women (Weissman and Klerman 1977, 108). "Depressions may occur not when things are at their worst, but when there is a possibility of improvement, and a discrepancy between one's rising aspirations and the likelihood of fulfilling these wishes" (Weissman and Klerman 1977, 108). Thus the inability of social and economic measures to keep pace with women's higher expectations is believed to cause an increase in women's vulnerability to psychological distress.

A final variant of the stress–strain model is suggested by researchers who posit that women's *work conditions* are hazardous to their health (Hibbard and Pope 1987; Lennon 1987; Muller 1986a, 1986b). Women usually hold jobs with lower quality, fewer benefits, and lesser remuneration than do men. Their work is repetitive, predictable, governed by deadlines, supervised closely—frequently by nonsupportive superiors—and dead-end. These negative dimensions of women's occupations are said to be frustrating and stressful and thus detrimental to women's health.

In sum, proponents of the stress–strain model posit that working attacks women's physiological and psychological integrity, thereby making them vulnerable to illness. Researchers who provide this seemingly plausible explanation, however, do not explain why some women are able to adapt to adverse stimuli whereas others are not. Portions of the literature suggest an answer to this question. The research on stress and coping, for example, posits either that social support buffers the impact of social stress (Parry 1986; Thoits 1984; Wethington and Kessler 1986) or that certain behavioral and cognitive strategies attenuate stress (Folkman and Lazarus 1980; Kobasa, Maddi, and Courington 1981; Pearlin and Schooler 1978; Wheaton 1985). Yet this work leaves another question unanswered: Why do women's coping styles vary? The following sections present material that suggests an answer.

Development in Taiwan

When the Nationalist government retreated to Taiwan in 1949, it found a primarily agricultural island marked by conditions not wholly favorable to development. The policies it adopted to foster economic growth have been documented in detail elsewhere (Ho 1978; Lin 1973). It is sufficient to say here that the government initially strengthened agriculture to provide a base for industrialization, pursued a strategy of import substitution for a brief period during the 1950s, and in the 1960s adopted a policy of export-oriented industrialization.

The last-mentioned policy produced dramatic changes in Taiwan's economic structure. Agriculture's contribution to the net domestic product (NDP) declined from 36 percent in 1952 to 7 percent in 1986, while the contribution of industry rose from 18 percent to 47 percent over the same period (Lu 1987, 2). As might be expected, industrialization brought about rapid urbanization and migration from rural areas to the cities. Incentives to take jobs away from the land were powerful; family farms proved too small to support the expanding rural population. A sizable income differential between the agricultural and the industrial sectors also spurred migration to urban areas.

Industrialization, however, was not restricted to a few urban centers. During the late 1960s, industry began to disperse to the countryside to gain access to labor and raw materials. By 1971, 50 percent of the industrial and commercial establishments and 55 percent of the manufacturing firms in Taiwan were located in rural areas, and the proportion of farm households with members working off-farm grew (Ho 1979).[3] Although the response of farm households to these changing conditions varied, most reacted in ways that were consonant with traditional Chinese culture and the Chinese family system.

The Traditional Chinese Family

The economic family, the *chia*, is the basic socioeconomic unit in China. Such a family takes one of three forms: conjugal, stem, or joint. The conjugal family consists of a husband, wife, and their unmarried children; the joint family adds two or more married sons, their wives, and their children to this core group. The stem family—a form that lies somewhere between the conjugal and the joint types—includes parents, their unmarried offspring, and one married son with his wife and children.

China's patrilineal kinship structure recognizes only male children as descent-group members with rights to family property. In the past (and to a large extent today), residence was patrilocal; when a woman married, she left her natal home to live as a member of her husband's family, severing her formal ties with her father's household. Parents considered daughters a liability: they were household members who drained family resources as children and who withdrew their assets (domestic labor and earning power) when they married. Sons, in contrast, contributed steadily to the family's economic security during its growth and expansion and provided a source of support in old age. Not surprisingly, parents strongly preferred male children.

Members of the older generation also strongly favored arranged marriages. Marriage brought a new member into the household, joined two individuals to produce children, and established an alliance between families. Therefore the needs of the family took precedence over the individual's desires in the selection of a mate. When parents arranged marriages, they attempted to recruit women who would be compliant, capable workers; who would produce heirs; and who came from families willing to forge bonds of cooperation and obligation.

Traditionally, all members of the family lived under one roof, except for a few who worked outside to supplement or diversify the group income. Ideally, the family functioned as a single cooperating unit in all activities. Members of the household had clearly defined tasks, which were allocated primarily on the basis of gender. Men, dominating the public domain, worked outside the home in the fields or elsewhere. Women, who presided over the domestic sphere, managed the household and served its members, helped with agricultural chores, and frequently engaged in supplemental cottage industry. Men and women, in other words, performed different tasks as members of a cooperative enterprise in which all property belonged to the family as a whole, except for the personal items and clothing brought by a woman as part of her dowry.

An authoritarian hierarchy based on gender, generation, and age dominated life within the family. The eldest male had the highest status; a woman's status, although it increased with age and with the birth of sons, was lower than that of any man. Women's desires were subordinated to those of men, just as the wishes of the young were subordinated to those of the old. The older generation socialized women from birth to accept their inferiority and subordination to males and to observe the "three obediences": to father, husband, and sons. Even though women's work was necessary for the maintenance of the household, family members took this labor for granted. Reproductive capacity, rather than hard work or economic contributions, defined women's status. Women were brought into the family for the purpose of bearing and rearing a new generation; whatever their other achievements were, their position in the family depended on fulfilling this expectation. In short, women had no real control over their lives; social and economic marginality marked their experience.

Hsin Hsing Village

Hsin Hsing is a nucleated village approximately 125 miles southwest of Taipei, Taiwan's capital city, and is located beside a road that runs between two market towns, Lu-Kang and Ch'i-hu. Its people are Hokkien (Minnan) speakers, as are most in the area; their ancestors emigrated from Fukien, China, several hundred years ago.

One travels by bus from Lu-kang to Hsin Hsing on a cement road flanked by clusters of village houses, farmland, and more than thirty factories. These factories are labor-intensive; they include large establishments that manufacture textiles and furniture, medium-sized enterprises that build bamboo and wood products, and small satellite factories (or family workshops) that perform piecework for larger firms. In addition to the factories situated along the road, the area is dotted with others that produce articles for local and foreign consumption. Many are located in or next to their owners' homes, as are the seven small satellite factories, the three artisans' workshops, and the twenty-six retail and service shops and small businesses located in Hsin Hsing.

In 1979, 382 people lived in the village, although the villagers considered the population to include 543 people in seventy-three households (see Table 2-1). More than four-fifths (85 percent) of these households derived their income from off-farm employment—a reflection of the unprofitability of agriculture—but households engaged both in off-farm work and in farming were by far the most common.[4] Further, fully 18 percent of families (34 percent of the population) were of the joint type, almost three times as many as in the late 1950s, when we first studied Hsin Hsing (B. Gallin 1966; Gallin and Gallin 1982a). This increase reflected the villagers' belief that the joint family provided the means for socioeconomic success in a changing world (Gallin and Gallin 1982b). A family that included many potential wage workers, as well as members

TABLE 2-1. Population of Hsin Hsing Village, by Family Type
(January–June 1979)

Family Type		Number	Percentage
CONJUGAL			
Households		33	45.0
Persons		163	30.0
Average number of persons per household	4.9		
STEM			
Households		27	37.0
Persons		194	36.0
Average number of persons per household	7.2		
JOINT			
Households		13	18.0
Persons		186	34.0
Average number of persons per household	14.3		
TOTAL			
Number of households		73	
Number of persons		543	
Average number of persons per household	7.3		

Source: Field interviews.

who could manage the household, supervise children, and care for the land, had a better chance of diversifying economically than did a small family.

The organization of the joint family facilitated the employment of women in Hsin Hsing; as Table 2-2 shows, twelve of the twenty-one women who were both under forty years of age and belonged to stem or joint families engaged in remunerative activities. These women had mothers-in-law resident in the household who could assume some of

TABLE 2-2. Work Status of Hsin Hsing Married Women, by Family Type and Age
(January–June 1979)

Family Type/Age	Work Status					
	Working for Remuneration		Not Working for Remuneration		Totals	
	Number	Percentage	Number	Percentage	Number	Percentage
CONJUGAL						
20 to 39	2	12.5	14	87.5	16	100.0
40 and older	10	33.3	20	66.7	30	100.0
STEM/JOINT						
20 to 39	12	57.1	9	42.9	21	100.0
40 and older	2	8.7	21	91.3	23	100.0
TOTAL	26	28.9	64	71.1	90	100.0

Source: Field interviews.

their role responsibilities during the day—for example, supervising their children or working the family land. Women without available mothers-in-law, by contrast, were far less likely to pursue paid employment. Only two of the sixteen women who were under forty years of age and were members of conjugal families worked for wages.

It is obvious, then, that women's access to wage work was affected directly by the existence of a supportive family structure in which mothers-in-law took over some of the younger women's tasks. Accordingly, some villagers used the joint-family strategy to attain socioeconomic mobility for the family. This goal, however, often was attained at the expense of daughters-in-law, who assumed double work loads and achieved security only through the social mobility of the family as a whole (R. S. Gallin 1984).

Village families employed other strategies as well to promote their well-being or to secure their subsistence. Wives of men who considered farming neither their primary nor their secondary activity took to the fields, replacing their husbands as principal agricultural workers. Further, to the extent that working was compatible with their child-care responsibilities, married women joined their unmarried daughters and daughters-in-law in the wage-labor force to earn income that supported families, helped to pay bills, and created educational opportunities for children, especially sons.[5]

Women's entry into the public sector can be seen from the fact that

TABLE 2-3. Primary and Secondary Activities of Hsin Hsing Married Women, by Age (January–June 1979)

	Age					
	20 to 39		40 and Older		Totals	
Activity	Number	Percentage	Number	Percentage	Number	Percentage
PRIMARY ACTIVITY						
Wage laborer	10	27.0	11	20.7	21	23.3
Enterpreneur	4	10.8	1	1.9	5	5.7
Worker in family business	1	2.8	1	1.9	2	2.2
Farmer	8	21.6	14	26.4	22	24.4
Housekeeper	14	37.8	26	49.1	40	44.4
Total	37	100.0	53	100.0	90	100.0
SECONDARY ACTIVITY						
Wage laborer	5	25.0	6	22.2	11	23.4
Worker in family business	2	10.0	3	11.1	5	10.6
Farmer	11	55.0	9	33.3	20	42.6
Housekeeper	2	10.0	9	33.3	11	23.4
Total	20	100.0	27	100.0	47	100.0

Source: Field interviews.

in 1979 more than half (55.6 percent) of the married women in the village identified their primary activities with roles nontraditional for women: one-quarter said they were wage laborers or entrepreneurs, and one-quarter listed themselves as farmers or as assistants in a family business (see Table 2-3). Although it might be argued that farming and helping with a family business fall within a broad definition of the female role, such activities were traditionally secondary to women's primary responsibility for managing and maintaining the household.

Among women thirty-nine years of age and younger, only sixteen identified housekeeping as one of their activities. This finding does not mean that the other twenty-three did not manage and maintain the household and care for their children. It means that 62 percent of these married women performed dual roles: they were both nondomestic workers and housekeepers. In the next section I discuss this double burden and the women's attitudes toward it.

Women's Work in Hsin Hsing

The daily routine of married women who work off-farm is typified by that of thirty-nine-year-old Mrs. Chen, whose day begins when she rises at 6:00 A.M. to prepare breakfast for her family of nine (five children ranging in age from eight to sixteen years, herself, and her husband and her in-laws). Before leaving for work, Mrs. Chen tends to the few chickens and ducks she raises for the family's consumption and does the daily shopping, buying her food from itinerant merchants who come to the village early in the morning. "Sometimes," she says, "if I am busy I will give my mother-in-law money and she will buy the food for me." More often, however, her mother-in-law helps only by looking after the children when they come home from school.

Mrs. Chen works in a local factory eight hours a day. She earns $230 NT (New Taiwan equals $8.36 U.S.) a day and works twenty-eight days a month. The factory is a ten-minute bicycle ride from the village, and Mrs. Chen makes the trip four times a day: at 8:00 A.M.; at noon, when she returns home for lunch; at 1:00 P.M., when she resumes work; and at 5:00 P.M., when her factory day ends. Mrs. Chen says: "I have to punch in on a timeclock four times a day: in the morning, in the evening, and before and after lunch. If I punch in one minute late, I lose [NT]$3–4 plus the [NT]$300 bonus that a worker receives for perfect attendance throughout the month."

Mrs. Chen's job involves placing precut baseball bats on a spindle for finishing. She processes approximately fifty bats per day, a task that she says "requires a lot of strength." Because the factory is owned by Japanese manufacturers and the workers neither speak nor understand the language, the owners have hired a translator to supervise the workers. Mrs. Chen describes the supervisor as "very bad."

> He does not allow us to talk to each other while we work. If he sees us talking he comes over and tells us to stop talking. Once I became very angry and argued with him. I told him, "The workers you hired are not deaf-mutes." Now his impression of me has deteriorated and he has threatened to fire me because of my attitude.

Mrs. Chen says she was not frightened by this threat: "I am tired of the work." She also admitted, however, that she has not argued since with the supervisor. Working in the factory, she says, "is not bad [although] the noise from the machinery is very loud. I do get tired, but I am used to it. I have to work to make money for the household necessities and to pay the children's school expenses. I was born to do these things. I must do these things."

At home in the evening, Mrs. Chen cooks, cleans, does the laundry, and tends to the children. Her husband does not share in these tasks. He does, however, take part in farming activities; apparently this division of labor explains Mrs. Chen's statement that only during the busy agricultural season does she "often get up, go to the fields, return home to cook breakfast, go to work, return home, go to the fields, and then finally return to cook the evening meal." Usually, however, her husband takes care of the field tasks, if there are any, and then joins other village men to chat. Mrs. Chen, in contrast, has little time to chat because her domestic chores usually occupy her until she goes to bed at 11:00 P.M.

I chose the above excerpts from my field notes for several reasons. First, they illustrate the extent to which the conditions of the women's work are stressful; their jobs involve highly predictable and repetitive activities paced by external controls, all of which make them vulnerable to ill health. Second, these excerpts illustrate the extent to which time pressures and role overload associated with the women's double burden (as paid workers and as unpaid housekeepers) expose them to repeated stressors that are associated with negative health outcomes. Third, they illustrate the women's attitudes toward their situation.

The excerpts show that the women saw their work as neither rewarding nor stressful. They acknowledged the negative consequences of their *work conditions* but thought that factory jobs were a welcome alternative to agricultural work (which they defined as "bitter"). They said they had too much to do (*role overload*) but did not consider their lives to be governed by incompatible norms (*role conflict*). They saw *no discrepancy* between their expectations and their life options but believed that what they were doing was what they should be doing.

The women of Hsin Hsing, in short, viewed their situation in ways different from those suggested by the literature. They considered paid employment as neither a positive nor a negative activity but instead viewed their work experience through the refracting prism of traditional ideology. How the women saw their employment—what it meant to them—was shaped by the context in which they lived.

Women's Employment and Health in Political, Economic, and Social Contexts

The political economy of Taiwan is involved inextricably in the world capitalist system. Therefore, its economy depends heavily on foreign capital and trade and is extremely vulnerable to international market fluctuations. Accordingly, the government must maintain (1) a favorable investment climate, including political stability and low wage rates, to ensure that capital does not seek a cheap labor force elsewhere; and (2) an elastic labor force responsive to the demands of business cycles. Thus, to ensure its advantage in the world economy, the government pursues policies to create a political, economic, and ideological environment attractive to foreign investors.

Since its arrival in Taiwan, the government has passed a series of laws and has implemented policies to restrict workers' rights.[6] The Labor Union Law, for example, includes provisions that limit severely the right to organize and to bargain collectively; the Labor Dispute Law prohibits strikes. The Labor Standards Law, in contrast, guarantees workers' rights such as minimum wages, pensions, benefits, pay equity, and occupational safety and health. Yet this law covers less than half the island's workers, primarily because it exempts workplaces with fewer than thirty employees. Moreover, passage of the law in 1984 did little to improve workers' conditions. The minimum wage it mandates—$8,000 NT ($290 U.S.) per month—is less than the amount needed to maintain a minimally adequate standard of living; the benefits it guarantees apply only to workers and not to dependents.

Provisions for pay equity and pensions included in the Labor Standards Law are rarely enforced. The government relies on management's voluntary compliance; only extremely light fines are imposed for infractions of the law. In combination, government regulations and guidelines erect powerful barriers to equitable labor relations, thereby creating an attractive environment for investment.

Other laws and policies enhance the attractiveness of this environment by affirming the ideological precepts of traditional Chinese culture. Equal rights for women are incorporated in the constitution, but family law places women at a decided disadvantage (Chiang and Ku 1985, 12–21). Women's rights are subordinated to those of men, and a woman has no legal claim to a share in family decisions. This subordination is reinforced through the ideological messages delivered by the educational system and the media. Women's primary roles are defined as wife and as mother; the purpose of their education (which is limited in relation to men's) is to produce obedient individuals who believe that paid employment is a temporary phase in their life cycle.[7] In sum, the law and the government's ideological apparatus create the conditions necessary to shape women into the kind of labor force that industry requires: a docile, minimally trained, tractable labor force willing to accept low pay, lackluster jobs, and irregular work according to the exigencies of the economy.

The creation of an attractive environment for investment, however, is a necessary but not a sufficient condition for economic growth. The requisite labor force also must be supplied to industry. Accordingly, the government in Taiwan adopted yet other policies that had profound consequences for family production and reproduction and spurred people's movement from farm to industry. These consequences have been described in detail elsewhere (Gallin and Gallin 1982a; Huang 1981). It is sufficient to say that state agricultural and industrial policies resulted in the stagnation of the farm sector, the spread of industry to the rural areas, and the commodification of the domestic economy.

In the absence of income from the land and in the presence of the need for cash, rural residents turned to off-farm employment to earn the money needed to support families or to secure their futures.[8] A household in Taiwan, however, requires more than one wage earner to maintain a minimum or relatively comfortable standard of living. Thus married women are propelled into the paid labor force to satisfy the family's need for money. Their employment is part of a household strategy—a strategy predicated on the knowledge that women will accept the double burden of wage labor and domestic responsibilities demanded by the patriarchal family. Women have no choice: socialized in norms of subordination and family responsibility, they accept the expectation that they will sell their labor power to reproduce the family group. Provided with only a modicum of education, they subscribe to the belief that they will obtain security and perhaps upward mobility through their contributions to the family economy.

The meanings that the women of Hsin Hsing attributed to their work were not produced in a vacuum. They were a product of the context in which they lived—a context defined by state policy in articulation with the culture of patriarchal familism. The long-term consequences of these meanings will be difficult to assess.

On the one hand, the women of Hsin Hsing showed little of the frustration or resentment purported to increase women's susceptibility to disease. In this sense, traditional culture may protect their physiological and psychological integrity. By sustaining and reinforcing women's position within the social structure, the culture may mediate the effects of situational stressors and may help to vitiate the influence of employment on their health. On the other hand, it must be recognized that the employment of the women of Hsin Hsing exposes them to physical and chemical hazards that are detrimental to health, and that it forces them to carry dual responsibilities that increase their susceptibility to disease.[9] Yet although the women complained of fatigue; muscle pains; and skin, eye, and respiratory problems, they neither stayed home from work nor visited health care providers for these ailments. If the effect of their tradition-bound socialization is to decrease their awareness and attention regarding symptoms, such socialization may have negative effects on their morbidity and mortality in the long run.

In short, the relationship of employment to these women's health is problematic. Detailed, longitudinal data are not available to assess the impact of wage labor on the women's well-being. Yet the synchronic data collected here suggest that an explanatory model of the effects of employment on women's health must move beyond existing models and must tie macro- and micro-phenomena into a dynamic whole that allows for contextual effects and variations. Such a model is necessary because the Taiwan data suggest that this relationship depends on the context in which women live.

In Taiwan, that context reflects the province's semiperipheral position in the world economic system. Because of that position, the industrial sector exhibits the features of competitive capitalism. In the United States, by contrast, that context reflects America's core position in the world system and its monopoly capitalist economy (Baran and Sweezy 1966; O'Connor 1973).

Each form of capitalism—competitive capitalism and monopoly capitalism—implies separate economic imperatives that are expressed culturally and politically in differing ways. In Taiwan, traditional culture is reinforced to sustain values that cement the integrity of the family as a work unit and to reproduce workers who satisfy the needs of the economy. In the United States, by contrast, new wants, standards, and norms are created (Baran and Sweezy 1966, 128) to produce a body of consumers who identify self-respect, status, and recognition with material possessions and individual achievement.

The penetration of these sharply contrasting views into Taiwanese and American families has different consequences for the meanings that women of each culture attach to their work and, in turn, to their health. Women in Taiwan are not faced with incompatible cultural pressures— their self-worth remains determined primarily by a matrix of values emanating from traditional familial culture—and the social aspects of their work appear to have no psychological repercussions that can be linked to illness. In contrast, many women in the United States are caught in a dilemma. If their employment conflicts with conservative definitions of female roles, they may find themselves in a particularly stressful situation that ultimately undermines their health. If their work is congruent with the cultural imperative of personal achievement, however, their employment may have no harmful effects on their health.

To trace the links between employment and women's health, then, we must understand how global forces and national political economies impinge on culture and how cultural constructs relate to cognitive and bodily responses. An explanatory model of the linkage must take into account the historical stage of a country's economic development, the institutional influences that are associated with different stages of capitalism, and the socialization process, along with its psychological repercussions. In sum, we must understand how macro- and microphenomena interact to produce health and illness.

NOTES

Acknowledgement: Research for this paper was carried out in collaboration with Bernard Gallin, whose insights helped me immeasurably. We acknowledge with thanks the organizations that provided financial assistance over the years and made possible our field trips to Taiwan. Specifically, funding was provided by a Foreign Area Training Fellowship, a Fulbright-Hays Research Grant, the Asian Studies Center at Michigan State University, the Mid-Western Universities Consortium for International Activities, the Social Sciences Research Council, and the Pacific Cultural Foundation.

1. During our six field trips we collected data using both anthropological and sociological techniques, including participant observation, in-depth interviews, surveys, censuses, and collection of official statistics contained in family, land, school, and economic records.

2. "Health" is not a conceptually coherent category. It has been operationalized through objective indexes of biochemical function (Haynes and Feinleib 1980) and through subjective measures of physical and mental well-being (Hibbard and Pope 1987; Powell and Reznikoff 1976; Woods and Hulka 1979). This paper makes no distinction between physiological and psychological health; nor does it distinguish between clinically defined and self-defined health (i.e., disease and illness)—a limitation found in much of the literature reviewed.

3. Ho's data are not disaggregated by area, but our observations suggest that throughout the 1960s industry penetrated mainly towns and rural areas within commuting distance to cities, rather than areas of the more distant countryside such as the village studied here.

4. Village families continued to cultivate the land because (1) it was a source of food, specifically rice; (2) the mechanization and chemicalization of agriculture obviated the need for either a large or a physically strong labor force; and (3) the small size of family farms—in 1979 the average acreage tilled per farming household was .63 hectares—required little labor. See Bernard Gallin and Rita S. Gallin (1982a) and Rita S. Gallin and Anne Ferguson (1988) for a detailed discussion.

5. The proportion of married women working in industry is higher in rural areas than in the city because of the imbalance between supply and demand in the countryside (i.e., a small pool of available single women combined with a large demand for

low-cost labor). Married women accordingly are recruited into the labor force to meet employers' needs. For discussion of young working women in Taiwan's cities, see Linda G. Arrigo (1980, 1985); Norma Diamond (1979); Lydia Kung (1976, 1981).

6. Until July 15, 1987, Taiwan was under martial law on the grounds that the province was engaged in civil war. The lifting of "emergency controls" and the changes in labor laws, however, have not changed "the basic pattern of industrial relations" (Cohen 1988, 128). Additional information on government policy and on its impact on workers can be found in Marc J. Cohen (1988, 127–38), the source of the material that follows on the laws governing workers.

7. According to Susan Greenhalgh (1985, 272), the government, "well aware of the links between education and development, in 1953 . . . made six years of primary education free and compulsory, and in 1968–69 . . . added three more years (junior middle school) of free schooling." Parents, however, practice "systematic discrimination against daughters" (Greenhalgh 1985, 303), and "educational investments vary by sex" (302). In 1985, for example, the ratio of female to male graduates was .85 at the junior level, .83 at the senior level, and .74 at the college level (DGBAS 1986, 132–33).

8. My comments in the discussion that follows apply only to women who are members of the petite bourgeoisie and the proletariat. According to Hill Gates (1979, 390–91), the petite bourgeoisie constitutes about 47 percent of Taiwan's population and includes almost all agricultural owner–operators and a large group of small businesspeople and artisans. The proletariat makes up about 20 percent of the population and includes factory and construction workers, sales clerks, hired artisans, and landless agricultural workers. On the role and status of women in the "new middle class," see Norma Diamond (1975).

9. Illness and disability reduce the likelihood that a woman will enter or remain in the labor force (Waldron, Herold, and Dunn 1982), an issue not discussed in this paper.

REFERENCES

Arber, Sara, G. Nigel Gilbert, and Angela Dale. 1985. "Paid Employment and Women's Health: A Benefit or a Source of Role Strain?" *Sociology of Health and Illness* 7:375–400.
Arrigo, Linda G. 1980. "The Industrial Work Force of Young Women in Taiwan." *Bulletin of Concerned Asian Scholars* 12:25–38.
———. 1985. "Economic and Political Control of Women Workers in Multinational Electronics Factories in Taiwan: Martial Law Coercion and World Market Uncertainty." *Contemporary Marxism* 11:77–95.
Baran, Paul A., and Paul Sweezy. 1966. *Monopoly Capitalism.* New York: Monthly Review.
Barnett, Rosalinda, and Grace Baruch. 1985. "Women's Involvement in Multiple Roles and Psychological Distress." *Journal of Personality and Social Psychology* 49:135–45.
Cassell, John. 1976. "The Contribution of the Social Environment to Host Resistance." *American Journal of Epidemiology* 104:107–23.
Chiang, Lan-hung Nora, and Yenlin Ku. 1985. "Past and Current Status of Women in Taiwan." Monograph 1, Women's Research Program. Taipei: National Taiwan University, Population Studies Center.
Cohen, Marc J. 1988. *Taiwan at the Crossroads.* Washington, D.C.: Asia Resource Center.
Diamond, Norma. 1975. "Women under Kuomintang Rule: Variations on the Feminine Mystique." *Modern China* 1:3–45.

———. 1979. "Women and Industry in Taiwan." *Modern China* 4:317–40.

Directorate-General of Budget, Accounting and Statistics (DGBAS). 1982. *Monthly Bulletin of Labor Statistics, Republic of China, December.* Taipei: Executive Yuan.

———. 1986. *Report on the Vocational Training Survey in Taiwan Area Republic of China,* 1985. Taipei: Executive Yuan.

———. 1987. *Statistical Yearbook of the Republic of China.* Taipei: Executive Yuan.

Folkman, Susan, and Richard S. Lazarus. 1980. "An Analysis of Coping in a Middle-Aged Community Sample." *Journal of Health and Social Behavior* 21:219–39.

Gallin, Bernard. 1966. *Hsin Hsing, Taiwan: A Chinese Village in Change.* Berkeley: University of California Press.

Gallin, Bernard, and Rita S. Gallin. 1982a. "Socioeconomic Life in Rural Taiwan: Twenty Years of Development and Change." *Modern China* 8:205–46.

———. 1982b. "The Chinese Joint Family in Changing Rural Taiwan." In *Social Interaction in Chinese Society,* ed. Richard W. Wilson, Sydney L. Greenblatt, and Amy Wilson, 142–50 New York: Praeger.

Gallin, Rita S. 1984. "The Entry of Chinese Women into the Rural Labor Force: A Case Study from Taiwan." *Signs* 9:383–98.

Gallin, Rita S., and Anne Ferguson. 1988. "The Household Enterprise and Farming System Research: A Case Study from Taiwan." In *Gender Issues in Farming Systems Research and Extension,* ed. Susan Poats, Marianne Schmink, and Anita Spring, 223–35. Boulder, Colo.: Westview.

Gates, Hill. 1979. "Dependency and the Part-Time Proletariat in Taiwan." *Modern China* 5:381–407.

Gove, Walter R., and Michael R. Geerken. 1977. "The Effect of Children and Employment on the Mental Health of Married Men and Women." *Social Forces* 56:66–76.

Greenhalgh, Susan. 1985. "Sexual Stratification: The Other Side of 'Growth with Equity' in East Asia." *Population and Development Review* 11:265–314.

Haw, Mary A. 1982. "Women, Work and Stress: A Review and Agenda for the Future." *Journal of Health and Social Behavior* 23:132–44.

Haynes, Suzanne G., and Manning Feinleib. 1980. "Women, Work and Heart Disease: Prospective Findings from the Framingham Heart Study." *American Journal of Public Health* 70:133–41.

Hibbard, Judith H., and Clyde R. Pope. 1987. "Employment Characteristics and Health Status among Men and Women." *Women and Health* 12:85–102.

Ho, Samuel P. S. 1978. *Economic Development in Taiwan, 1860–1970.* New Haven: Yale University Press.

———. 1979. "Decentralized Industrialization and Rural Development: Evidence from Taiwan." *Economic Development and Cultural Change* 28:77–96.

House, James S., Victor Strecher, Helen L. Metzner, and Cynthia A. Robbins. 1986. "Occupational Stress and Health among Men and Women in the Tecumseh Community Health Study." *Journal of Health and Social Behavior* 27:62–75.

Huang, Shu-min. 1981. *Agricultural Degradation: Changing Community Systems in Rural Taiwan.* Washington, D.C.: University Press of America.

Kandel, Denise B., Mark Davies, and Victoria H. Raveis. 1985. "The Stressfulness of Daily Social Roles for Women: Marital, Occupational and Household Roles." *Journal of Health and Social Behavior* 26:64–78.

Kessler, Ronald C., and James A. McRae. 1982. "The Effects of Wives' Employment on the Mental Health of Married Men and Women." *American Sociological Review* 47:216–27.

Kobasa, Suzanne C., Salvatore R. Maddi, and Shiela Courington. 1981. "Personality and Constitution as Mediators in the Stress–Illness Relationship." *Journal of Health and Social Behavior* 22:368–78.

Kung, Lydia. 1976. "Factory Work and Women in Taiwan: Changes in Self-Image and Status." *Signs* 2:35–58.

———. 1981. "Perceptions of Work among Factory Women in Taiwan." In *The Anthropology of Taiwanese Society*, ed. Emily Ahern and Hill Gates, 184–211. Stanford: Stanford University Press.

Lennon, Mary Clare. 1987. "Sex Differences in Distress: The Impact of Gender and Work Roles." *Journal of Health and Social Behavior* 28:290–305.

Lewin, Ellen, and Virginia Olesen. 1985. "Occupational Health and Women: The Case of Clerical Work." In *Women, Health, and Healing*, ed. Ellen Lewin and Virginia Olesen, 53–85 New York: Tavistock.

Lin, Ching-yuan. 1973. *Industrialization in Taiwan, 1946–1972*. New York: Praeger.

Lu, Min-jen. 1987. "Promotion of Constitutional Democracy Government's Goal." *Free China Journal* (October 5):2.

Makosky, Vivian Parker. 1982. "Sources of Stress: Events or Conditions?" In *Lives in Stress: Women and Depression*, ed. Deborah Belle, 35–53 Beverly Hills: Sage.

Miller, Joanne, Carmi Schooler, Melvin L. Kohn, and Karen A. Miller. 1979. "Women and Work: The Psychological Effects of Occupational Conditions." *American Journal of Sociology* 85:66–94.

Muller, Charlotte. 1986a. "Health and Health Care of Employed Women and Homemakers: Family Factors." *Women and Health* 11:7–26.

———. 1986b. "Health and Health Care of Employed Adults: Occupation and Gender." *Women and Health* 11:27–47.

Nathanson, Constance A. 1980. "Social Roles and Health Status among Women—The Significance of Employment." *Social Science and Medicine* 14:463–71.

O'Connor, James. 1973. *The Fiscal Crisis of the State*. New York: St. Martin's.

Parry, Glenys. 1986. "Paid Employment, Life Events, Social Support, and Mental Health in Working-Class Mothers." *Journal of Health and Social Behavior* 27:193–208.

Pearlin, Leonard I., and Carmi Schooler. 1978. "The Structure of Coping." *Journal of Health and Social Behavior* 192:2–21.

Powell, Barbara, and Marvin Reznikoff. 1976. "Role Conflict and Symptoms of Distress in College Educated Women." *Journal of Consulting and Clinical Psychology* 44:473–76.

Ross, Catherine E., and Joan Huber. 1985. "Hardship and Depression." *Journal of Health and Social Behavior* 26:312–27.

Selye, Hans. 1976. *Stress in Health and Disease*. Boston: Butterworth.

Stellman, Jeanne M. 1977. *Women's Work, Women's Health*. New York: Pantheon.

Thoits, Peggy A. 1983. "Multiple Identities and Psychological Well-Being: A Reformulation and Test of the Social Isolation Hypothesis." *American Sociological Review* 48:174–87.

———. 1984. "Explaining Distributions of Psychological Vulnerability: Lack of Social Support in the Face of Life Stress." *Social Forces* 63:452–81.

Verbrugge, Lois M. 1984. "Physical Health of Clerical Workers in the U.S., Framingham, and Detroit." *Women and Health* 9:17–41.

Waldron, Ingrid. 1980. "Employment and Women's Health: An Analysis of Causal Relationships." *International Journal of Health Services* 10:435–54.

Waldron, Ingrid, Joan Herold, and Dennis Dunn. 1982. "How Valid Are Self-Report Measures for Evaluating Relationships between Women's Health and Labor Force Participation?" *Women and Health* 7:53–66.

Weissman, Myrna M., and Gerald L. Klerman. 1977. "Sex Differences and the Epidemiology of Depression." *Archives of General Psychiatry* 34:98–109.

Wethington, Elaine, and Ronald C. Kessler. 1986. "Perceived Support, Received Support, and Adjustment to Stressful Life Events." *Journal of Health and Social Be-havior* 27:78–89.

Wheaton, Blair. 1985. "Models for the Stress-buffering Functions of Coping Resources." *Journal of Health and Social Behavior* 26:352–64.

Woods, Nancy F., and Barbara S. Hulka. 1979. "Symptom Reports and Illness Behavior among Employed Women and Homemakers." *Journal of Community Health* 5:36–45.

Chapter 3

Urgency and Utilization of

Emergency Medical Services in

Urban Indonesia:

A Report and Reflection

PETER CONRAD

Modernization is having a variety of effects on developing countries. Among these are increased urbanization and the development of Western-influenced biomedical systems. It has been estimated that, by the year 2000, 51 percent of the population of developing countries will be living in urban areas (Rossi-Espangnet 1984). Most research on medical care in the Third World has rightly focused on public health, maternal and infant care, and, more recently, primary care (especially rural health care). As developing societies become more urbanized, however, the needs of their medical systems shift. One aspect of this shift is that the use of emergency medical services becomes more important and visible, both in terms of managing accidents, trauma, and urgent care and as an accessible portal into the medical system.

In spite of the thousands of articles published on health care in the developing societies, there has been little research done on emergency services. The few extant articles tend to be programmatic, focusing on how to organize emergency medical services (e.g., Ali and Naraynsingh 1987; Silva 1973). This neglect is partly a result of government and funding agencies' understandable emphasis on the major health problems in developing societies, especially infectious disease and maternal and infant health. This has led to an abundance of research on public health and primary and rural health services, with very little on emergency medical services. In addition, only relatively recently has emergency medicine become a recognized speciality in Western countries, and most developing countries do not have fully developed or elaborate emergency medical systems, as are found in North America.

Epidemiological studies, however, show that accidents, trauma, and injury are becoming important causes of morbidity and mortality in developing societies (Jacobs and Cutting 1986). In Indonesia, for example, accidents have become the seventh leading cause of death (Committee on Health Statistics 1988). Injuries are now the third most frequent reason for admission to hospitals (Suparnadi 1988). Throughout the country, traffic- and motor vehicle-related trauma patients comprise 10 percent of the hospital inpatient population (cited in Suparnadi and Hermansyur 1986). The severity of accidents in developing countries is high: for example, fatality rates are two to four times higher than in France and six to twelve times higher than in the United Kingdom (WHO Study Group 1989). A recent World Health Organization (WHO) Study Group (1989) suggested that this was at least in part "a consequence of the lack of or inadequacy of emergency services." As societies become more urbanized and modes of travel more motorized, the need for emergency medical services increases.

From research in Western countries we know that emergency departments (EDs) are not used only for emergencies. EDs are often used as a source of primary care, mostly by patients in the lower socioeconomic classes (Bohland 1984). Because EDs are open for twenty-four hours with "no appointment necessary," they provide a convenient location for medical care (Roth and Douglas 1983). Studies have shown "that 40–60% of all ED patients could well be taken care of at out patients clinics or primary health care centres" (Andren and Rosenqvist 1987, 828). Paul Torrens and Donna Yedvab (1970) suggest that EDs perform three functions: they treat trauma cases, they substitute for private physicians when they are not available and they serve as family physician for the urban poor. The latter two functions are clearly related to the widespread nonemergency use of EDs reported in North America (Bohland 1984) and Europe (Reilly 1981; Andren and Rosenqvist 1987).

This chapter examines the utilization of emergency medical services in an urban area in a developing society. Using data from a study in Yogyakarta, Indonesia, I present an analysis of the utilization of EDs in terms of the "urgency" of the patients' problems. In ED terms, urgency means how quickly medical assessment or intervention must be made so as not to compromise a patient's life or potential recovery. By focusing on the patients in terms of urgency, we can obtain some understanding of the role of emergency services in developing societies and begin to examine how EDs operate in the medical care system.

Method

The Yogyakarta Emergency Medical Services Study (YEMSS) is a collaborative study between American and Indonesian researchers. The investigators included an American emergency-medicine specialist, an Indonesian neurologist, an American medical sociologist, and an Indonesian medical anthropologist. Thus the focus of data collection is both social-scientific and medical. The overall goal of the study is to examine utilization of the entire emergency system, not just the emergency services of individual hospitals.

Although many studies of emergency services rely on medical records, we thought it essential to collect our own data. Medical records often do not include data in a form that is useful for sociomedical research, and in developing countries they are often inconsistent and incomplete. Furthermore, because we would be collecting data in four different EDs, it would be important to have a systematic and consistent method of collection.

We collected data on all patients who utilized emergency medical services in Yogyakarta during the month of February 1990. This meant collecting data twenty-four hours a day, seven days a week, for four weeks in four EDs in Yogyakarta. To accomplish this task we, along with a bilingual research coordinator, developed an observational survey questionnaire and hired and trained twenty-two research assistants (RAs) who gathered data on every patient coming for ED services. These RAs were advanced social science and medical students who worked around-the-clock on eight-hour shifts.

The survey included a wide range of questions on demographic, medical, and social issues. Additional specific data were collected on all trauma and "emergency" (as defined in this study) patients. Survey data were gathered by observation and by interviewing patients, family, and medical staff. Investigators and RAs also collected some qualitative observational and interview data. Although during very busy times the RAs might have missed a few patients, random checks against ED logs suggest we probably obtained data on over 95 percent of the patients using the EDs.

Our total sample included 4,527 patients who used EDs in Yogyakarta in February 1990. In addition, under the supervision of the emergency physician on the team, we collected follow-up data from the medical records on the 577 trauma or "emergency" ED patients who were hospitalized.

In terms of this paper, a major difficulty the RAs had was designating whether a presenting problem was an emergency, urgent, or nonurgent. To achieve greater accuracy and consistency, the emergency-physician investigator reviewed all the surveys and designated the problem status from the complaint, diagnosis, treatment, and disposition, as well as from the RA's perception. Although these designations are a judgment call, we think there is both some face validity and internal consistency to our categories. In general, we used categories that aligned with those presented by the WHO task force (Cara 1981). Medical emergency requires prompt action within a few hours to prevent loss of life or disability; urgent care requires intervention within twenty-four hours; nonurgent care does not require medical treatment within twenty-four hours.

Setting

Indonesia is the fourth most populous country in the world, with 175 million people. The Indonesian archipelago contains over three thousand islands, with 60 percent of the population living on densely populated Java. Although over 70 percent of the population lives in rural areas, there are several dozen densely populated urban areas. Indonesia's population is rather young; approximately 60 percent is under twenty-four years old (Department of Information 1988). Roughly 85 percent of the population is Muslim. Indonesia's per capita income in 1983 reached $530, which places it economically in the middle of the range of developing countries (World Bank 1989).

The Indonesian health care system has expanded and developed over the past two decades, largely as part of governmental five-year plans. In 1970, Western medical care was only available in the larger cities. During the 1970s, a system of *Puskesmas* (public health centers) was developed, so that now over five thousand such centers are spread (albeit unevenly) throughout the country, along with twelve thousand auxiliary health posts. In the majority of cases, the health center is staffed by paramedical staff and a recent medical-school graduate who serves two to five years of compulsory government service. The number of physicians has grown steadily over two decades, now including over twenty-two thousand trained doctors. Because of Indonesia's large population, however, this translates to only 1.3 doctors per ten thousand persons (compared to 15.7 in Japan, 9.5 in the Philippines, and 3.5 in Malaysia), with a large concentration in the urban areas (Committee on Health Statistics 1988).

Indonesia spends about 2.7 percent of its gross domestic product on the health sector, which is considerably below the 5 percent recommended by the World Bank for developing countries. Overall, the government contributes about one-third of health care costs, which means the government spends about four dollars per capita on health care. Even though by world standards the medical system is not adequate in terms of investment and accessibility, there is nevertheless considerable evidence that "modern medical care" is underutilized in Indonesia, at least in terms of doctor visits and hospital admissions (Berman 1985).

Yogyakarta (known locally as Yogya) is a city with a metropolitan population of about 800,000 people. It is located in central Java and considered by some to be the cultural capital of Indonesia because of its rich heritage of Javanese court dance, *gamelon* music, *wayang* shadow puppets, and other traditional as well as modern arts. It is also an educational center, the location of Indonesia's largest university and many smaller universities and academies. Estimates suggest that 80,000 to 100,000 college and university students live in Yogya. While Yogya only ranks in the middle of the range of Indonesian cities in terms of income, it has a relatively low cost of living. In addition, its population ranks among the highest in education and health indexes (e.g., low infant mortality) in Indonesia.

There are four major hospitals in Yogya, each with its own emergency service. For the purposes of this study we call them government hospital (GH), Catholic hospital (CH), Protestant hospital (PH), and Muslim hospital (MH); the latter three are privately sponsored by religious organizations but used by the general public. The first three hospitals are located in the northern section of the city; the fourth, farther south (see Figure 3-1). GH is connected with the medical school and serves as a teaching and referral hospital. The hospitals vary in terms of number of beds and occupancy rate: GH—650 beds, 64 percent occupancy rate; CH—342 and 70 percent; PH—658 and 61 percent; MH—175 and 80 percent. PH has the longest-standing ED, which began as an "accident room"; GH opened its ED in 1981; and the other two opened theirs in the middle 1980s. The patient volume for the EDs varies also: GH sees about thirty patients per day; CH, approximately fifty; PH, between sixty and eighty; and MH, between forty and sixty. All EDs are staffed by general physicians and nurses; GH also has residents and medical students. The basic fees are lowest at the government hospital (approximately U.S. $.50 per visit); the others fees are similar (approximately U.S. $1.10 to U.S. $1.50 per visit).

Findings

Utilization of Emergency Medical Services in Yogyakarta

We recorded a total of 4,527 patient visits to Yogyakarta EDs during the month of February 1990. Average patients per day in each hospital ED ranged from 30.4 to 49.9.

If we consider the four EDs together as the emergency medical care system (EMCS) in Yogya, we can examine the community's use of emergency services rather than look at individual hospitals. In this light, there were 161.1 patients per day seen in the EMCS. Assuming that there are

FIGURE 3-1. Location of Hospitals in Yogyakarta with EDs

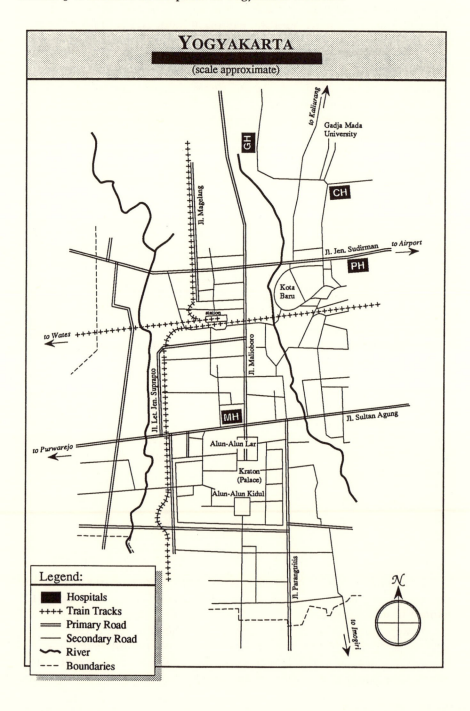

TABLE 3-1. Emergency Department Use, Distance, and Trauma, by Hospital and System in Yogyakarta, Indonesia, 1990

	Hospitals				
	GH	PH	MH	CH	Total
A. USE					
Number of Patients in Month	851	1,396	1,201	1,078	4,526
Avg. Number of Patients/24 hrs.	30.4	49.9	42.3	38.5	161.1
System/% to Each Hospital	18.8	30.8	26.5	23.8	99.9
B. DISTANCE FROM HOSPITAL (IN PERCENTAGES)					
< 3 km.	18.4	25.8	48.0	46.7	
3–7 km.	31.4	29.3	27.3	29.3	
8–15 km.	24.3	29.4	10.5	12.1	
16–50 km.	27.8	9.7	9.0	8.4	
> 50 km.	7.3	3.3	1.1	1.1	
Mean	23.1	17.2	11.5	10.5	
Median	8.0	6.0	4.0	4.0	
C. DISTRIBUTION OF TRAUMA SYSTEM (IN PERCENTAGES)					
Total Trauma	12.2	52.0	23.5	12.3	
Traffic Accidents	12.8	52.3	22.4	12.5	
Falls	15.2	50.1	24.9	9.2	

4,527 patients who want or need ED care, how are they dispersed throughout the system? As Table 3-1 shows, patients are not equally distributed among the hospitals: PH receives 30.8 percent of the patients, MH receives 26.5 percent, CH receives 23.8 percent, and GH receives 18.8 percent.

What are the characteristics of the patients seen in the EMCS? They are 56 percent male, generally young (62 percent under thirty years of age, 8 percent over sixty), and relatively well educated (highest education: 26.2 percent high school, 23.7 percent university). The largest occupational groups are not in the regular work force: college students (22.9 percent), school pupils (15.3 percent), preschool children and babies (13.2 percent), and housewives (11.8 percent). Thus slightly more than half the patients who come to EDs are not in the regular work force. Nearly one-fifth of the patients (19.5 percent) are white-collar and professional workers. The remainder are mostly blue-collar, farm, and unemployed workers (see Table 3-2).

The most common mode of transportation to the ED was by automobile (37 percent), followed by motorcycle (29 percent), *becak* or three-wheeled pedicab (13 percent), and bus or minibus (12 percent). (See Table 3-3.) Only 3 percent of patients arrived by ambulance, and a large portion of these (60 percent) were transfers from other hospitals. What is of note here is the large percentage of patients who arrived by automobile in a city that has only fifteen thousand registered cars, compared to one-hun-

TABLE 3-2. Occupations of Emergency Department
Patients in Yogyakarta, Indonesia, 1990

Occupation	Percent
College Student	22.9
School Pupil	15.3
Child/Baby (before school)	13.2
Housewife	11.8
White-Collar (incl. gov't.)	11.1
Professional	8.4
Blue-Collar/Service	7.4
Farmer	6.1
Pensioner	4.2
Trader	3.3
Unemployed	3.8
Other	2.0
Foreigner/Tourist	0.5

Note: N = 4,476

dred fifty thousand motorcycles. It is also interesting how few patients
came by ambulance.

Distance from hospital appears to be a factor in utilization of ED
services. Over one-half of the patients lived within seven kilometers of
the hospital where they sought care. As Table 3-1 shows, the four hospitals presented slightly different profiles in terms of patient catchment
areas. MH and CH were more "neighborhood" hospitals, with almost
three-quarters of ED patients living within seven kilometers and fewer
than 10 percent living beyond fifteen kilometers from the hospital. GH's
profile is different: only about 50 percent of ED patients lived within
seven kilometers of the hospital, whereas about 35 percent came from
beyond fifteen kilometers. This reflects GH's role as a referral hospital for
smaller government hospitals in provincial areas. PH falls someplace in
between these two patterns.

TABLE 3-3. Modes of Transportation to Emergency
Department (rounded to nearest percent)

Method of Transport	Percent
Automobile	37
Motorcycle	29
Pedicab (Becak)	13
Bus	12
Walking	3
Taxi	1
Bicycle	1
Others[1]	1

Note: N = 4,469
1. Truck, mixed modes of transport

An overwhelming majority of patients are "self-referred" (i.e., referred by self, family, or friends), roughly 81 percent, compared to 17 percent who were "medically referred" (by doctor, health center, or other hospital). Slightly over 1 percent were police-referred. In a society where few people have any type of health insurance, 76.2 percent paid for ED services by self-payment (including family or friends); 16.1 percent had services paid for by a "third party" (government or school insurance or employer); a surprising (to us) 3.7 percent of the cost for ED services was paid by the *penabrak* ("crasher"), the person culpable in a traffic accident; and about 2 percent of patients either didn't pay or didn't know how the bills were paid.

Of all patients coming to EMCS in Yogya, 38.7 percent were defined as trauma cases. Of these, the largest categories were traffic accidents (49.5 percent) and falls (23 percent), with few burns (2.3 percent) and poisonings (0.3 percent). The trauma cases were not evenly distributed among the EDs in Yogya (see Table 3-1), with over half of such cases going to PH and fewer than one-eighth going to GH or CH.

If we divide the day into three eight-hour shifts, then it is during the afternoon–evening shift (14:00 to 22:00) when 53 percent of the patients are seen. The night shift (22:00 to 06:00) sees the fewest patients, about 13 percent. The morning–noon shift (06:00 to 14:00) sees about 34 percent of the patients. Figure 3-2 shows the changes in distribution during the day. Note the biggest hump is from 17:00 to 21:00. This time distribution of patients is affected by several factors: the health centers and hospital polyclinics close at 14:00, leaving EDs and private physicians as the only available sources of medical care; and large numbers of patients may come later in the day, after work (see Figure 3-2).

Emergency, Urgency, and Nonurgency

An EMCS by definition has to be concerned with the issue of "urgency." Many patients come to EDs because they perceive an urgency for their problem. Medical staff need to be ready to respond to all "emergencies" that may come through the door. In this section we examine urgency in three ways: first, by examining the issue of prehospital time for all trauma patients, with an emphasis on transport; second, by looking at the management of patients with medically designated "emergencies"; and third, by analyzing patients' views on using the ED.

In each case, the issue of time is a significant variable in medical care. With serious emergencies, time is often a critical factor in treatment: to maximize survival and minimize potential of disability, severe injuries or sudden changes in condition need to be brought to medical attention quickly. Once in the ED, all "emergency" cases must receive immediate and appropriate treatment. Although our analysis does not

FIGURE 3-2. Time Patients Arrive in Emergency Department

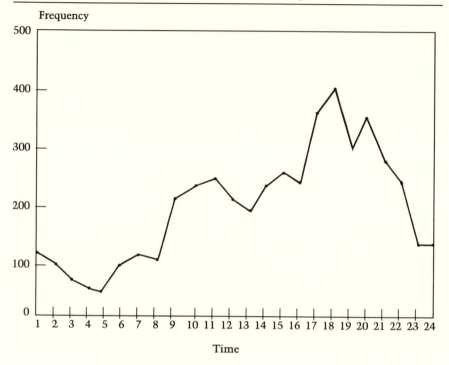

focus on the immediacy and appropriateness of treatment, we do high-light characteristics that differentiate patients with a medical emergency from others who seek care in the ED.

PREHOSPITAL TIME FOR TRAUMA PATIENTS. Prehospital care for trauma patients has become a major policy issue for emergency medical services (EMS) in developed countries. The time between incident and treatment for trauma patients can be of critical importance; therefore elaborate systems for rapid stabilization and transport have already been created in developed countries. Most developing countries do not have the resources to create such elaborate systems, but prehospital time remains a critical health-related issue. The issue of time and transport from site of trauma (e.g., accident) to the ED is just as significant a factor in the EMCS in developing countries as in the developed countries.

Nearly 39 percent (N = 1,749) of all ED patients in Yogyakarta's EMCS are trauma injuries. In our data collection, we logged in the time each patient arrived at the ED and asked each trauma patient (or the accompanying person) the time of the accident or incident. For patients where we had this self-report (N = 1,455), we were then able to calculate how long it took for them to arrive in the ED. Overall, 42 percent of the

TABLE 3-4. Time from Accident Site to Emergency Department, by Type of Accident

Type of Accident[1]	Median	Within 30 Min.	Within 60 Min.	
Motorcycle	23 min.	66%	82%	N = 436
Automobile	50 min.	52%	76%	N = 21
Pedestrian	20 min.	69%	81%	N = 80
Fall	45 min.	39%	59%	N = 279
"Emergency" Trauma Patients	30 min.	50%	75%	N = 90

1. Excluding transfers

trauma patients arrived within thirty minutes of the accident, 64 percent within sixty minutes, and 72 percent within ninety minutes. Twenty-eight percent of the trauma patients took more than ninety minutes to reach the ED. (These figures exclude the fifty-two patients that were transferred from other hospitals.)

Traffic accidents compromised nearly half the trauma cases, with falls nearly another quarter. Table 3-4 shows the prehospital time for these different types of accidents. Note that the median prehospital time for pedestrian accidents (twenty minutes) and motorcycle injuries (twenty-three minutes) is very short, whereas for falls it is considerably longer (forty-five minutes).

A large proportion of the traffic injuries come by car (44 percent) or motorcycle (25 percent) to the ED; this is in part because the vehicles are already on the scene, since the accident takes place on the road, and the injured party is put into a vehicle and brought directly to the ED. A somewhat smaller percentage of falls arrives by automobile (36 percent), although a larger percentage arrives by motorcycle (40 percent).

It is interesting to note here that less than 2 percent of the trauma patients arrive by ambulance (excluding transfers from other hospitals). Automobiles rather than ambulances are the major trauma transporters. Yet trauma injuries seem to arrive at the ED rather quickly. The informal "system" of emergency transport, where a person with a car available brings the injured party to the hospital, seems to work well in Yogya, at least to the extent that it produces very short prehospital times for these injuries. We have not yet examined specifically whether the most seriously injured patients arrive at the hospital in such short times. To a degree, this issue is reflected in our discussion of prehospital times of emergency patients.

EMERGENCY PATIENTS. The avowed rationale for hospital EDs is to handle medical emergencies. But only a relatively small percentage of patients who come for care in EDs are true emergencies. In this section, we attempt to separate the emergencies from the other cases and to analyze what characteristics we can discern about emergency patients.

To designate particular patients as medical emergencies, we need to categorize their problems in terms of the urgency of the need for care. Here we use medical definitions of urgency rather than patients' definitions. Often a patient, family members, or friends see the patient's need as urgent, but medical personnel may define it differently. These particular judgments about urgency have been made by the investigators, based on RAs' evaluations and careful review by a project physician.

To categorize the urgency of patients' problems, we used a modified version of the classification presented in a WHO report (Cara 1981). This classification is based on the rapidity of negative (often fatal) outcomes for different pathologies; in essence, how quickly the medical intervention must be made. In this context, we consider the following to be our definitions:

1. emergency: assessment or intervention must be made within one hour (e.g., patient in coma, in respiratory distress, or with major hemorrhage);
2. urgent: assessment or intervention should be made within twenty-four hours (e.g., patient with laceration requiring suturing or with abdominal pain);
3. nonurgent: may require medical attention but not necessarily within twenty-four hours (e.g., patient with sore throat or with bronchitis).

This classification encompasses "distress" (needing immediate medical intervention) within the emergency category, because patients requiring rapid medical attention are the raison d'être for emergency services. It also leaves a generous category for urgency (within twenty-four hours) so as to distinguish them from nonurgent patients who present in the ED. While we were careful in categorizing the patients, we recognize that some distinctions were judgment calls. Thus we feel most confident in differentiating emergency and nonurgent cases, allowing the placement of all questionable cases in the urgent category.

Using this definition, 7 percent of the patients were emergencies, 66 percent were urgent, and 26 percent were nonurgent. In this analysis we focus on the emergency, with some comparisons to other categories.

Emergency patients tended to be male (60 percent), older than other patients (mean = thirty-six years), somewhat less educated (47 percent primary school or lower, 14 percent academy–university), and more likely to be unemployed or working in lower-level occupations. For example, these patients were four times as likely as nonurgent patients to be unemployed or pensioners (15 percent); twice as likely to work in blue-collar, service, or farm occupations (23 percent); and less than half as likely to be students (22 percent). The mean distance of the hospital from home was for emergency patients the same as for urgent patients (sixteen kilometers) but considerably farther than for nonurgent patients (seven kilometers).

Emergency patients were most likely to be medically referred (32 percent), to arrive by automobile (52 percent) or ambulance (13 percent), and to arrive in the 14:00–22:00 shift (53 percent). The majority of ambulance arrivals (60 percent) were transfers from other hospitals. In terms of pre-hospital time, trauma and emergency patients' median time from incident to ED was thirty minutes, with a mean of roughly eighty-four minutes (excluding the transfers). As expected, emergency patients by far were most likely to be admitted (90 percent, compared to 39 percent for urgent and 7 percent for nonurgent).

Forty percent of emergency patients had trauma or injuries. Of the emergency patients with nonintentional trauma, 68 percent of the cases arose from traffic accidents, 16 percent from falls, and 16 percent from other causes, with very few burns and poisonings. There were relatively few cases of intentional trauma (N = 72). The Injury Severity Scores (ISS) (Copes et al. 1988), a widely used scaler (single-number) measure of anatomic injury, were similar for admitted emergency and urgent patients with trauma, with most emergency patients' injuries in the mild (ISS = 1–8, 53 percent) and moderate (ISS = 9–15, 26 percent) ranges, although there were also significantly more serious or severe injuries among the emergency patients (ISS = 16–40, 18 percent for emergency to 6 percent for urgent). Fifteen percent of emergency patients had surgical intervention; 21 percent of urgent, and 4 percent of nonurgent.

There were significantly more deaths among the emergency patients. Of the nonadmitted emergency patients, eight died in the ED (2.5 percent, compared to 0 percent for urgent and nonurgent). Of the admitted patients fifty-four emergency patients died (19 percent), compared to two for urgent (.7 percent) and none for nonurgent. It is clear that the death rate among emergency patients is much higher than for the other categories; what factors are involved with this high death rate will be analyzed in a subsequent paper.

In terms of urgency, most came by automobile, with a small percentage by ambulance. It seems that emergency patients arrive at the ED rather quickly, at least as indicated by trauma patients, the only group for whom we have such time data.

PATIENTS' PERSPECTIVES ON URGENCY. For the second two weeks of our study, we asked patients why they came to the ED for care. Table 3-5 summarizes responses to this question. If we assume that responses 1 and 2 refer to patient-perceived urgency, then over half the patients came to the ED because they defined their problems as urgent. Roughly one-quarter of the patients came to the ED because of patient-perceived conve-

Table 3-5. Most Important Reason for Coming to ED for Medical Care

Response[1]	Total[3]	Percent of Emergency	Percent of Urgent	Percent of Nonurgent
1. Can't Wait; Worried	32	25	32	33
2. Urgent Problem	20	26	25	3
3. Open Long Hours	20	9	17	32
4. Referred	13	25	13	8
5. Others Suggested	7	6	6	9
6. Always Use ED	3	1	2	5
7. Need Second Opinion	2	1	3	1
8. Other[2]	4	5	4	6

N = 1,932

1. Respondents were asked to give the single most important reason for coming to the ED. We coded the response in these categories:
    1. The sickness or injury can't wait; worried about this sickness or injury.
    2. Sickness is already critical or injury has just occurred.
    3. ED is open for long hours (always open).
    4. Referred by doctor, hospital, health center, or clinic for follow-up.
    5. Others (nonmedical) suggested coming to ED for care.
    6. Always come to ED for health care.
    7. Came for second opinion.
    8. Other.
2. Most common response in this category was "fast service."
3. Totals may vary from 100%, due to rounding.

nience in terms of long hours, fast service, or familiarity with using the ED for care (responses 3, 6, and 8). About 15 percent came for doctor-related reasons, specifically referrals (including follow-ups) or second opinions (responses 4 and 7).

Among the emergency and urgent patients, patient-perceived urgency is fairly consistent (51 percent and 57 percent, respectively). Among nonurgent patients it drops to 36 percent, with over 90 percent of these worried about their illness or injury but not actually defining it as an urgent problem. Perceived convenience provided the reason for about 44 percent of the nonurgent patient's responses to the question (compared to 15 percent of emergencies and 23 percent of urgents).

Although these findings are only suggestive, it appears that patients have a fairly good sense of whether or not their problem is urgent, but many patients come to the ED because they are "worried" (regardless of urgency) and many of the nonurgent patients use the ED because it is a convenient source of medical care.

In this section we used three strategies to examine urgency in the ED. It should be noted that while there are overlaps among the patient groupings, essentially three different subgroups were used: trauma patients, emergency patients, and all patients in the third and fourth weeks of the study. Because the patients all came from the same cohort of ED patients, however, it seems likely that together they reflect accurately on the urgency issue in the Yogya EMCS.

Discussion

Western industrialized countries such as the United States have created elaborate prehospital (EMS) systems of care that include 911 emergency telephone systems, ambulances with sophisticated equipment, two-way radio communication, paramedics and emergency medical technicians, helicopters, designated trauma centers, and sophisticated ED medical equipment. Developing countries usually cannot afford these medical technologies and have to be modest in what they offer as emergency medical care. In Indonesia, most hospitals provide emergency care, with many having specified emergency rooms (*Unit Gawat Darurat*) and ambulances with drivers.

Although the medical problems that arrive in the average ED in Indonesia may be similar to those in Western countries (e.g., a large proportion of trauma cases, of which half are traffic accidents, and a significant proportion of nonurgent cases), the situation with regard to EMS is quite different. At least in Yogya, a medium-sized city, prehospital care differs from the Western model. There are relatively few telephones in Yogya (public or otherwise), and so they are rarely used to summon aid. Although hospitals have ambulances (there are at least eighteen hospital-based ambulances), they are overwhelmingly used to transfer patients or transport medical personnel, rather than to respond to emergency situations. In addition, in a society where few have any medical insurance, ambulances are an expensive mode of transport. A recent Dutch report on EMS in Jakarta, Indonesia's capital city of eight million, noted that although the city has six hundred ambulances and a 118 emergency phone system (equivalent to 911), the EMS system is underutilized by accident and injury patients because of lack of public knowledge about using the system, an unreliable phone system, limited ambulance stations, and the perception of the cost of ambulance transport (Ministry of Welfare, Health, and Cultural Affairs 1989).

As noted above, most patients in Yogya arrive by private motor vehicle (car or motorcycle) or public transport (pedicab or bus). Only a tiny fraction (3 percent) use ambulances. If we can use the emergency patients as an indicator of severity (and therefore urgency), even among these patients 52 percent arrive by car, compared to 13 percent by ambulance. What is remarkable is how rapidly people seem to reach the ED without ambulance service. Among trauma patients, 42 percent report arriving within thirty minutes and 64 percent within an hour after the injury incident. If we again take the emergency trauma patients as an indicator of severity, from incident to arrival, 50 percent arrived within thirty minutes and 75 percent within sixty minutes. Twenty percent of the emergency patients' prehospital times exceeded ninety minutes, and several of these times were much longer; the overall mean time was eighty-four minutes. Of the ninety emergency patients, four died after hospital admission; the prehospital time for two of these was over 60 minutes—one 65 and the other 250 minutes. In general, however, the prehospital times seem surprisingly short, given the location of the hospitals (e.g., three are within a two-mile area of the city) and lack of a developed telephone or ambulance system.

There seems to be some type of informal system of transport that more or less works in getting sick and injured patients to the ED. Because there are only fifteen thousand private cars and over 800,000 people in Yogya, it appears that a considerable amount of cooperative use of cars must exist for 37 percent of all ED patients and 52 percent of the emergency patients to arrive by auto. Two examples illustrate this. In the first case, an American man was severely injured in a motorcycle accident about twelve miles outside of Yogya. After some discussion about the severity of the injury, a man who owned a nearby store volunteered his car and drove the man to the hospital. As a further example, during our research I was driving home when I saw a small crowd of young people on the side of the road. I noticed a young man lying on the side of the road, next to an overturned motorcycle. One or two people were in the street, trying to flag down vehicles; within a few minutes a pickup truck stopped and the injured person was placed in the back and driven to the hospital (which was less than one-third of a mile away).

Similar to the case with EDs in many developed countries, we found relatively few patients are true emergencies (7 percent) and a fair proportion are nonurgent cases (25 percent). We were not able to ascertain how many genuine emergency cases did not reach the EDs for treatment, but anecdotal evidence suggests rather few. The nonurgent users (and some in the urgent category as well) use the ED as a source of primary care, in part because it is more accessible than the health centers and polyclinics, which close at 14:00. After this hour, only doctors' private practices or EDs are available for medical care. Such use of EDs as primary care facilities has been found in the United States (Bohland 1984), Israel (Carmel, Anson, and Levin 1990), and Sweden (Andren and Rosenqvist 1985), among other countries. In these countries, social class differences have been found to be significant factors relating to primary care use of EDs. A recent study suggests that social class is also significant in using EDs for primary care in Indonesia (Gish, Malik, and Sudhart 1988), although in our study students constituted the largest group of nonurgent users.

The finding that patients with a range, in terms of urgency, of medical problems and needs come to the ED in part reflects the dual role of EDs in the medical system: that of "rescuing" the critically ill or injured and that of providing convenient access to hospital care. While on one level it is a policy question whether in a medical system EDs ought to be a major source of primary care, in practice they are called upon to be just that. In this sense they are an important part of a community medicine system (this issue will be addressed in a subsequent paper).

This chapter has only begun to examine issues of medical urgency in developing countries. As societies become more urbanized and the number of motor vehicles increases—as, consequently, will traffic problems— EMS will become a more significant topic in developing countries. Given the limited resources available for health services, it is questionable whether these countries should be developing EMS systems similar to those in Western industrialized countries. In Yogya, for example, it is not at all clear that an investment in expensive emergency vehicles and ambulances would substantially improve prehospital time; most trauma patients arrive at the ED in a short time frame. Although spiffy ambulances are attractive to the rescue mission of emergency medicine, they may not be the best way to invest scarce health dollars in these countries. It may be more useful to invest small amounts of money to investigate whether and how indigenous medical and "cultural" emergency systems currently operate and then to formulate strategies for supporting these systems.

In the long run, emergency medicine in developing countries will need to develop its own EMS models, based on limited medical resources, existing emergency systems, indigenous social and cultural predilections, and with a public health emphasis on prevention and injury control. Perhaps expensive Western EMS systems could then learn from the more socially-based developing-society models how to deliver more economical emergency care.

A Reflection on a Research Report

After I completed a draft of this chapter, I had a sense it somehow was different from most of the papers and books I have written in the past twenty years. This left me a bit uneasy, but I simply assumed that this was a more "applied" piece of work than I had previously done and left it at that. I gave it to a few colleagues for their reactions and comments (as is my usual style) and their responses led me to consider the chapter further. Most of the comments were to the effect that, while the paper was competent and the findings somewhat interesting, it seemed narrow, lacking an explicit theoretical framework, less "sociological" than my usual writings, and seemed too much like a straight research report (which I assume meant less interesting than a standard sociological analysis). At first I thought, How am I going to revise this to meet my colleagues' criticisms? I puzzled over this for a few weeks, rereading the paper several times, considering alternative frameworks and various paths to revision. I even outlined revision strategies: perhaps I should be more explicit about the utilization framework and develop some type of "illness behavior" framework or examine more well established sociological factors, such as the effect of social class or networks on utilization; or perhaps I should make the paper more explicitly cross-national, comparing my Indonesian data to, for example, the United States; or perhaps it would be better if I framed this as a "policy" paper and shifted the focus to injury control and ED policy in the Third World. As I considered these, none seemed to me exactly the right strategy.

As I often do, I went with this dilemma to my friend and departmental colleague Irving K. Zola. We discussed how I was stuck, unsure of how to revise or where to go with the paper. He concurred with issues raised about the paper but suggested that instead of embarking on a major revision—whose direction was not clear to me anyway—I should somehow use it to identify difficulties and dilemmas of doing research on Third World health care. Let the discomforts with the chapter become a focus for a reflection on the research and presentation of the findings.

From the outset, this study was different in orientation from my previous work. The motivation behind this study was my desire to spend my sabbatical year learning about health and health care in the Third World. After focusing on Indonesia as an appropriate and interesting locale for examining Third World health care and after securing a teaching position in an Indonesian university through a World Bank project, I began to consider what type of research I wanted to do during my year's stay. The choice of studying EMS was a pragmatic one: it would be an opportunity to do collaborative research with my wife, who is an emergency physician. So from the outset this research had a "sociomedical" orientation, rather than a predominantly sociological one. We agreed that, given our role as visitors and the developing-society context, we wanted our research eventually to be "useful" to those working in the Indonesian medical system. Therefore we, along with our Indonesian colleagues, settled on examining utilization in the ED, with special attention to trauma. This meant that a good portion of our research would focus on more practical medical care questions: Who comes to the ED? With what purpose and problem? How do they get there? Who treats them? and so forth. From the outset, although loosely deemed a "sociology-in-medicine" study, the research didn't focus on a specific sociological problem.

Another problem in developing this research from the beginning involved language. Although both my wife and I studied Indonesian and developed a limited fluency, it always remained limited. Some of the language problems manifested themselves in the construction of our data-collection instrument (which was written in Indonesian), although most of these were eventually overcome with the aid of our Indonesian collaborators and research coordinator. The biggest problem with language for me, however, was my inability to have adequate access to the subjective social world I was studying. This limited my ability to develop the qualitative portion of the study. I could speak with people who spoke English reasonably well, but these were limited to a few physicians in the EDs and less than half of our RAs. Thus no nurses, auxiliary staff, or patients were included. While my Indonesian was good enough to make small talk with people, when it came to ethnographic interviewing my language reached the level where I could ask all the questions I needed to but didn't always understand the answers. Our RAs gathered some qualitative data for us, but it was, frankly, limited in quantity and quality. It was difficult to get them to see the importance of writing down conversations and subjective perspectives as data. Even though this was not an ethnographic study, stronger language ability would have allowed me to penetrate Indonesian medical culture more deeply and to use such data to interpret our more systematic and quantitative data with more cultural sensitivity.

This was a big lesson for me. The limits of language pushed the focus of the study in a more structured and quantitative direction than I had taken in my previous studies and had me spending more time reading and coding our structured surveys than doing participant observation and interviewing, to which I was more accustomed. Having done fieldwork in the United States, I had taken for granted how much I relied on the cues and context of language for understanding the social world I studied. Here the limits of language only allowed me glimpses of social meaning and process, which are the grist of most of my sociological work.

Although the project proceeded with an inductive research orientation (as have virtually all my studies), I encountered some dilemmas different from any in my previous research. For lack of a better term, I can call it an absence of "context." Before we began the study, I already knew there was almost no previous research on EDs in the Third World and little work by sociologists on EDs in general. As I more thoroughly reviewed the extant literature, however, I was surprised at how little data there was on the utilization of EDs in developed countries. This made it more difficult to develop a comparative orientation for analysis. While there were studies on patients who come to the ED with nonurgent problems or studies on some specific aspects of trauma, there were few that presented comparative data on ED utilization. Thus, in a general paper like this one, it is difficult to find a context in which to anchor the analysis. This is why I chose the twin themes of utilization and "urgency," without being able to compare them directly to other situations.

It is perhaps a combination of these three factors—a sociomedical orientation, the limitations of language, and the lack of comparative context—that implicitly conspires to make this appear to be a "straight research report" and a study less sociological than the rest of my writings.

NOTE

Acknowledgments: I want to acknowledge my intellectual and practical debt to my coinvestigators Rusdi Lamsudin, Ylisabyth Bradshaw, and Nanniek Kasniyah, without whose collaboration this research would not have been possible. The Clinical Epidemiology Unit of Gadjah Mada University provided a stimulating and supportive atmosphere for the research; special thanks to Director Tonny Sadjimin. Thanks also to Yanri Subronto and our twenty-two research assistants and to Ninik, Diwi, and Stephen Fielding for assistance in the analysis. Gene Gallagher, Stephen Fielding, and Irving K. Zola provided helpful comments on earlier drafts. This project was supported by grants from the Center of International Studies at Brandeis University, the Mazur Faculty Fund at Brandeis, and the Rockefeller Foundation.

REFERENCES

Ali, J., and V. Naraynsingh. 1987. "Potential Impact of the Advance Trauma Life Support (ATLB) Program on a Third World Country." *International Surgery* 72:179–84.

Andren, Kjerstin Genell, and Urban Rosenqvist. 1985. "Heavy Users of an Emergency Department: Psycho-social and Medical Characteristics. Other Health Care Contacts and the Effect of a Hospital Social Worker Intervention." *Social Science and Medicine* 21: 761–70.

———. 1987. "Heavy Users of the Emergency Department—A Two Year Follow-up Study." *Social Science and Medicine* 25:825–31.

Berman, Peter. 1985. *Equity and Cost in the Organization of Primary Health Care in Java, Indonesia*. Ithaca, N.Y.: New York State College of Agriculture and Life Sciences, Cornell University.

Bohland, James. 1984. "Neighborhood Variations in the Use of Hospital Services for Primary Care." *Social Science and Medicine* 19:1217–26.

Cara, M. 1981. "Tentative Classification of Emergency Situations." In *Planning and Organization of Emergency Medical Services*, compiled by WHO Technical Group, 21–28, EURO Reports and Studies 35. Copenhagen: WHO Regional Office for Europe.

Carmel, Sara, Ofra Anson, and Mordechai Levin. 1990. "Emergency Department Utilization by Two Subcultures in the Same Geographical Region." *Social Science and Medicine* 31: 557–63.

Committee on Health Statistics, South East Asian Medical Information Center. 1988. *Seamic Health Statistics, 1988*. Tokyo: International Medical Foundation of Japan.

Copes, Wayne S., Howard R. Champion, William J. Sacco, Mary M. Lawnick, Susan L. Keast, and Lawrence W. Bain. 1988. "The Injury Severity Score Revisited." *Journal of Trauma* 28:69–77.

Department of Information, Republic of Indonesia. 1988. *Indonesia*. Jakarta: Department of Information.

Gish, Oscar, Ridwan Malik, and Paramita Sudharto. 1988. "Who Gets What? Utilization of Health Services in Indonesia." *International Journal of Health Planning and Management* 3:185–96.

Jacobs, J. D., and C. A. Cutting. 1986. "Further Research on Accident Rates in Developing Countries." *Accident Annals and Prevention* 18:119–29.

Ministry of Welfare, Health, and Cultural Affairs, The Netherlands. 1989. *Emergency Medical Services with the City of Jakarta, Indonesia: Recommendations for Future Development*. Jakarta: Republic of Indonesia.

Reilly, P. M. 1981. "Primary Care and Accident and Emergency Departments in an Urban Area." *Journal of the Royal College of General Practice* 31:223–28.

Rossi-Espangnet, A. 1984. *Primary Health Care in Urban Areas, Reaching the Poor in Developing Countries: A State-of-the-Art Report by UNICEF.* WHO.SH8–84–4. Geneva: World Health Organization.

Roth, Julius A., and Dorothy J. Douglas. 1983. *No Appointment Necessary: The Hospital Emergency Department in the Medical Services World.* New York: Irvington.

Silva, J. Francis. 1973. "The Organization of Accident and Emergency Services in a Developing Country." *Medical Journal of Malaysia* 28:19–22.

Suparnadi Praptasuganda. 1988. "Kasus Cedera di Indonesia." ("Injury Cases in Indonesia.") *Bulitin Penelitian Keseshatan [Bulletin of Health Studies]* 16(2):48–55.

Suparnadi Praptasuganda, and Hermansyur Kartowisastro. 1986. "An Analysis of Traffic Accident Deaths in a Hospital in Jakarta." *Bulitin Penelitian Kesehatan [Bulletin of Health Studies]* 14(4):10–17.

Torrens, Paul, and Donna G. Yedvab. 1970. "Variations among Emergency Room Populations: A Comparison of Four Hospitals in New York City." *Medical Care* 8:60–75.

World Bank. 1989. *World Development Report 1989.* New York: Oxford University Press.

WHO Study Group. 1989. *New Approaches to Improve Road Safety.* WHO Technical Report Series, 781. Geneva: World Health Organization.

Chapter 4

Ethnicity, Health Behavior,

and Modernization:

The Case of Singapore

STELLA R. QUAH

The world has entered the final decade of the twentieth century amid the piping notes of an ethnic symphony. This has been an unexpected phenomenon. Modernization, with its high technology and scientific outlook, has shrunk the distances between peoples by increasing the speed and quality of their communication to levels never before thought possible. Yet, contrary to the educated calculations of intellectuals, modernization and improved knowledge of one another has not reduced peoples' consciousness of and pride in their differences. If anything, the determination of numerous ethnic communities to go back to their roots and to demand national and international recognition of their particular cultural features has reached a higher pitch around the globe during recent years.

The importance of ethnic identity and its accompanying set of cultural values and beliefs in determining people's behavior has been highlighted by social scientists, particularly sociologists and anthropologists, throughout this century. There were indications, however, that we were also tempted to expect an eventual decline in ethnic identity, especially among urban populations who are more exposed to the influence of modernization. This expectation was popularized by the "melting pot" assumption. Empirical signs of it could be found in large host countries (that is, countries seen as the final destination for large groups of immigrants) such as the United States. Today, however, the awakening of ethnic identity is undeniable. More important, in some Third World societies ethnic identity has never reached the melting pot state. For these reasons, I believe that the analysis of health behavior in Singapore provides a unique opportunity to examine the role of ethnic identity. Singapore is basically a metropolis that enjoys the status of independent republic and the prestige of being one of Asia's "economic miracles." At the same time, Singapore is located in the center of Southeast Asia and is home for a multiethnic population of 2.68 million, whose ancestries or cultural roots are Chinese (76 percent of the population), Malay (15.2 percent), Indian (6.5 percent), and a combination of other ethnic communities (2.4 percent) (Ministry of Communications and Information 1990, 3).

The objective of this discussion is to explore the persistent influence of ethnic identity upon health behavior, using Singapore, a society that is at once modern and traditional, as an illustration. I accomplish this in three steps. I first deal with the concepts of ethnicity and health behavior as they have been analyzed in the relevant literature. I then illustrate the link between ethnicity and health behavior with empirical evidence from Singapore, making comparisons with other societies whenever possible. The final section of this chapter is a summary of the main findings.

Ethnicity and Health Behavior

The social science literature is abundant with studies linking ethnicity and health-related behavior. There is a basic agreement in most of these studies with the premise that ethnic-group membership "is a matter of social definition" (Horowitz 1975, 113). Indeed, one of the most accurate definitions of ethnicity has been provided by S. H. King (1962), precisely because he emphasizes its social meaning. King speaks of ethnic boundaries delimiting a cultural setting where people share "common backgrounds in language, customs, beliefs, habits and tradition, frequently in racial stock and country of origin," in addition to a "consciousness of kind" (1962, 79).

Margaret Mead stresses the importance of differences among the patterns of behavior of people with different ethnic backgrounds in the analysis of health-related behavior (1956, 260). She was referring to the work of Mark Zborowski (1952), Lyle Saunders (1954), and Benjamin Paul (1955), among others. Mead's view differs from King's in that she assumes that ethnic differences cut across class, racial, and religious lines.

Paul sees the cultural setting of an ethnic group as an integral phenomenon: "a group's design for living, a shared set of socially transmitted assumptions about the nature of the physical and social world, the goals of life and the appropriate means of achieving them" (1963, 34). He collected ample evidence of the impact of ethnic differences on people's health-related behavior and identifies the "cultural gap" as one of the four obstacles "impeding prevention programs" (1963; and in Lynch 1969, 32–36). Furthermore, two decades ago Paul stressed a view that has been confirmed today: he argued that regardless of the pace and diversity of social change, "the degree to which [people's] actions are influenced by their respective cultures" is a constant factor (1977, 234). He agreed with Steven Polgar (1963) that people's health beliefs are an integral part of other beliefs and values that guide their daily life.

These pioneer ideas underlining the resilience of ethnic identities have been incorporated and expanded in recent conceptual work in sociology addressed to our understanding of health behavior. Whether the conceptual framework applied is the structural–functional model, the interactionist perspective, the conflict approach, the labeling theory, or still another theoretical perspective, there is a keen awareness among sociologists of the importance of the ethnic dimension of health behavior (McHugh and Vallis 1986; Bates and Linder-Pelz 1987; Gerhardt 1989; Fox 1989; Freeman and Levine 1989).

Following a general emphasis on the outcome of illness, empirical research on the association between ethnicity and health behavior has been primarily concerned with responsive rather than preventive behavior. That is, more attention has been given to ways in which people respond to illness (illness behavior or sick-role behavior) than to what people do to avoid falling ill. Some examples of this emphasis on responsive behavior are: the problems of patient–physician interaction in mixed cultures (Saunders 1954); the differences in responses to pain among different ethnic groups (Zborowski 1952); differences in symptom-reporting among ethnic groups (Zola 1966); the ethnic differences in the incidence of chronic diseases (Graham 1956; Graham and Reeder 1972, 80–89); ethnic differences in the utilization of medical services (Babson 1972); ethnic variations in the perception of symptoms (Sanborn and Katz 1977); and ethnic variations in the response to medical treatment (Yamamoto and Steinberg 1981; Good 1986) and to disease in general (Owen 1987).

Reviewing the work of Edward Suchman (1964, 1965) on health behavior and ethnicity, Reed Geertsen and his colleagues confirm the association between these two variables. They found that "group closeness and exclusivity increases the likelihood of an individual's responding to a medical problem in a way that is consistent with his subcultural background" (1975, 232). More detailed findings on the link between ethnicity and health behavior are provided by David Mechanic (1978). He lists studies of infant mortality, child socialization and health, high blood pressure, obesity, perceived desirability of mental conditions, illness behavior, and utilization of medical services, among others. A similar account is provided by Leon Robertson and M. C. Heagarty (1975); John Kosa and I. K. Zola (1975); and C. L. Estes and L. E. Gerard (1979). Useful references to health-related practices in various ethnic communities around the world are offered by Charles Leslie (1976), David Landy (1977), Arthur Kleinman (1980), N. G. Owen (1987), H. B. Kaplan (1989), and R. C. Kessler and C. B. Wortman (1989). The wealth of contributions to the study of the link between ethnicity and health behavior is so extensive that Mechanic declared as early as twelve years ago that "cultures are so recognizably different that variations in illness behavior in different societies hardly need demonstration" (1978, 261).

Mechanic's opinion, however, refers to responses to illness in the form of sick-role behavior or illness behavior. The latter is defined by S. V. Kasl and Sidney Cobb as behavior relevant to "any condition that causes or might usefully cause an individual to concern himself with his symptoms and to seek help" (1966, 246; Mechanic 1978, 249). Consequently, while there is abundant empirical evidence of ethnic differences in illness behavior and sick-role behavior, the impact of ethnicity on preventive health behavior has not yet been sufficiently demonstrated.

But the research mentioned above provides a strong basis for the assumption that ethnic differences also affect preventive health behavior—actions taken to avoid illness, by a person who considers himself or herself healthy. A few interesting studies already provide evidence of ethnic differences in preventive health behavior. Among the most important are those examining body management among the Japanese (Caudill 1976); food and food habits among the Zulu people (Cassel 1977); rituals and domestic sanitation in a North Indian village (Khare 1977); knowledge of cancer prevention among black women in the United States (Manfredi et al. 1977); medical and food beliefs among Chinese fishermen (Anderson and Anderson 1978) personal health behavior among the Malaysian Chinese (Dunn 1978); coronary risk factors among aborigines in Australia (Simons et al. 1981); and food habits that may be linked to cancer in South Africa (Randeria 1981). These and similar studies usually focus on the description of preventive practices among small groups of individuals. What is needed now is a detailed analysis of the factors that may explain differences in preventive health behavior in large, multiethnic populations. This brings me to the subject of Singapore.

Health Behavior and Ethnicity in Singapore

As indicated at the beginning of the this chapter, Singapore is an appealing setting for the study of the link between ethnicity and health behavior because of the multiethnic composition of its population, the interesting combination of tradition and modernity in its society, and the influence of ethnic identity on that society. These three factors deserve elaboration, albeit briefly.

First, Singapore has a predominantly urban and multiethnic population. When British ships arrived in 1819, the island had only a small fishing village with 150 people, about 30 of whom were Chinese "engaged in pepper and gambier planting"; the rest were Malay fishermen and their families, many of them immigrants from Indonesia. The first population records indicate that by January 1824 the population had increased to 10,683, of whom 31 percent were Chinese, 60 percent Malay, 7 percent Indian, and 2 percent from other ethnic groups (Ministry of Communications and Information 1989, 26–27). The influx of immigrants to Singapore ran parallel to the development of the island into a busy trading port under British rule. Singapore became attractive as a place of economic opportunity not only to the islanders from the region but especially to the Chinese. Within the span of four decades, the Chinese shifted from being a minority to constituting 65 percent of the Singapore population. The Chinese position as an ethnic majority has been maintained since then. As indicated earlier, by 1989, 76 percent of the population of 2.68 million were Chinese. Malays became an ethnic minority (15.1 percent). The proportions of Indians (6.5 percent) and other minorities (2.4 percent), however, have remained relatively stable. In contrast to the Chinese, who came on their own initiative as traders or in search of jobs and ways to earn a living, the first waves of Indians arrived in Singapore in a more formal role, as part of the British armed forces and civil administration. Their command of the English language and the experience of India as a British colony made Indians very suitable, from the British perspective, to assist in the administration of their other Asian colonies.

Second, Singapore provides a good setting for the study of ethnicity and health behavior because of its interesting combination of tradition and modernity. Although modernization and high technology rule Singapore's economic development, the people's everyday life is at the crossroads between tradition and modernization. Differences in traditional values and beliefs among the three main ethnic groups are clearly discernible, particularly because there is some overlap between ethnicity and religion: for example, practically all Malays are Muslims, and all Hindus are Indians. Yet, notwithstanding this awareness of ethnic boundaries, as Singaporeans most citizens share some basic values (for example, the conviction that an honest government is necessary, belief in the need for religious harmony, belief in the importance of education as the means to success in life), as well as some fundamental environmental features attained through economic development. Indeed, regardless of their ethnic origin, Singaporeans enjoy affordable and efficient housing, health services, schools and other educational institutions, modern services such as drinking water, modern sanitation, electricity, and modern transportation and communication facilities both local and international.

Third, ethnic identity in Singapore has not yet been superseded by a national identity. On the contrary, explicit efforts are made by the government and community leaders to foster the individual's interest in cultural matters concerning his or her own ethnic community, particularly for the three major ethnic groups. In the political landscape of Singapore, the numerical size of each ethnic group is not commensurate with each group's respective political significance. A good illustration of this point is the case of the Malays. Although they constitute only 15.1 percent of the population, they enjoy a separate legal system, the Muslim Law Act, and free education including, until 1990, free university education. Their political importance is underscored—as in the case of the Indian community—by Singapore's ideological commitment to racial and religious harmony.

These features of Singapore motivated me to study the preventive behavior of a random sample of the total population of Singaporean citizens and to explore the influence of ethnicity and social class upon preventive practices concerning cancer, heart disease, and tuberculosis (Quah 1980). I refer in this chapter to the main findings from that study on the impact of ethnicity as the empirical background to this discussion, as well as to more recent data on ethnic differences in morbidity and mortality.

Before dealing with health-behavior data, some comparative figures are required to appreciate the position of Singapore with respect to other countries in Asia. Table 4-1 compares Singapore with Japan and four of its Southeast Asian neighbors, that is, Indonesia, Thailand, the Philippines, and Malaysia, in terms of some key indicators of development and health care for the latest year available, 1986. Singapore stands second to Japan in high life expectancy, low infant mortality, and the availability of health services such as hospital beds, physicians, and nurses. Singapore ranks first, however, in proportion of households living in dwellings with piped water (99 percent) and flushable toilets (95 percent). Although there are no available figures for Japan on the proportion of household dwellings with electricity to make a comparison, still Singapore has a high proportion (95 percent). On the negative side, Singapore is second only to Japan in the rate of suicides, and its population density is significantly higher (4, 158 persons per square kilometer) than that of all five of the other countries.

There are other relevant indicators of Singapore's development among 1988 figures. Over 80 percent of the population are home owners; infant mortality was reduced from 12.6 per 1,000 live births in 1978 to 7 per 1,000 in 1988; the per capita indigenous gross national product in-

TABLE 4-1. Comparative View of Development and Health Statistics, 1986

	Indonesia	Japan	Malaysia[1]	Philippines	Singapore	Thailand
Population in millions	163,366	121,492	16,109	56,004	2,586	50,396
Population density (persons per square kilometer)	86	326	49	187	4,158	98
% urban population in 1980	22.4	76.2	34.1	37.3	100.0	17.0
Rate of suicides per 10,000 population	0.06	21.2	1.67	0.20	12.70	5.50
Infant mortality rate per 1,000 live births	7.9	5.9	—	6.9	7.8	7.8
Life expectancy (years from birth)						
Males	58.8	75.2	67.9	61.6	70.3	61.7
Females	62.5	80.9	72.9	65.2	75.7	67.5
% Households in dwellings with piped water	10.8	94.0	65.0	71.4	99.0	18.9
% Households in dwellings with flushable toilets	14.9	58.5	56.4	67.9	95.0	4.2
% Households in dwellings with electricity	30.5	—	64.4	—	95.0	43.0
Persons per hospital bed	1,498	79	489	3,273	259	622
Persons per physician	8,486	6,362	986	1,046	930	5,564
Persons per nurse	6,255	190	661	369	302	1,286

Source: SEAMIC 1987.
1. The figures on suicide rates and life expectancy refer only to peninsular Malaysia. All other figures include the Malaysian states of Sabah and Sarawak.

TABLE 4-2. Principal Causes of Death in Singapore

Rank	1948[1]	1979[1]	1988[2]
1	Tuberculosis	Cancer	Cancer
2	Pneumonia	Heart Disease	Heart Disease
3	Gastroenteritis	Cerebrovascular Disease	Cerebrovascular Disease
4	Infections of Newborn	Pneumonia	Pneumonia
5	Heart Disease	Accidents, Poisonings, and Violence	Accidents, Poisonings, and Violence

1. Ministry of Health 1980, 7.
2. Ministry of Health 1989, 4.

creased from S $6,303 in 1978 to S $15,999 in 1988; the annual number of international telephone calls increased from 1,760 in 1978 to 43,672 in 1988, that is, from 0.8 international calls per 1,000 people in 1976 to 16.5 calls per 1,000 people in 1988; and in 1988 there were 2 persons per telephone, 5 persons per television set, 297 persons per public bus, and 253 persons per taxi (Ministry of Communications and Information 1989; Department of Statistics 1989).

Turning to the question of ethnic differences among Singaporeans of Chinese, Malay, and Indian descent, studies have reported significant variations in important aspects of life such as political attitudes, religious beliefs, employment, housing, fertility behavior, occupational status, and the utilization of curative health services (see, e.g., Ooi and Chiang 1969; Gwee, Lee, and Tham 1969; Quah 1975; Hassan 1976, 1977; Quah 1983, 1984; Hughes et al 1984). Comparisons between these ethnic communities have also revealed variations in other health behaviors as well as in mortality and morbidity rates for cancer, heart disease, diabetes mellitus, peptic ulcers, and hepatitis B, among other disease (see, e.g., Oh 1975; Chen 1980; Goh 1980; Lun and Lee 1981 ; Lee and Lun 1982; Shanmugaratnam, Lee, and Day 1983; Cheah et al. 1985; Kang et al. 1986; Hughes et al. 1987; Lee, Lee, and Shanmugaratnam 1987; Lee 1989; Emmanuel 1989; Hughes et al. 1989; Chua et al. 1990).[1]

The consistent ethnic differences in morbidity and mortality that all these medical studies discuss are best exemplified by the cases of cancer, heart disease, and tuberculosis. The principal causes of death in Singapore have changed over the years, but, as shown in Table 4-2, the predominance of cancer and heart disease as the two major "killer" diseases in Singapore has remained constant during the past decade. These two diseases are also the two "most important causes of death" in every one of the twenty-four nations in the Organization for Economic Cooperation and Development (OECD), comprising all Western European countries,

Australia, New Zealand, Turkey, Japan, Canada, and the United States (OCED 1987, 45). The seriousness of cancer and heart disease as principal causes of death justifies their selection in this discussion of ethnic differences. In contrast, tuberculosis has been successfully controlled in Singapore to the point where its mortality rate was only 7.1 per 100,000 population in 1987, even though it was the top leading cause of death during the 1940s. Table 4-3 provides evidence on the persistence of ethnic differences by showing the mortality rates for cancer, heart disease, and tuberculosis in 1970, 1980, and 1987.

It is opportune to recall at this point that the ethnic composition of the Singapore population is 76 percent Chinese, 15.1 percent Malay, and 6.5 percent Indian; the remaining 2.4 percent includes a variety of other ethnic communities. According to the figures on Table 4-3, there is a clear ethnic pattern in mortality rates for all three diseases, but, as the incidence of tuberculosis is declining and it is considerably lower, the ethnic differences for tuberculosis are not as significant as those found for cancer and heart disease.

Cancer mortality rates show that, of the three major ethnic groups, the Chinese are the most affected whereas the Malays are the least affected; the mortality rate for Indians falls in between these two ethnic groups. The most serious types of cancer are, in descending order, cancer of the lung, colorectal cancer, stomach cancer, and liver cancer (Ministry of Health 1989, 4). Following the International Classification of Diseases (ICD), the term "cancer of the lung" covers "malignant neoplasm of trachea, bronchus and lung" (Registrar-General of Births and Deaths) 1988, 82); the disease is said to have reached "epidemic proportions in all developed countries and many of the urban centres of the developing world" (Lee 1985, 485). In fact, the 1985 mortality rate for cancer of the lung in Japan was 36.1 deaths per 100,000 persons, which was the same rate for Singapore in 1986 (SEAMIC 1987, 30–31). In a detailed study of dialect-group differences in lung cancer among the Singaporean, Chinese, H. P. Lee found that "the Hokkien and Teochew males had one of the highest age-standardized rates in the world—73.2 and 67.0," while among the Chinese women, "the Cantonese had about double the risks compared to other dialect groups with an age-standardized rate at 28.5 (1985, 487)." The incidence of colon and rectal cancers for the period 1968 to 1982 followed the same pattern of the overall cancer mortality rates, that is, it was highest among the Chinese of both sexes and lowest for the Malays (Lee, Lee, and Shanmugaratnam 1987, 398–99).

Significant ethnic variations are also evident in the mortality rates for heart disease presented in Table 4-3. However, the ethnic pattern for heart disease is different from that of cancer. Since 1980, the highest heart disease mortality rates are found among Indians; the second highest rates are found among the group "others," followed by Malays; and the

TABLE 4-3. Singapore Mortality Rates for Cancer, Heart Disease, and Tuberculosis by Ethnicity, 1970, 1980, and 1987 (rates per 100,000 population)

		1970	1980	1987
CANCER				
Only Malignant Neoplasm[1]	Chinese	89.9	121.9	137.4
	Malay	27.3	46.1	57.1
	Indian	42.0	67.3	82.2
	Other ethnic groups	76.1	62.0	55.5
	Total population	76.9	106.1	119.8
All Types[2]	Chinese	—	124.4	138.9
	Malay	—	48.9	58.9
	Indian	—	69.8	82.8
	Other ethnic groups	—	64.0	55.5
	Total population	—	108.6	121.3
HEART DISEASE				
Ischemic Heart Disease[3]	Chinese	33.9	69.4	83.6
	Malay	27.6	80.2	94.2
	Indian	99.9	216.7	217.6
	Other ethnic groups	149.6	127.9	104.4
	Total population	39.7	81.7	94.3
All Types[4]	Chinese	—	88.3	98.3
	Malay	—	98.7	107.9
	Indian	—	236.0	234.2
	Other ethnic groups	—	145.4	156.6
	Total population	—	100.5	109.9
TUBERCULOSIS[5]				
	Chinese	25.6	10.7	6.9
	Malay	9.0	7.1	7.1
	Indian	15.9	9.7	10.6
	Other ethnic groups	5.2	3.9	4.9
	Total population	22.1	9.9	7.1

1. Ministry of Health 1990. Includes all malignant neoplasms under the International Classification of Diseases. (ICD) List, Ninth Revision (ICD codes 147–208, but excludes "other and unspecified neoplasm, carcinoma in-situ" (ICD codes 210–39).
2. Calculated from Registrar-General of Births and Deaths 1981, 80; 1988, 82. Includes all malignant and benign neoplasms (ICD codes 147–239).
3. Ministry of Health 1990. Includes acute myocardial infarction and other forms of ischemic heart disease (ICD codes 410–14).
4. Calculated from Registrar-General of Births and Deaths 1981, 81; 1988, 83. Includes acute myocardial infarction, other forms of ischemic heart disease, and diseases of pulmonary circulation and other forms of heart disease (ICD codes 410–29).
5. Ministry of Health 1990 and Registrar-General of Births and Deaths 1981, 80; 1988, 82. Includes ICD codes 010–18.

Chinese have the lowest mortality rates. Making an international comparison of mortality rates for ischemic heart disease among men in the age cohorts thirty-five to sixty-four for the period 1980 to 1984, Kenneth Hughes and his colleagues (1989, 246) report the following descending order: Singaporean Indians, 613 per 100,000; Singaporean Malays, 306; England and Wales, 276; the United States, 228; Singaporean Chinese,

162; and Japan, 33. The same order is found for the corresponding death rates among women in these populations, although the rates are much lower: Singaporean Indians, 214 per 100,000; Singaporean Malays, 133; England and Wales, 68; the United States, 68; Singaporean Chinese, 57; and Japan, 10.

These figures underscore the high risk of ischemic heart disease faced by Singaporean Indians, compared not only to other ethnic groups in Singapore but also to other populations abroad. The same fact is emphasized with respect to coronary heart disease:

> The ravaging effect of Coronary Heart Disease on the Indian male
> . . . manifests its effect at a younger age group compared with
> that for the national average, with Indian males aged 40 to 49 . . .
> already experiencing an age-specific mortality rate of 359 per
> 100,000 population . . . three and a half times that of Malay
> males and seven times that of Chinese males [of] the same age.
> (Emmanuel 1989, 21)

Thus there is sufficient evidence of ethnic differences in morbidity and mortality rates for the two major causes of death, cancer and heart disease: Chinese face the highest risk of cancer and Indians have the highest risk of dying of heart disease. The challenging question before researchers is: Why do people who call the same country home and basically share the same political, economic, social, and physical environments differ so significantly in their risks of getting cancer and heart disease? There are two kinds of answers, the medical answers and the answers provided by social science, particularly by sociology. Both are tentative to various degrees, but they do contribute to our understanding of the problem and, most importantly, to the planning of prevention programs. I will briefly review the medical perspective before proceeding to the sociological perspective.

Physicians worldwide tend to agree on some primary risk factors for cancer and heart disease. Concerning cancer, the most accepted risk factors appear to be cigarette smoking, whether active or passive (e.g, the risk faced by the spouses of smokers); prolonged exposure to radioactive agents, asbestos, certain chemical agents such as mustard gas, arsenic, and chromium; severe air pollution; solar radiation; alcohol drinking; and the side effects of certain drugs (Lee 1985, 488–489; Whelan 1977, 51–175). Other risk factors whose effects are less certain are diet, genetic predisposition, and the possible causal link between some nonfatal diseases and cancer (Whelan 1977; Glucksberg and Singer 1982; Lee 1985). The uncertainty among medical researchers moved two cancer specialists at the University of Washington to caption the title of one of their chapters "Eating, Drinking, Working and Breathing Can Be Dangerous"

(Glucksberg and Singer 1982, 15). The impact of two other factors, age and gender, are evident in terms of cancer morbidity and mortality figures. However, medical researchers have not found solid explanations for variations between men and women.

The situation surrounding the medical identification of risk factors for heart disease is similar. There are some causal factors that have been well tested in other countries, but there is uncertainty about their effect in Singapore. Among the factors that medical professionals, including local physicians, agree upon are cigarette smoking, high blood pressure, and high cholesterol levels (Emmanuel 1989, 22; Hughes et al., 1989, 246–47). Nevertheless, it has been found in Singapore that although Indian men have the highest mortality rates for heart disease, it is the Malays that show the highest prevalence of hypertension and the highest proportion of smokers (Emmanuel 1989, 22; Hughes et al. 1989, 246–47); furthermore, the differences in hypertension found among the three major ethnic groups were not statistically significant, and the "mean serum cholesterol concentrations in Singapore showed no differences by ethnic group in either sex" (Hughes et al. 1989, 247).

Taken together, the medical identification of risk factors does not explain why there are differences among ethnic groups. S. C. Emmanuel concludes that her study did not have "the specific purpose" of analyzing "the reasons for the trends" in the mortality rates for coronary heart disease, and she appeals for more research on this (1989, 22). In a similar vein, Hughes and his colleagues state that "as the much higher mortality from ischemic heart disease in Indians cannot be explained by conventional major risks factors, research on this is needed" (1989, 249). These pleas for more research suggest the need for multidisciplinary investigations. As medicine faces limitations, other fields of knowledge such as sociology and anthropology take up this challenge.

What could sociology contribute to the explanation of ethnic differences in mortality rates for cancer and heart disease? The contribution of sociology rests upon the fact that some of the principal risk factors identified by medical experts as associated with cancer, heart disease, and many other diseases—including (AIDS)—are behavioral factors, that is, life-style and daily activities such as smoking, alcohol drinking, exercise, and diet. A basic sociological assumption is that values and beliefs characteristic of a person's ethnic community influence personal decisions and choices concerning the individual's life-style and daily activities. Ethnic or cultural values—which often overlap religious values and beliefs—influence, directly and indirectly, a person's attitudes and values about intangible issues such as the purpose of life, competition, success, wealth, thriftiness, and power, as well as more prosaic aspects of daily life such as food preferences, ways of relaxing, and patterns of entertaining. Abundant sociological and anthropological research supports the assumption that a link exists between ethnicity and behavior, especially health-related behavior.

An empirical illustration of this basic assumption is provided by the findings from a larger study on preventive behavior in Singapore, focusing on cancer, heart disease, and tuberculosis. The first phase of the study (Quah 1980) was based on a survey of attitudes, beliefs, and behavior among the total population of Singapore concerning the prevention of these three diseases. Personal interviews were conducted with a stratified random sample of 1,271 Singaporeans in 1977. Only the findings on ethnic differences are discussed here.

During the personal interviews with each of the subjects, five types of activities involving personal choices and life-style were analyzed. Two of these were on general health practices, namely, keeping medicines at home for eventualities and practicing at least one activity to protect against the onset of illness. The other three were specific activities, selected because they have been medically identified as being directly connected with the prevention of cancer and heart disease. These activities were regular smoking, regular exercise, and regular alcohol drinking. A summary of the findings on the practice of the five health-related activities is presented in Table 4-4.

As may be seen in Table 4-4, the two general preventive activities were practiced more by Malays than by Chinese and Indians. Malays were more likely to keep medicines at home. More important, about seven out of every ten Malays indicated they did something to protect themselves from illness regularly, in contrast to only four out of every ten Chinese and Indians. With respect to the three specific preventive activities linked to risk factors, two—exercise and moderation of alcohol drinking—presented a statistically significant difference among the three main ethnic groups in Singapore. Regular exercise was reported more by Malays (59 percent) than by Chinese (34 percent) and Indians (29 percent). Following the same preventive pattern, the lowest proportion of alcohol drinkers was found among Malays (5 percent), compared to Chinese (35 percent) and Indians (36 percent). The only exception in statistically significant differences across ethnic groups was smoking, although a higher proportion of smokers (35 percent) was found among the Malays than among the Indians (28 percent) and the Chinese (27 percent).

Smoking is also the exception in the otherwise preventive health orientation manifested by the Malays. Some figures provide the relevant background. Given the aggressive public educational campaigns and legislation against smoking pursued during the past decade, the overall proportion of smokers in the Singapore population has been decreasing steadily, from 28 percent in 1977 to 19 percent in 1984; 16 percent in 1986; and 13 percent in 1987 (Quah 1988, 213; Emmanuel, Phe, and Chen

TABLE 4-4. Health-related Activities by Ethnic Group (in Percentages)

Percentage of Respondents Answering "Yes" to Five Questions on Health-related Activities	Ethnic Groups			Total Sample
	Chinese	Malays	Indians	
GENERAL PREVENTIVE ACTIVITIES				
Keep medicines at home[1]	50.0	62.0	56.0	52.0
(N)[2]	(963)	(167)	(122)	(1,252)
Practice at least one activity to prevent illness[3]	44.0	74.0	45.0	48.0
(N)	(975)	(167)	(125)	(1,267)
SPECIFIC ACTIVITIES				
Preventive				
Exercise regularly[4]	34.0	59.0	29.0	37.0
(N)	(974)	(167)	(126)	(1,267)
Risk factors				
Smoke regularly[5]	27.0	35.0	28.0	28.0
(N)	(972)	(166)	(126)	(1,264)
Drink alcohol regularly[6]	35.0	5.0	36.0	31.0
(N)	(971)	(166)	(124)	(1,261)

Source: Quah 1980.
1. Statistically significant difference among the three ethnic groups at p > .01, based on the Chi-Square test.
2. N stands for the number of interviewees answering each question. Nonresponses were excluded from the calculations.
3. p > .00001.
4. p > .00001.
5. No statistically significant difference at p > .05.
6. p > .00001.

1988, 236). Most smokers are men. Only 4.5 percent of women were smokers in 1977; 3.4 percent in 1984; and 2.0 percent in 1987. The corresponding figures for men are 42 percent in 1977; 34.9 percent in 1984; and 25.3 percent in 1987 (Emmanuel, Phe, and Chen 1988; Emmanuel, Chen, and Phe 1986). Against this backdrop of a decline in cigarette smoking and its characteristic as a male habit, another significant and constant factor is the overrepresentation of Malay men among male smokers. In 1984, 46.3 percent of the Malay men were smokers, compared to 32.9 percent of the Chinese men and 31.8 percent of the Indian men. Similarly, in 1987, 36.7 percent of the Malay men smoked regularly, compared to 23.4 percent of the Chinese men and 23.8 percent of Indian men (Emmanuel, Phe, and Chen 1988, 236). This interesting difference in smoking between Malays on the one hand and Chinese and Indians on the other hand will be discussed in more detail.

In addition to the variations among the general and specific health-related activities, the three ethnic communities also vary in other aspects such as information on the etiology of disease, beliefs in personal responsibility when falling ill, level of disruption caused by the disease, per-

TABLE 4-5. Respondents' Information, Beliefs, and Attitudes about Cancer, Heart Disease, and Tuberculosis by Ethnic Group

Information, Beliefs, and Attitudes on Cancer, Heart Disease, and Tuberculosis	Ethnic Group			Total Sample
	Chinese	Malay	Indian	
(Total respondents in each group)	(977)	(167)	(126)	(1,270)
Percentage with accurate information on the causes of[1]				
Cancer	28	39	30	30
Heart Disease	60	68	76	63
Tuberculosis	52	56	69	54
Percentage agreeing that a person should be held responsible for contracting[2]				
Cancer	5	26	18	9
Heart Disease	14	26	35	18
Tuberculosis	16	32	34	20
Percentage believing that the disease causes serious disruption of normal activity[3]				
Cancer	56	23	52	52
Heart Disease	47	20	35	41
Tuberculosis	20	16	25	20
Percentage believing that they were highly susceptible to getting[4]				
Cancer	81	82	90	82
Heart Disease	71	74	78	72
Tuberculosis	36	41	44	37
Any Disease, to Fall Ill	13	40	25	18
Percentage believing strongly in the benefits of preventive action against disease[5]	47	65	68	52
Percentage with postsecondary school education[6]	9	2	9	8

Source: Quah 1980.
1. Statistically significant differences, based on Chi-Square, were found for cancer $(p = .012)$, heart disease $(p = .002)$, and tuberculosis $(p = .00001)$.
2. Cancer $(p = .00001)$; heart disease $(p = .00001)$; tuberculosis $(p = .00001)$.
3. Cancer $(p = .00001)$; heart disease $(p = .00001)$; tuberculosis $(p = .0002)$.
4. Cancer $(p = .0044)$; tuberculosis $(p = .0336)$; disease in general $(p = .00001)$.
5. $p = .00001$.
6. $p = .03$.

sonal susceptibility to illness, and benefits of preventive action. Table 4-5 presents the relevant figures.

It is not unusual to find uncertainty about the causes of diseases such as cancer among medical experts. It is therefore expected that lay people may also feel uncertain about what causes a particular disease. The level of available knowledge or information about the etiology of disease changes in the light of new medical discoveries. Among the numerous interpretations of how diseases come about, different ethnic communities have their own folk or traditional beliefs—the role of spirits, black magic used by one's enemies, bad luck, or even a breach in a rule of moral conduct (Quah 1989).

My earlier study (Quah 1980) supported the conclusion that lay people are uncertain about the causes of disease. A diversity of answers, including traditional beliefs and medical causes, were given to the questions on why a person gets cancer, heart disease, or tuberculosis. Table 4-5 presents the percentage of respondents who could mention at least one medically identified risk factor associated with cancer, heart disease, and tuberculosis. As expected, people were most uncertain about cancer, with only 30 percent of all respondents able to mention a risk factor. In contrast, 63 and 54 percent of all respondents, respectively, were acquainted with risks factors concerning heart disease and tuberculosis. Comparing the three ethnic groups, Malays were the least uncertain about the etiology of cancer, 39 percent of them knew about risk factors, in contrast to 30 percent of the Indians and 28 percent of the Chinese. Indians, however, were more informed about the causes of heart disease (76 percent) and tuberculosis (69 percent), compared to Malays (68 and 56 percent) and Chinese (60 and 52 percent).

Whether a person should be held responsible for falling ill is a moot question. In the classical Parsonian tradition, "a sick person . . . is not held morally accountable for being sick—it is not considered his 'fault'" (Fox 1989, 19).[2] The basic assumption is that every sick person is an innocent victim of his or her genetic makeup or social and physical environments. This assumption is undergoing reassessment, however, in the light of medical research findings during the past twenty years—particularly because of the current international AIDS epidemic. In both the medical and social science fields, experts are collecting irrefutable evidence that personal choices about one's daily activities and life-style are directly and indirectly linked with the onset of diseases such as cancer, heart disease, and AIDS. This has been known for decades with respect to venereal diseases.

As R. C. Fox puts it, the perception of personal responsibility concerning illness "is significantly influenced by the cognitive, belief and value systems of the society or group within which it occurs" (1989, 18). This assumption is corroborated in Table 4-5. Only a minority of all respondents were prepared to attribute responsibility to people suffering from cancer, heart disease, and tuberculosis. Still, significant differences were found across ethnic groups. Malays were more inclined (26 percent) than Indians (18 percent) to think that a person is responsible for getting cancer, and Chinese were the least likely to agree with this view (5 percent). With respect to heart disease, Indians were the most inclined (35 percent) to agree with personal responsibility, followed by Malays (26 percent). The Chinese (14 percent), again, were the most reluctant to blame the patient. The same pattern was found for tuberculosis: Indians (34 percent) and Malays (32 percent) were more likely than Chinese (16 percent) to see the sick person as responsible for contracting tuberculosis.

Interestingly, the three ethnic groups differed as well in their perception of the seriousness of each disease, as indicated by their beliefs in how disruptive of normal activity these diseases are. While all the three ethnic groups saw cancer as most disruptive and tuberculosis as least disruptive of daily life, there are significant variations among them. Malays were the most optimistic in assessing the disruption caused by cancer, heart disease, and tuberculosis. The percentage of Malays believing in serious disruption were only 23 percent, 20 percent, and 16 percent, respectively. Chinese and Indians differ only slightly from each other in their perceptions of cancer and tuberculosis: both Chinese (56 percent) and Indians (52 percent) were more inclined than the Malays (23 percent) to consider cancer as likely to cause serious disruption. Both groups see tuberculosis as less disruptive than cancer: only 25 percent of the Indians and 20 percent of the Chinese saw tuberculosis as highly disruptive of normal daily activities. The perception of the seriousness of heart disease was more varied. Chinese were the most likely (47 percent) to see heart disease as highly disruptive, compared to Indians (35 percent) and Malays (20 percent).

The perception of personal susceptibility to illness is yet another aspect related to the beliefs and value systems of each ethnic community. The data in Table 4-5 corroborates this assumption in the case of cancer, tuberculosis, and the perception of vulnerability to disease in general. But there was no statistically significant difference across ethnic groups in their belief in personal susceptibility to heart disease. Confronted with the three diseases, eight out of every ten respondents felt they were personally susceptible to cancer; seven out of every ten believed they were personally susceptible to heart disease; about four of every ten believed in their personal susceptibility to tuberculosis; and just about two out of every ten declared they felt susceptible to falling ill in general. This pattern in the respondents' perception of personal susceptibility is realistic. The actual mortality rates, as mentioned earlier, show cancer and heart disease as the two main causes of death in Singapore. In terms of ethnic differences, Indians were the most likely to feel susceptible to cancer and tuberculosis, followed by the Malays. However, Malays were significantly more inclined (40 percent) to feel susceptible to disease in general than were Indians (25 percent) and Chinese (13 percent).

One's belief in the benefits of preventive action appears to be related to the cultural values and beliefs characteristic of one's ethnic community. The main difference was found between the Indians and Malays on the one hand, who were more inclined to believe that preventive action is beneficial (68 percent and 65 percent respectively), and the Chinese on the other hand, who were less inclined (47 percent) to believe in the benefits of preventive action against disease.[3]

The final set of figures in Table 4-5 deals with formal education and presents the percentage of respondents with postsecondary education.

Following the basic premise that one of the best vehicles of modernization is formal education, it was expected that a respondent's level of formal education could act as a "buffer" with respect to ethnic beliefs and value systems on health and illness. That is, one of the original assumptions guiding this study was that people with lower levels of education would be more inclined to follow traditional values and beliefs on health without question, whereas people with higher levels of education were expected to be more discerning or critical of folk traditions. If such an assumption were correct, then ethnic differences in health behavior, attitudes, and beliefs would disappear or become negligible as people's level of education increased. This, however, was not the case. The same differences in health-related activities, information, beliefs, and attitudes between Chinese, Malays, and Indians—described in Tables 4-4 and 4-5—were found when the subjects' level of education was examined. Highly educated Chinese, Malays, and Indians differed from each other just as much as their less educated counterparts.

An overview of preventive health behavior in the three ethnic communities is provided in Table 4-6. Malays had a stronger inclination to-

TABLE 4-6. Overview of Preventive Health Behavior in the Three Ethnic Groups (in Percentages)

	Ethnic Group			
Preventive Activities Observed	Malay	Indian	Chinese	Total Sample
(Total respondents)[1]	(167)	(108)	(976)	(1,251)
GENERAL[2]				
None	10.2	30.6	31.7	28.7
Only one	44.3	44.4	44.0	44.1
Both	45.5	25.0	24.3	27.2
Total	100.0	100.0	100.0	100.0
SPECIFIC[3]				
None	1.8	8.3	8.3	7.3
Only one	12.6	25.9	26.7	24.8
Only two	50.3	52.8	50.5	50.7
All three	35.3	13.0	14.5	17.2
Total	100.0	100.0	100.0	100.0

Source: Quah 1980.
1. Twenty respondents did not answer one or more of the questions on the practice of the five preventive activities.
2. The general activities involved keeping medicines at home and taking general care of one's health. The most frequently mentioned activities were having "proper" and regular meals, "enough" rest, and trying "not to worry too much." The association between general preventive behavior and ethnicity was statistically significant, based on the Chi-Square test ($p = .00001$).
3. The specific preventive activities were regular exercise and abstention from smoking and alcohol. There was also a statistically significant association between specific preventive behavior and ethnicity, based on the Chi-Square test ($p = .00001$).

ward preventive behavior than did the Indians and Chinese. Whereas nearly one out of every two Malays reported practicing both of the general preventive activities, only one out of every four Indians and Chinese did the same. Similarly, 35 percent of the Malays practiced all three specific preventive activities, in contrast to only 13 percent of the Indians and 14.5 percent of the Chinese.

The comparison of behavior among the three ethnic groups is, essentially, a comparison of implied cultural differences. In the larger study (Quah 1980), a set of twenty-seven variables—including those in Table 4-5, which form part of the Health Belief Model (Rosenstock 1974; Becker 1974)—was tested by means of factor analysis as a possible explanation for differences in preventive behavior. But ethnic variations persisted. With the exception of gender, none of the other variables or clusters of factors explained more than 10 percent of the observed variations in behavior. Gender differences in behavior are based on ethnic traditions that dictate "appropriate" conduct for men and women (the impact of gender is discussed in more detail in Quah 1990). Exercising, lighting up a cigarette, or taking a hard drink—these are all personal and private decisions that one may or may not make at any time during a regular day. These everyday decisions tend to be influenced by the internalized patterns of conduct learned in one's ethnic community and reinforced by social pressure.

In connection with this, a relevant feature of the cultural setting of Singapore is religion. As mentioned earlier, religious affiliation is closely linked to ethnicity. The overwhelming majority (90.2 percent) of Muslims are Malay; practically all the Buddhists (98 percent) and Taoists (99.96 percent) are Chinese; and just about all the Hindus (99.7 percent) are Indian. The closest overlap between religion and ethnicity is found among Malays: 99.4 percent of the Malays are Muslim. Among the Chinese and Indians, however, one may find Muslims, Christians, and a variety of adherents to other faiths (Department of Statistics 1981; Ministry of Communications and Information 1989, 28).

The importance of religion is best illustrated by the influence of Islam upon the Malays' inclination toward preventive health behavior. The majority of Muslims (68.5 percent) reported general preventive practices against illness. A larger proportion of Muslims practiced regular exercise (53.5 percent) than did other believers, for example, Buddhists (27.9 percent) and Hindus (21.2 percent). Muslims were more inclined than Buddhists, Hindus, Christians, and agnostics to place the responsibility for getting cancer on the patient—and to see themselves as susceptible to falling ill. Thus religious beliefs may well constitute a key distinguishing feature between Malays and other ethnic groups with regard to preventive health behavior.

Among Malays, religious, cultural, and social values are closely intertwined, so that Islam is their way of life (Colson 1970; Syed Ali Husin 1981, Clammer 1981, 21). Furthermore, the cultural values associated with Islam among the Malays support traditional indigenous beliefs (possibly stronger than indigenous beliefs among the Chinese and the Indians) that connect illness with the work of "many formless spirits of disease" (Winstedt 1981, 21); bad spirits or devils "entering a person as a result of sorcery" (Syed Ali Husin 1981, 44); or as a result of actions of the person, particularly deviant or inappropriate behavior (Colson 1970, 34). The last explanation of disease harmonizes with more orthodox religious beliefs in God's punishment for wrongdoing. This blending of indigenous and orthodox religious beliefs helps to explain the characteristic preventive orientation of the Malays. Religion, together with other aspects of the Malay culture, influences preventive health actions.

There is another set of features, however, mentioned earlier, that deserves attention at this juncture. The available data from this and other studies indicate that Malay men over the past decade have consistently displayed a stronger inclination to smoke than men from other ethnic groups. At the same time, Malay smokers are more aware of their personal susceptibility to cancer and tuberculosis than nonsmokers. At least two significant questions therefore arise from these findings: (1) Why do smokers, who see themselves susceptible to disease, smoke? (2) Why is this seemingly contradictory situation found only among the Malays?

Let us take question 1 first. The Malay data clearly rebut the findings from other studies (e.g., Kegeles 1963; Suchman 1964; Becker et al. 1975) that report that people who believe they are susceptible to disease are more inclined than others to take preventive measures. Still, the problem may be in the concept of perceived susceptibility. In his review of studies on health behavior, M. K. Becker (1979, 225–60) points to a related finding that may throw some light on this matter. As explained by Becker, "For the asymptomatic individual, very low levels of perceived severity [of the disease] are not sufficiently motivating, while very high levels (including fear), are inhibiting." (1979, 260).

The Malay data suggest that the perception of personal susceptibility may act in the same manner as described by Becker in the case of perceived severity. More specifically, low levels of perceived personal susceptibility to cancer and tuberculosis may not impede Malays from smoking. A high level of perceived personal susceptibility, by contrast, may lead to a fatalistic attitude on the part of smokers, rather than triggering abstention. The smoking habit appears to provoke the perception of personal susceptibility to disease. This chain of events is not as unusual as it might seem. Indeed, the Malay smokers' situation resembles that of recidivist "ex-smokers," reported by S. V. Kasl. He indicates that recidivists not only share with successful ex-smokers a belief in the health hazards of smoking but also have a "greater sense of susceptibility to lung cancer and emphysema" than successful ex-smokers (Kasl 1974, 117).

This leads us to question 2, regarding the uniqueness of this situation to the Malays. Perhaps the most ready explanation comes from the strong tendency toward prevention, particularly general prevention and exercise, found among the Malays and explained mostly in terms of religious beliefs and practices closely intertwined in the traditional Malay way of life. Within the Malay community, the individual is expected to comply with strict religious and cultural demands guiding his or her conduct, including health-related activities. Hence the individual who smokes may undergo social pressure to stop smoking. This is particularly true in Singapore, where smoking has been publicly identified as a health hazard by the government; active public education campaigns and legislation reinforce this position. If a person defines his or her smoking habit as a personality trait that is difficult to overcome, the social pressure to comply with community antismoking standards would produce a higher level of perceived susceptibility to disease but not sufficiently strong motivation to give up smoking.

The situation of the Malay man who smokes may further be seen as a case of cognitive dissonance, which is defined by L. A. Festinger as "the existence of nonfitting relations among cognitions," that is, "among knowledge, opinion or belief about the environment, about oneself, or about one's behavior" (1957, 3). In the 1950s, Festinger was already using the example of smoking to illustrate his concept: "A person may know that smoking is bad for him and yet continue to smoke"; but the smoker would rarely accept the inconsistency between his or her behavior and beliefs and would instead make attempts to rationalize it. Such effort is due, according to Festinger, to the fact that the presence of inconsistencies or dissonance causes psychological discomfort.

However, the Malay findings do not indicate clearly that, as Festinger proposed, the existence of dissonance prompts the person "to reduce the dissonance and to avoid increases in dissonance" (1957, 31). In fact, there are reasons to believe that individuals may be desensitized to dissonance, as suggested by Morton Deutsch and R. M. Krauss (1965, 69–70). The Malay smokers who believed they were susceptible to disease may have become desensitized to cognitive dissonance by culture or personality elements yet to be identified.

The stress caused by underachievement may be yet another answer to the question of why high perceived susceptibility and smoking are features found together only among Malays, not among Chinese or Indians. In his study of the social dynamics of cigarette smoking among high-school students, I. M. Newman (1968) found that smoking was a compensatory behavior for underachievers. This finding was later supported by

E. J. Stone (1978) in her study of the effects of antismoking programs in schools. In terms of underachievement, the Singaporean Malays are, as a group, overrepresented at the lower level of the socioeconomic ladder (Saw 1981; Chiew 1991). Moreover, considering that the traditional role of economic provider for the family is primarily or exclusively assigned to men, it is understandable that the pressure to improve one's social status in this competitive society may be high for the Malays. It is revealing to note that the national figures on drug abuse—perhaps another compensatory behavior—also show an overrepresentation of Malays: although the proportion of Malays in the total population has remained around 15 percent during the past decade, the proportion of Malay heroin addicts in the total number of addicts arrested in 1983 was 32 percent, and it increased to 47 percent in 1987 (*Sunday Times*, 1988).

With respect to the third specific activity, abstention from alcohol, the case of Malays is again interesting because the picture found is rather different from that of smoking. Following the trend found in the practice of general preventive activities and exercise, Malays were again more inclined to exhibit preventive behavior than Chinese or Indians. While 35 percent of the Chinese and 36 percent of the Indians reported that they drank alcohol regularly, only 5 percent of the Malays did the same.

Why were the Malays so obviously different from the other ethnic communities in alcohol abstention? As in the case of other preventive health activities, the findings suggest the strong influence of cultural and religious values. Alcohol drinking is prohibited among orthodox Muslims. Besides Islam, other indigenous beliefs may be at work. Ali Syed Husin (1981) sees two powerful forces shaping the cultural environment of the Malays. One of these forces is a set of traditional beliefs based on animism, which was the belief system preceding the arrival of Islam to the region. Ali Syed Husin explains:

> In animism it is believed that there exist many types of supernatural powers which inhibit or protect everything surrounding man—the mountains, hills, even molehills, lakes, rivers and streams, the sea and the sky, trees, and even a worm-eaten tree trunk. Man makes all kinds of requests to these supernatural powers through persons who have expertise in supernatural affairs, and who resort to all kinds of rituals in which members of the community concerned sometimes participate. (1981, 43).

The other force is Islam. Ali Syed Husin considers that Islam influences the Malays' way of life not only religiously but also politically and socially (1981, 42). More important, as suggested earlier, Islam and traditional beliefs have found a way of coexisting. Both sets of beliefs influence the realm of health and illness. Traditional beliefs dictate that "the way to cure illness is by chasing away spirits" that caused the disease when invading the body. Islam dictates that God is the cause of everything, including health and illness.

The coexistence of these sets of beliefs rests upon the interpretation of the boundaries of traditional beliefs. There is a subordination of indigenous traditions to Islam, or, as explained by Ali Syed Husin, "The powers that the spirits and ghosts possess are limited, and whether they are effective or not, depends on the Power and Will of Allah" (1981, 46). This subordination applies as much to the cause of illness as to its cure. In contrast to smoking, which does not constitute a serious breach of Islamic guidelines of behavior, the case of alcohol abstention illustrates further a social setting where both forces, those of Islam and traditional beliefs, appear to reinforce each other, thus setting the Malays apart from the Indians and Chinese as far as their preventive health behavior is concerned.

Conclusion

The main point of this chapter has been to illustrate the influence of ethnic values and beliefs on preventive health behavior in a rapidly modernizing society. Data from personal interviews with a representative sample of Singaporeans, as well as other studies and analyses of mortality rates from 1970 to 1987, confirm persistent differences among Singaporeans of Chinese, Malay, and Indian descent concerning their preventive actions, beliefs, and attitudes with regard to cancer, heart disease, and tuberculosis. The data reveal a consistent pattern: Malays, who among the three ethnic groups are the most inclined toward preventive behavior, are not afflicted by cancer or by heart disease with the same severity as Chinese, who have the highest mortality rates for cancer, and Indians, who have the highest mortality rates for heart disease.

Two questions, one general and one specific, have guided this discussion. The general question is: What can we learn from Singapore—a modern metropolis, proud of its multiethnic population—about the links between ethnicity, health behavior, and modernization? The specific question is related to the first: Why are the Indians affected so strongly by heart disease and the Chinese by cancer, whereas the Malays are significantly less affected by these two diseases?

Concerning the first question, the Singapore case suggests that, as far as preventive health behavior is concerned, the process of modernization does not necessarily influence the steadiness of ethnic identity, particularly when ethnicity and religion overlap. The ethnic values and beliefs of the communities involved tend to be both resilient enough to secure their transmission across generations and flexible enough to adapt to changing conditions in the socioeconomic, political, and physical environments. Furthermore, some ethnic and religious values and beliefs in certain communities may actually reinforce, rather than hinder, preventive health behavior.

These findings are significant, considering the process of modernization and interaction enjoyed by Singaporeans. People from all ethnic communities interact daily at work, in school, and in the neighborhood. Constant interethnic communication is supported by many factors, including the high population density, the open labor market, the open educational system, the meritocratic system of rewards, and a conscious official effort to discourage ethnic residential enclaves while supporting ethnic cultural activities. Moreover, after passing through the common educational system, the compulsory national service scheme brings all young men together for a two-year intensive military training and communal living in military barracks. Thus, technically, modernization and economic development provide the right conditions for ethnic integration rather than differentiation, which makes Singapore a good testing ground for the ethnic differentiation assumption. Contrary to expectations, the evidence presented here suggests that the conjunction of ethnic and religious values that shape the cultural landscape of Singapore still exerts a strong influence upon what people do (or neglect to do) to prevent illness. Concerning illness prevention, the most favorable combination of ethnic and religious values and beliefs is found in the Malay community.

The second question is more challenging: Why are the Indians affected so strongly by heart disease and the Chinese by cancer? Attitudinal and behavioral information throw some light on ethnic differences in mortality rates. The Malay community is doing something right. Nevertheless, the data collected thus far do not provide satisfactory answers. The attitudinal and behavioral data point in the general direction of a looser orientation toward disease prevention among Chinese and Indians than among Malays, but this finding does not explain the differences in mortality rates between Chinese and Indians. Medical research has focused on risk factors associated with both cancer and heart disease, such as smoking, alcohol drinking, and diet. The only explicit behavioral finding from the survey was on alcohol consumption, which was higher among the Indians and the Chinese than among the Malays. Smoking, another behavioral risk factor, was found to be more common among the Malays than among Indians and Chinese.

Dietary habits were not explored in the larger study and could well be worth careful analysis. Singaporeans from all ethnic communities frequently treat themselves with dishes from one another's folk cuisines, but their daily menu is dominated by their own ethnic foods. Generally speaking, the most basic dietary differences among the three ethnic communities are: nonvegetarian Chinese are more inclined to include pork and pork-based foods in their daily meals; pork is a forbidden meat for Muslims; nonvegetarian Indians prefer mutton; and coconut milk is a very popular ingredient in Singaporean dishes, particularly in Malay cuisine. Dietary differences are more complex than this, however, and need to be studied in a systematic manner. The drawback is that medical research has produced inconclusive findings on what constitutes the optimum preventive diet and what types of food are harmful; a good illustration is the cholesterol controversy.

Stress is another risk factor for cancer and heart disease that is mentioned often but has not been analyzed systematically. Nevertheless, if a stressful life-style makes a person more susceptible to such diseases as cancer and heart disease, then it is useful to note that conventional wisdom in Singapore indicates that, compared to the Malays, the Chinese and Indians are more inclined to join in the bustle of modern life and are more attracted to competition in Singapore's dynamic socioeconomic system.

In sum, there is no conclusive explanation for differences in cancer and heart disease mortality rates between Chinese and Indians; but the differences between these two ethnic groups and the Malays tend to be clearer. It is to be hoped that this discussion will stimulate further investigation into more specific behavioral and attitudinal factors that may support preventive actions in different ethnic communities. This point differs from the position held by M. H. Becker and I. M. Rosenstock, who, in the conclusion to their review of studies on preventive health behavior, state that "attempts to target interventions to 'high-risk' subpopulations should be avoided since the population does not for the most part sort into high- and low-risk groups" (1989, 300). Although their idea may be applicable to countries considered "Western" in culture, I suggest that the same proposition may not be valid for countries with "non-Western" cultures, or where ethnic identities predominate.

There is, however, a qualification to my suggestion. There are limitations to the generalization of findings from Singapore to other nations. The active emphasis of the government on health education, the constant improvement in the standard of living, and the level of health awareness among its increasingly educated population may set Singapore's population apart from other societies, both Western and non-Western. This assumption remains to be tested empirically through comparative investigation.

NOTES

1. Although these and other studies have identified subgroups within each of the three major ethnic groups, their tendency is to revert to the classification of Chinese, Malays, and Indians as the focus of analysis. The main reason for the widespread use of

this trichotomy is the obvious difficulty involved in conducting systematic research on the relatively diffused subcommunities within each of the three main ethnic groups. Nevertheless, differences across Chinese dialect groups have been investigated in cancer research (e.g., Lun and Lee 1981, Lee and Lun 1982; Shanmugaratnam, Lee, and Day 1983; Lee 1985). In a study of lung cancer, the highest incidence was found among the Chinese, particularly in the Hokkien and Teochew dialect groups (Lee 1985).

2. The same principle is also postulated by other theoretical approaches. Indeed, several important perspectives in medical sociology tend to place the blame for illness upon societal forces that may cause negative outcomes for the individual: for example, "a loss of role capacity," according to the structural–functionalist theory; or a "breakthrough of dependency needs," according to the deviance approach; or a "stigmatizing label or role," as suggested by the interactionist framework; or, as the phenomenologists see it, a breakdown of "the trouble–trust cycles of taken-for-granted everyday life"; or, as explained by the conflict theory, "a loss of illness-buffering protective support" or the "ill-effects of pathological social structures" (Gerhardt 1989).

3. The proportion of the population accepting the benefits of preventive action against cancer, heart disease, and tuberculosis is expected to be higher today. During the past ten years, the Ministry of Health and some professional organizations have made considerable efforts in educating the public through health campaigns on the risk factors associated with cancer and heart disease (Quah 1988). These efforts have included AIDS during the past three years.

REFERENCES

Anderson, E. N., and M. L. Anderson, 1978. "Folk Dietetics in Two Chinese Communities, and Its Implications for the Study of Chinese Medicine." In *Culture and Healing in Asian Societies*, ed. Arthur Kleinman, Peter Kunstadter, E. Russell Alexander, and James L. Gale, 69–100. Cambridge, Mass.: Schenkman.
Babson, J. H. 1972. *Health Care Delivery Systems: A Multinational Survey*. London: Pitman.
Bates, E. M., and S. Linder-Pelz. 1987. *Health Care Issues*. Sydney: Allen & Unwin.
Becker, M. H. 1979. "Psychological Aspects of Health-Related Behavior." In *Handbook of Medical Sociology*, 3d ed., ed. H. E. Freeman, Sol Levine, and L. G. Reeder, 253–74. Englewood Cliffs, N.J.: Prentice-Hall.
———, ed. 1974. *The Health Belief Model and Personal Health Behavior*. Thorofare, N.J.: Charles B. Slack.
Becker, M. H., and I. M. Rosenstock. 1989. "Health Promotion, Disease Prevention, and Program Retention." In *Handbook of Medical Sociology*, 4th ed., ed. H. E. Freeman and Sol Levine, 284–305. Englewood Cliffs, N.J.: Prentice-Hall.
Becker, M. H., M. M. Kaback, I. M. Rosenstock, and M. V. Ruth. 1975. "Some Influences on Public Participation in a Genetic Screening Program." *Journal of Community Health* 1:3–14.
Cassel, John. 1977. "Social and Cultural Implications of Food and Food Habits." In *Culture, Disease and Healing Studies in Medical Anthropology*, David Landy, 236–42. New York: Macmillan.
Caudill, William. 1976. "The Cultural and Interpersonal Context of Everyday Health and Illness in Japan and America." In *Asian Medical Systems: A Comparative Study*, ed. Charles Leslie, 159–77. Berkeley: University of California Press.
Cheah, J. S., P. B. Yeo, A. C. Thai, K. F. Lui, K. W. Wang, Y. T. Tan, Y. K. Ng, and B. Y. Tan. 1985. "Epidemiology of Diabetes Mellitus in Singapore: Comparisons with Other ASEAN Countries." *Annals of the Academy of Medicine, Singapore* 13:542–47.

Chen, A. J. 1980. "Recent Trends in the Mortality and Morbidity of Cardiovascular Diseases." *Annals of the Academy of Medicine* 9:411–15.

Chiew, S. K. 1991. "Ethnic Stratification." In *Social Class in Singapore*, by S. R. Quah, S. K. Chiew, Y. C. Ko, and M. C. Lee. Singapore: Times Academic.

Chua, T. S. J., C. C. Khoo, A. T. H. Tan, and C. K. Ho. 1990. "Mortality Trends in the Coronary Care Unit." *Annals of the Academy of Medicine, Singapore* 19:3–8.

Clammer, John. 1981. "Malay Society in Singapore: A Preliminary Analysis." *Southeast Asian Journal of Social Science* 9:19–32.

Colson, A. C. 1970. "The Prevention of Illness in a Malay Village: An Analysis of Concept and Behavior." Ph.D. diss., Stanford University.

Department of Statistics. 1981. *Census of Population 1980 Singapore: Release No. 9. Religion and Fertility*. Singapore: Department of Statistics.

———. 1989. *Yearbook of Statistics Singapore 1988*. Singapore: Department of Statistics.

Deutsch, Morton, and R. M. Krauss. 1965. *Theories in Social Psychology*. New York: Basic Books.

Dunn, F. L. 1978. "Medical Care in the Chinese Communities of Peninsular Malaysia." In *Culture and Healing in Asian Societies*, 143–72. *See* Anderson and Anderson 1978.

Emmanuel, S. C. 1989. "Trends in Coronary Heart Disease Mortality in Singapore." *Singapore Medical Journal* 30:17–23.

Emmanuel, S. C., A. J. Chen, and Aylianna Phe. 1986. "Cigarette Smoking in Singapore." *Singapore Medical Journal* 29:119–24.

Emmanuel, S. C., Aylianna Phe, and A. J. Chen. 1988. "The Impact of the Anti-Smoking Campaign in Singapore." *Singapore Medical Journal* 29:233–39.

Estes, C. L., and L. E. Gerard. 1979. "Social Research in Health and Medicine: A Selected Bibliography." In *Handbook of Medical Sociology*, 3d ed., 475–503. *See* Becker 1979.

Festinger, L. A. 1957. *A Theory of Cognitive Dissonance*. Evanston, Ill.: Row Peterson.

Fox, R. C. 1989. *The Sociology of Medicine: A Participant Observer's View*. Englewood Cliffs, N.J.: Prentice-Hall.

Freeman, H. E., and Sol Levine. 1989. *Handbook of Medical Sociology*. 4th ed. *See* Becker and Rosenstock 1989.

Geertsen, Reed, M. R. Klauber, M. Rindflesh, R. L. Kane, and R. Gray. 1975. "A Re-Examination of Suchman's Views on Social Factors in Health Care Utilization." *Journal of Health and Social Behavior* 16:226–37.

Gerhardt, Uta. 1989. *Ideas about Illness: An Intellectual and Political History of Medical Sociology*. London: Macmillan.

Glucksberg, Harold, and J. W. Singer. 1982. *Cancer Care*. New York: Charles Scribner.

Goh, K. T. 1980. "Hepatitis B Surveillance in Singapore." *Annals of the Academy of Medicine, Singapore* 9:136–41.

Good, Byron. 1986. "Explanatory Models and Care-Seeking: A Critical Account." In *Illness Behavior: A Multidisciplinary Model*, ed. Sean McHugh and T. M. Vallis, 161–72. New York: Plenum.

Graham, Saxon. 1956. "Ethnic Background and Illness in a Pennsylvania County." *Social Problems* 4:76–82.

Graham, Saxon, and L. C. Reeder. 1972. "Social Factors in the Chronic Illnesses." In *Handbook of Medical Sociology*, 3d ed., 63–107. *See* Becker 1979.

Gwee, A. L., Lee Y. K. Lee, and N. B. Tham, 1969. "A Study of Chinese Medical Practice in Singapore." *Singapore Medical Journal* 10:2–7.

Hassan, Riaz. 1976. *Singapore: Society in Transition*. Oxford and Kuala Lumpur: Oxford University Press.

———. 1977. *Families in Flats*. Singapore: Singapore University Press.

Horowitz, D. L. 1975. "Ethnic Identity." In *Ethnicity, Theory and Experience*, ed. Nathan Glazer and D. P. Moynihan, 111–40. Cambridge: Harvard University Press.

Hughes, Kenneth, P. P. B. Yeo, K. C. Lun, S. P. Sothy, A. C. Thai, K. W. Wang, and J. S. Cheah. 1984. "Risk Factors for Ischaemic Heart Disease in the Ethnic Groups of Singapore." *Proceedings of the International Epidemiological Association 10th Scientific Meeting*. Helsinki: IEP.

———. 1989. "Ischaemic Heart Disease and Its Risk Factors in Singapore in Comparison with Other Countries." *Annals of the Academy of Medicine, Singapore* 18:245–49.

———. 1987. "Cardiovascular Diseases in the Ethnic Groups of Singapore." *Proceedings of the International Epidemiologic Association 11th Scientific Meeting*. Helsinki: IEP.

Husin Ali Syed. 1981. *Malay Peasant Society and Leadership*. Oxford and Kuala Lumpur: Oxford University Press.

Kang, J. Y., S. J. LaBrooy, Ivy Yap, Richard Giuan, K. P. Lim, M. V. Math, and H. H. Tay. 1986. "Racial Differences in Peptic Ulcer Frequency in Singapore." *Digestive Diseases and Sciences* 13:825–28.

Kaplan, H. B. 1989. "Health, Disease, and the Social Structure." In *Handbook of Medical Sociology*, 4th ed., 46–68. See Becker and Rosenstock 1989.

Kasl, S. V. 1974. "The Health Belief Model and Behavior Related to Chronic Illness." In *The Health Belief Model and Personal Health Behavior*, 106–27. See M. H. Becker, ed. 1974.

Kasl, S. V., and Sidney Cobb. 1966. "Health Behavior, Illness Behavior and Sick-Role Behavior." *Archives of Environmental Health* 12:246–66; 12:531–41.

Kegeles, S. S. 1963. "Why People Seek Dental Care: A Test of a Conceptual Formulation." *Journal of Health and Human Behavior* 4:166–73.

Kessler, R. C., and C. B. Wortman, 1989. "Social and Psychological Factors in Health and Illness." In *Handbook of Medical Sociology*, 4th ed., 69–86. See Becker and Rosenstock 1989.

Khare, R. S. 1977. "Ritual Purity and Pollution in Relation to Domestic Sanitation." In *Culture, Disease and Healing*, 242–50. See Cassel 1977.

King, S. H. 1962. *Perception of Illness and Medical Practice*. New York: Russell Sage Foundation.

Kleinman, Arthur. 1980. *Patients and Healers in the Context of Culture*. Berkeley: University of California Press.

Kosa, John, and I. K. Zola. 1975. *Poverty and Health: A Sociological Analysis*. Rev. ed. Cambridge: Harvard University Press.

Landy, David, ed. 1977. *Culture, Disease and Healing*. See Cassel 1977.

Lee, H. P. 1985. "The Epidemiology of Lung Cancer in Singapore." *Annals of the Academy of Medicine, Singapore* 14:485–90.

———. 1989. "Patterns of Smoking among Singaporeans." *Annals of the Academy of Medicine, Singapore* 18:286–88.

Lee, H. P., and K. C. Lun. 1982. "Standardised Mortality Ratios for Some Cancer Sites among the Main Ethnic and Chinese Dialect Groups in Singapore, 1970." *Singapore Medical Journal* 23:85–89.

Lee, H. P., James Lee, and K. Shanmugaratnam. 1987. "Trends and Ethnic Variation in Incidence and Mortality from Cancers of the Colon and Rectum in Singapore, 1968 to 1982." *Annals of the Academy of Medicine, Singapore* 16:397–401.

Leslie, Charles, ed. 1976. *Asian Medical Systems*. See Caudill 1976.

Lun, K. C., and H. P. Lee, 1981. "Standardised Mortality Ratios for Some Selected Causes among Main Ethnic and Chinese Dialect Groups in Singapore, 1970." *Singapore Medical Journal* 22:144–49.

Lynch, L. R. 1969. *The Cross-Cultural Approach to Health Behavior*. Cranbury, N.J.: Fairleigh Dickinson University Press.

Manfredi, C., R. B. Warnecke, Saxon Graham, and S. Rosenthal. 1977. "Social Psychological Correlates of Health Behavior: Knowledge of Breast Self-Examination Techniques among Black Women." *Social Science and Medicine* 11:433–40.

McHugh, Sean, and T. M. Vallis, eds. 1986. *Illness Behavior. See* Good 1976.

Mead, Margaret. 1956. "Understanding Cultural Patterns." *Nursing Outlook* 4:260–62.

Mechanic, David. 1978. *Medical Sociology*. 2d Ed. New York: Free Press.

Ministry of Communications and Information. 1989. *Singapore 1989*. Singapore: Information Division, Ministry of Communications and Information.

———. 1990. *Singapore Facts and Pictures 1990*. Singapore: Information Division, Ministry of Communications and Information.

Ministry of Health (MOH). 1980. *Annual Report 1979*. Singapore: MOH.

———. 1989. *Annual Report 1988*. Singapore: MOH.

———. 1990. Figures provided by S. C. Emmanuel, Director, Research and Evaluation Department, 19 February. Singapore: MOH.

Newman, I. M. 1968. "The Social Dynamics of Cigarette Smoking in a Junior High School." Ph.D. diss., University of Illinois.

Oh, Winston. 1975. *Give Your Heart a Chance*. Singapore: Federal Publications.

Ooi, J. B., and H. D. Chiang. 1969. *Modern Singapore*. Singapore: SUP.

Organization for Economic Cooperation and Development. (OECD). 1987. *Financing and Delivering Health Care: A Comparative Analysis of OECD Countries*. Paris: OECD.

Owen, N. G., ed. 1987. *Death and Disease in Southeast Asia: Explorations in Social, Medical and Demographic History*. Oxford and Singapore: Oxford University Press.

Paul, Benjamin D., ed. 1955. *Health, Culture and Community*. New York: Russell Sage Foundation.

———. 1963. "Anthropological Perspectives on Medicine and Public Health." *Annals of the American Academy of Political and Social Science* 346:34–43.

———. 1977. "The Role of Beliefs and Customs in Sanitation Programs." Reprinted from *American Journal of Public Health* 48:1502–6. In *Culture, Disease and Healing*, 233–36. *See* Cassel 1977.

Polgar, Steven. 1963. "Health Action in Cross-cultural Perspective." In *Handbook of Medical Sociology*, 1st ed., ed. H. E. Freeman, Sol Levine, and L. G. Reeder. Englewood Cliffs, N.J.: Prentice-Hall.

Quah, S. R. 1975. *Utilization of Health Services and Self-Medication in Singapore*. Research report. Singapore: Department of Social Medicine and Public Health.

———. 1980. "Preventive Health Behaviour in Singapore." Ph.D. diss., University of Singapore.

———. 1983. "Social Discipline in Singapore: An Alternative to the Resolution of Social Problems." *Journal of Southeast Asian Studies* 14:266–89.

———. 1984. *Balancing Autonomy and Control: The Case of Professionals in Singapore*. Cambridge, Mass.: Center for International Studies, Massachusetts Institute of Technology.

———. 1988. "Private Choices and Public Health: A Case of Policy Intervention in Singapore." *Asian Journal of Public Administration* 10:207–24.

———. 1990. "Gender Roles, Family Roles, and Health Behavior." *Southeast Asian Journal of Social Science* 18:51–64.

———, ed. 1989. *The Triumph of Practicality: Tradition and Modernity in Health Care Utilization in Selected Asian Countries*. Singapore: Institute of Southeast Asian Studies.

Randeria, J. D. 1981. "Dietary Modulation in Cancer Prevention with Reference to Social and Cultural Food Habits." *Cancer Detection and Prevention* 4:141–48.

Registrar-General of Births and Deaths. 1981. *Report on Registration of Births and Deaths 1980.* Singapore: Registry of Births and Deaths.

——. 1988. *Report on Registration of Births and Deaths 1987.* Singapore: Registry of Births and Deaths.

Robertson, L. S., and M. C. Heagarty. 1975. *Medical Sociology: A General Systems Approach.* New York: Nelson Hall.

Rosenstock, I. M. 1974. "Historical Origins of the Health Belief Model." In *The Health Belief Model and Personal Health Behavior,* 1–8. *See* M. H. Becker, ed., 1974.

——. 1974. "The Health Belief Model and Preventive Health Behavior." In *The Health Belief Model and Personal Health Behavior,* 27–59. *See* M. H. Becker, ed., 1974.

Sanborn, K. O., and M. M. Katz, 1977. "Perception of Symptom Behavior across Ethnic Groups." In *Basic Problems in Cross-Cultural Psychology,* ed. Y. H. Poortinga, 236–40. Amsterdam: International Association for Cross-Cultural Psychology.

Saunders, Lyle. 1954. *Cultural Differences and Medical Care.* New York: Russell Sage Foundation.

Saw, S. H. 1981. *Demographic Trends in Singapore.* Census Monograph no. 1. Singapore: Department of Statistics.

Shanmugaratnam, K., H. P. Lee, and N. E. Day. 1983. *Cancer Incidence in Singapore, 1968–1977.* Lyon: International Agency for Research on Cancer.

Simons, L., P. Whish, B. Marr, A. Jones, and J. Simons. 1981. "Coronary Risk Factors in a Rural Community Which Includes Aborigines: Inverell Heart Disease Prevention Programme." *Australia–New Zealand Journal of Medicine* 11:386–90.

Southeast Asian Medical Information Center (SEAMIC). 1987. *SEAMIC Health Statistics 1987.* Tokyo: International Medical Foundation of Japan.

Stone, E. J. 1978. "The Effects of a Fifth Grade Health Education Curriculum Model on Perceived Vulnerability and Smoking Attitudes." *Journal of School Health* 667–71.

Suchman, E. A. 1964. "Socio-Medical Variations among Ethnic Groups." *American Journal of Sociology* 70:319–31.

——. 1965. "Social Patterns of Illness and Medical Care." *Journal of Health and Human Behavior* 6:2–16.

Sunday Times. 1988. "Alarming Rise in Malay Heroin Addicts." (February 21):1.

Whelan, Elizabeth. 1977. *Preventing Cancer.* New York: W. W. Norton.

Winstedt, R. O. 1981. *The Malays: A Cultural History.* Rev. ed. Singapore: G. Brash.

Yamamoto, J., and A. Steinberg. 1981. "Ethnic, Racial and Social Class Factors in Mental Health." *Journal of the National Medical Association* 73:231–40.

Zborowski, Mark. 1952. "Cultural Components in Response to Pain." *Journal of Social Issues* 8:16–30.

Zola, I. K. 1966. "Culture and Symptoms: An Analysis of Patients' Presenting Complaints." *American Sociological Review* 31:615–30.

Part III

Traditional

and

Modern

Medicines

Chapter 5

The Contribution of Modern

Medicine in a Traditional System:

The Case of Nepal

JANARDAN SUBEDI *and*
SREE SUBEDI

Modern medicine, or Western medicine, as it is known throughout the world, is closely identified historically with the germ theory of disease. This theory assumes that specific germs cause specific diseases in the human body, and that the cure for these diseases depends upon the efficacy of drugs or medicines to kill the germs. However, the drug must not seriously affect or impair the functioning of the normal physical system. Basically, a complex technological approach characterizes modern medicine. It is also heavily oriented toward control or cure of illnesses, rather than toward their prevention (Feagin 1989).

In most of the developing countries, modern health care systems are relatively recent phenomena. They are still in the early stages of elaboration, where the organization of the delivery system can be significantly determined by public policy (Berman 1985). Further, in most of these countries indigenous forms of health care exist and are widely used by the population. By and large, these indigenous systems do not utilize the germ theory to explain illness or develop treatment.

Various classification schemes have been used to explain the complexities of health care delivery. According to W. M. Gesler (1984), the simplest and most common scheme separates traditional or indigenous medicine from modern medicine. Arthur Kleinman (1980) distinguished between three social and health sectors within which people experience and seek health care. The first is the "popular" sector, which is the lay, nonprofessional, nonspecialist cultural arena involving family, social networks, and the community. The "folk" sector is composed of nonprofessional, nonbureaucratic "specialists," both natural and supernatural (i.e., not lay), who have developed a prescientific body of beliefs and practices. Finally, there is the "professional" sector, which comprises trained, professional, indigenous and modern health care practitioners.

F. L. Dunn's (1976) classification scheme described three types of health care services or systems. He distinguished between the "local" system, consisting of primitive, folk practitioners and health care services, and the "regional" system, involving codified, traditional health care services—for example, Ayurvedic, Unani, and Chinese medicines—delivered by trained professionals in the area. The third type of health care system referred clearly to the professional, bureaucratic, modern or "worldwide" system of health care service.

For the purpose of this paper, the use of Dunn's scheme is appropriate because it distinguishes not only between the indigenous and modern health care systems but also between nonprofessional and professional indigenous health care services. Therefore this chapter discusses the two types of indigenous services as folk (primitive, nonprofessional) and traditional (trained, professional) health care systems, while the modern health care system refers to trained, specialized, Western medicine.

Basically, this chapter attempts to assess the contribution of modern medicine in Nepal, a developing country where not only is the introduction of modern medicine fairly recent but where both folk and traditional forms of health care services are still commonly used.

The Case of Nepal: The Health Status of the Population

Due to the absence of reliable and comprehensive information, it is impossible to make an accurate assessment of the health status of the population of Nepal. By any standard, however, the health situation is extremely poor. Infectious disease and nutritional deficiency are widespread, and mortality rates, especially the infant mortality rate, are extremely high (UNFPA 1979). In Nepal, ill health in childhood, especially for children under the age of five years, ranks as the country's major health problem. The main causes of infant and child deaths are diarrhea, nutritional deficiencies, pneumonia, respiratory infections, malaria, measles, diphtheria, tetanus, tuberculosis, and accidents (Justice 1981). Table 5-1 provides a comparison between Nepal and other developing countries (and the United States) on certain key health status indicators.

As can be seen, the infant mortality rate in Nepal at present stands at 133.3 per 1,000 live births, which is higher than in neighboring developing countries. Similarly, general life expectancy is lower in Nepal than

TABLE 5-1. Some Indicators of Health in Nepal and Neighboring Developing
Countries

	Nepal	India	Bangladesh	Pakistan	Sri Lanka	U.S.A.
Public Expenditures per Capita (U.S.$)[1]	1	2	.05	1	6	439
Population per Physician[1]	30,780	2,910	9,780	3,630	7,220	550
Population per Hospital Bed[1]	5,865	1,312	4,602	1,844	343	171
Infant Mortality Rate (per 1,000)[2]	133.3	83.9	118.1	110	26.8	13.7
Crude Death Rate (per 1000)[2]	17.4	11.3	15.3	14.2	5.8	9.1
Life Expectancy (Years)[2]	47.7	57.1	50.5	51.9	70.6	75.1

1. 1980 figures. *Source:* Susser, Watson, and Hopper 1985.
2. 1985–90 figures. *Source:* My T. Vu. 1984. *World Population Projections 1984.*
Washington, D.C.: World Bank.

in the other countries. From every indicator, it is apparent that Nepal
has substantially poorer health status than even neighboring developing
countries.

The causes of Nepal's health problems can be divided into four major
categories: overpopulation, malnutrition, environmental factors, and infectious diseases (World Bank 1979). When the major causes of death
among developing and industrialized countries are compared, in Nepal
and several developing countries the major cause of mortality is the prevalence of infectious diseases, whereas in the United States and other af-
fluent countries the major causes of death are chronic diseases (Susser,
Watson, and Hopper 1985; Polednak 1989).

The Health Care Delivery System

As mentioned earlier, the health care system in Nepal is pluralistic (i.e.,
there are a number of competing systems related to health care, each of
which is distinctive by its set of ideas, practices, methods, and treatment
material). Details on the different health services in the system follow.

Folk Medicine

This medicine is practiced by witch doctors, religious healers, or
curers, who attribute particular diseases to either natural or supernatural
causes. For example, sources of illness are often attributed to the existence of spirit possession caused by disease goddesses, bad or impure
blood, or imbalances in the body due to extra consumption of "hot" or

"cold" foods (Beals 1976). According to Peter Streefland (1985), faith healing seems to be strongly rooted in the minds of most Nepali people. In its
organization, the folk-medicine enterprise is decentralized—each practitioner works in his or her own village or group of villages, with no cod-
ification of knowledge and no professional organization of healers.

Traditional Medicine

According to Carl E. Taylor (1976), in almost all countries there are
traditional methods of health care that have evolved within the local cultures, and in some instances these are linked with religious beliefs. In
Nepal this form of health care consists mainly of homeopathic, ayurvedic, and the unani systems of medicine, which are practiced all over
the country by various traditional practitioners and represent a vast human resource outside the government-sponsored health services.

HOMEOPATHIC MEDICINE. This form of medicine was discovered in
the nineteenth century by a German physician named Samuel Hahnemann. Building on the balance-based theories of Hippocrates and Aris-
totle, Hahnemann focused on the concept of "similars," but with a new
twist. The fundamental notion is that "like cures like" (Wolinsky 1988,
225). Hence homeopathy is based on the concept of creating resistance to
an illness by giving small doses of medicine that, in large doses, produces
symptoms similar to those of the treated illness (Leslie 1976, 1980).

AYURVEDIC MEDICINE. The science of medicine known as *ayurveda*
gives a clear idea of classical Indian medicine: "the science of (living to a
ripe) age" (Basham 1976). Its root meaning derives from two Sanskrit
words, *ayuh* (life or longevity) and *veda* (sacred knowledge or science).
Basically, it evaluates medical phenomena in terms of three humors:
wind, bile, and phlegm, of which everything in the universe is composed
and whose perfect balance constitutes health (Durkin-Longley 1982).

UNANI MEDICINE. The Muslim form of traditional medicine known
as unani medicine is classical Greek medicine, as modified by Arab
scholars. It is widely practiced in the Muslim-dominant areas by Muslim
Hakims (*Hakim* is an Arabic word meaning a person who practices unani
medicine). It is based on various aspects of humoral pathology and is
influenced by the religious and philosophical components of Islam (Foster and Anderson 1978; Lindsey 1983; Joseph, Desrochers, and Kalathil
1983).

Modern Medicine

Modern medicine, or allopathic medicine, as it is referred to throughout South Asia, was introduced in Nepal by Christian missionaries who
built the first hospitals and clinics and by Nepali medical practitioners
trained abroad (Justice 1981). In 1972, however, a major landmark in
modern health care in Nepal was the establishment of the Institute of

Medicine under Tribhuvan University. Thus, since the 1980s Nepal has begun to produce a few physicians trained in the country itself.

At present, the modern health care delivery system is composed of government and semigovernment (missionary) hospitals, health centers, and private clinics; and services are provided by a number of physicians, trained abroad or in Nepal; health assistants; nurses; and mostly middle-level workers and paraprofessionals, who help to serve the rural areas and supplement the severe inadequacy of trained professionals.

Growth of Modern Medicine

Unlike other South Asian countries such as India, Bangladesh, and Pakistan, Nepal was never colonized. Until 1951, it remained closed under the Rana regime to most outsiders. Due to this isolation, all attempts at modernization are relatively recent. A foreign health care system had never been imposed upon Nepal by a colonial power. Hence the concept of the modern health care system is relatively new (Justice 1981).

In 1951, Nepal had only a few mission and government hospitals located mainly in the Kathmandu Valley. At that time, the country had only twelve physicians trained in modern medicine and some compounders who gave medications, dressers, injections, and dressed wounds (USAID 1975).

In 1956, planned development of Nepali health services was initiated with His Majesty's Government (HMG) First Five Year Plan (1956–1961). At this time, Nepal had thirty-four hospitals with 625 beds, and twenty-four dispensaries. By mid-1977, the health service consisted of forty-seven government and fifteen other hospitals with 2,174 beds, 233 health centers, and 433 health posts. By 1983, the figure had risen to seventy-five hospitals with 2,993 beds, 277 health centers, and 744 health posts. Similarly, the total number of physicians participating in government and nongovernmental setting had increased to 645 (Nepal Janch Bujh Kendra 1976; UNICEF 1978; *Statistical Pocket Book*, 1984).

In Nepal, the growth and the development of modern medicine has been carefully planned and initiated. Besides being the officially sponsored medical system, it enjoys access to valuable resources and aid from the government and multiple foreign agencies. Hence, in spite of its being such a recent phenomenon in Nepal's pluralistic system of health care delivery, modern medicine has clearly come to be identified as the dominant medical system.

The Strength of Modern Medicine

As noted, modern medicine was introduced into the Nepali traditional system with the full support of the government and various international agencies.

TABLE 5-2. Some Indicators of Health of Nepal

Year or Period	CDR[3]	LE(M)[4]	LE(F)[5]	IMR[6]
1952–54[1]	37	27.1	28.5	—
1961[1]	27	35.4	37.4	—
1960–64[1]	—	—	—	182
1965–69[1]	—	—	—	168
1971[1]	21	37.0	39.9	—
1970–74[1]	—	—	—	156
1974–76[1]	21	44.7	41.8	—
1980–85[2]	18.6	46.6	45.1	144.6
1985–90[2]	17.4	48.3	47.3	133.3
1990–95[2]	15.8	49.9	49.5	123.3
1995–2000[2]	14.3	51.4	51.9	111.8

1. *Source:* Banister, Judith, and Shyam Thapa. 1981. *The Population Dynamics of Nepal.* Papers of the East-West Population Institute no. 78. Honolulu: East-West Population Institute.
2. *Source:* My T. Vu. 1984. *World Population Projections 1984.* Washington, D.C.: World Bank.
3. CDR = Crude Death Rate (per 1,000 persons)
4. LE(M) = Life Expectancy, Male (years)
5. LE(F) = Life Expectancy, Female (years)
6. IMR = Infant Mortality Rate (per 1,000)

Within the short period of time since its institution, there has been a drastic reduction in mortality rates and infectious diseases (World Bank 1979). Although this may be in part due to societal development (e.g., rising standard of living, better nutrition), it is clear that public health (e.g., sanitation, disease control) has made a significant contribution, and therefore much of the health improvement is attributed to modern medicine.

As can be seen in Table 5-2, the infant mortality rate has been reduced from 182 per 1,000 infants during the early 1960s to about 123 per 1,000 at present, and the crude death rate has been reduced from 37 per 1,000 persons in the early 1950s to 15.8 per 1,000 today. Similarly, the average life expectancy has improved from twenty-seven to twenty-nine years in the 1950s to almost fifty-two years in the early 1990s. Further, the widespread availability of modern drugs and immunizations has helped to strengthen many people's confidence and to improve attitudes toward the modern care system.

For most people with little or no understanding of diseases, a quick and effective cure is appealing. The strength of the modern medicine lies in that it can offer not only this quick and effective relief for certain specific categories—for example, cold, cough, diarrhea, and several respiratory and infectious diseases—but also scientific and logical explanations for each disease etiology and treatment, unlike folk or traditional medicine, which depends on culturally specific explanations.

According to Richard Burghart (1984), when people distinguish between modern and traditional medicine, they may understand the distinction differently from the medical scientist. Due to the fast and effective treatment offered by modern medicine for many acute illnesses,
many people have been convinced of the efficacy of modern medicine.
The connection between illness and treatment, however, is seen not only
in terms of efficacy but also in terms of appropriateness. Modern medicine works fast and is therefore appropriate for "fast" (acute) illnesses,
whereas traditional medicine works slowly and hence is particularly appropriate for "slow" (chronic) illnesses. Thus Surinder Bhardwaj (1975)
and H. K. Heggenhougen (1980) found that modern medicine was sought
for quick cures of "acute" illnesses, whereas slower, "chronic" problems
were taken to practitioners of traditional medicine for treatment.

The Weakness of Modern Medicine

In Nepal, however, modern medicine has not been able to achieve
universal acceptance and remains underutilized for several reasons. The
most important reason is that, to the vast majority of the people, modern
medicine is alien and foreign. They tend to accept and identify more with
the folk or traditional types of medicine because these forms of medicine
seem closer to them culturally and appeal to them emotionally. The folk
and traditional forms are also less expensive.

Modern health services in Nepal were expanded primarily through
the influence of international health assistance. The process was begun
in the 1950s when a number of Christian missions and Western charita-
ble foundations came to render service. Western drug companies also assisted. The primary contributors to public health and medical programs
during the early years were the U.S.A., India, the USSR, China, and the
World Health Organization. During the past twenty-five years, the number of donors has multiplied many times (Justice 1981). In spite of growth
in donations, however, the overall health situation in Nepal remains precarious.

Until recently, all doctors practicing modern medicine were trained
abroad, and only a handful of them were employed in public institutions.
Most preferred to live in Kathmandu, where basic amenities and comforts
were available. In contrast, most of the paramedical workers (i.e., nurses,
assistants, technicians) worked in rural areas, district hospitals, and various health-related projects. Even when functioning optimally, however,
the health posts and hospitals in rural areas, where over 93 percent of the
population resides, serve only 20 percent of the population (Durkin-Longley 1982).

Over 50 percent of the country's hospital beds are located in Kathmandu. The majority of hospitals are small, fifteen-bed units that are

relatively expensive to equip and staff and unable to provide comprehensive hospital services. Even where rural district hospitals, health centers, and health posts exist, they are generally understaffed and undersupplied. Often they are vacant.

Hence, despite the fact that modern medicine has had a direct impact on morbidity and particularly infant mortality in Nepal, the inadequacy of finances, facilities, and personnel constitutes a major problem for the modern health care delivery system.

Yet another extremely significant reason for the underutilization and lack of total acceptance of modern medicine is the incomplete differentiation of health care systems in Nepal, resulting in institutional pluralism.

According to the differentiation theory, the most significant feature of modern social change is the replacement of multifunctional structures by more specialized institutions and roles. For example, in simple societies, the family or kinship group is the one major social institution responsible for educational, economic, religious, political, legal, and a variety of other functions. As societies grow larger and more complex, progressive differentiation and specialization occur and functions are transferred from the family to more specialized, outside institutions. A major assumption of the theory, however, is a one-dimensional idea of complete differentiation, that is, of a society in which fully legitimate, multifunctional traditional structures have been replaced by fully legitimate modern institutions responsible for a number of limited, specialized functions (Colomy 1986, 1990). Furthermore, it is assumed that the specialized institutions are indicative of the society's dominant values (Smelser 1959).

Regarding medical evolution, Renee Fox (1976) points out that modern society is marked by the relative differentiation of medicine from the kinship or family system. The primary agents who define, certify, and treat illness in modern societies are technically specialized medical professionals who belong to one institution—the modern scientific medical institution.

In the case of Nepal, however, this is not so. The health care system or the medical institution is structurally pluralistic, that is, there are three legitimate medical systems providing essentially similar health care services. In other words, there are no boundaries between the different types of health care system, specifying when or for what problems a particular kind of service may be sought. Hence it is a society where differentiation is finished but "incomplete" (Surace 1992), because health care service is not provided by one major medical institution but shared by three overlapping, conflicting, and sometimes competing institutions—the folk, traditional, and modern medical systems. The result is a pluralistic institutional configuration (Subedi 1989a; Subedi and Subedi 1990).

Further, full legitimation of modern medicine in Nepal is problematic because it is an exogenous and culturally foreign institution, premised on a significantly different cultural belief system. Hence it is not based upon or legitimated by the dominant values of the society and faces competition for "cultural authority" (Starr 1982, 13).

Thus modern medicine has to compete with folk and traditional medicines to create conditions wherein people can identify, trust, and feel satisfied with it, so that in spite of the presence of folk and traditional medical systems providing basically similar health care functions, people will seek modern health care services. As long as people are free to decide which type of health care service appeals and seems beneficial to them, the probability of turning to either folk or traditional health care remains high.

A number of studies in Nepal have suggested that individuals use the folk, traditional, and modern health care systems exclusively, simultaneously, or alternatively (Durkin-Longley 1982), based on their perceptions and beliefs regarding the illness problem.

According to Streefland (1985) and M. S. Durkin-Longley (1982), in Nepali society traditional bias and superstition play a dominant role. Hence folk healers are widely used, especially in rural areas (Achard 1983). Similarly, *Midterm Health Review 2035* (Ministry of Health 1979) finds traditional healers to be the most frequent providers of health care. According to Shah, Shrestha, and Parker (1978), over three-fourths of all illnesses in Nepal are treated by the traditional health care system.

Studies (e.g., Justice 1981; Subedi 1986b) have also reported that individuals generally favor and turn to indigenous health care services or systems before seeking modern medicine. The typical progression for an illness problem begins with the use of traditional home remedies and is followed by seeking traditional health care services if the illness persisted. Modern health care services were for the most part sought only as a last resort.

Therefore, in a study conducted by Tribhuvan University's Institute of Medicine in 1978, the researchers concluded that modern medical practitioners face fairly strong competition from indigenous practitioners when it comes to utilization of services.

The Contribution of Modern Medicine

In spite of these shortcomings, modern medicine has made a tremendous contribution in the context of Nepal. According to G. G. Grenholm (1983), the modern medical approach has little concern for the relationship of physical and social environments to health care. But in spite of this criticism, it may be noted that in Nepal, where the modern health care delivery system has been developed through international aid and assistance, modern health services are integrated with public health development measures. Up to 1975, public health care in Nepal was largely delivered through five separate projects: the Family Planning and Maternal and Child Health Care Project, the Malaria Eradication Project, the Tuberculosis Project, the Leprosy Control Project, and the Expanded Program of Immunization. In 1975 these five projects were integrated to improve their implementation and cover the entire population (UNFPA 1979; World Bank 1979). Thus the aim of modern medicine in Nepal has been not only to treat and cure diseases but to prevent the various factors that cause them. This has helped to reduce the morbidity and mortality rates substantially.

Moreover, because modern medicine means big business for several industries—for example, drug manufacturers and pharmacies—huge sums of money have been invested by these agencies to advertise modern medicines through the mass media and thereby popularize it. All this has contributed to developing and increasing people's knowledge and understanding of health problems and of the availability of different types of drugs associated with various types of problems, without individuals having to spend time or money in appointments or consultations with medical practitioners. Thus today in Nepal, for many of the common health problems nonprescription medicines such as aspirin, Alka-Seltzer, cough syrups, eyedrops, nasal drops, and various lotions and ointments have become a part of the regular home treatment used by the people.

Also due to the influence of modern medicine, there appears to be a growing awareness among people regarding proper nutrition, hygiene, sanitation, and environmental conditions. For example, even in rural areas uneducated persons have been heard to discuss how important "protein" and "vitamins" were for strength and health, although they did not have any knowledge or understanding about the nature of these essential elements or about which food items supplied them.

According to W. M. Gesler (1984), the modern medical system is usually received favorably where it does exist. It is criticized, however, for not being emotionally gratifying and for its inability to cater to the majority of the people. In recent years, critics of modern medicine have extolled traditional medicine because of its social and cultural relevance.

In spite of this, modern medicine remains the predominant government-sponsored and promoted health care service, and goals are to increase its availability throughout the population. This has led to a realization among traditional practitioners that, if they are to continue successfully, they have to compete with the modern health care system on equal terms. That is, if they do not enhance or modernize their treatment approach to keep pace with the changing expectations of the clients, they may be viewed negatively. For example, Wen-Hui Tsai (1988) found that in Taiwan, modernization has led to the labeling of traditional

Chinese medicine as "backward" in comparison to modern medicine, resulting in rejection of it by many people. Therefore in Nepal, following the example of the practitioners of modern medicine, the practitioners of traditional medicine have modified their treatment to the rising expectations of their patients who are adapting to the modern world. They have also formed a number of associations and have created drug manufacturing concerns along modern lines (e.g., Dabur, Baidhnath, and Charak are three leading multinational ayurvedic pharmaceuticals, whose products are widely available and used throughout South Asian countries), as well as advertising through the mass media. At present, not only are a variety of traditional lotions, ointments, and medicines for a number of health problems and health maintenance available over the counter, but these are constantly being commercially advertised and thereby made familiar. Thus traditional practitioners have directed attention to the availability and efficacy of traditional drugs for specific health problems, so that people do not have to rely on modern medicine alone. Hence the people now have access to more information and can shop around for the health care source that they consider most suitable.

Concluding Remarks

Although the availability of different types of health care services provides people with more options, it is becoming apparent that both the modern and the indigenous, traditional health care systems have certain strengths and weaknesses, advantages and disadvantages, within a pluralistic health care context. Therefore many suggestions have been made in recent years to find ways and means of integrating aspects of the traditional health care into the modern health care system, thereby addressing many of the drawbacks (e.g., cultural, labor, and identification issues) faced by modern medicine. This problem requires serious and careful consideration by policymakers, planners, and the health administrators. Integrated with the indigenous forms of health care and public health development measures, modern medicine could make a significant contribution to the health status of the people. The example of China has shown this. Ben Zeichner (1988) found that in China traditional psychiatric approaches have been effectively combined with modern psychiatric treatment to enhance acceptance and cost-effectiveness.

In Nepal the government is actively promoting the ayurvedic system of medicine by establishing clinics and firms manufacturing ayurvedic medicine. It has also established a modern drug manufacturing establishment. Even though the two systems are yet to be integrated, both systems are developing simultaneously.

REFERENCES

Achard, Thomas. 1983. *Primary Health Care in the Hills of Nepal.* Kathmandu: HMG/
Swiss Association for Technical Assistance (SATA), Development Project (IHDP).
Basham, A. L. 1976. "The Practice of Modern Medicine in Ancient and Medieval In-
dia." In *Asian Medical Systems: A Comparative Study,* ed. Charles Leslie, 18–43.
Berkeley: University of California Press.
Beals, A. R. 1976. "Strategies of Resort to Curers in South India." In *Asian Medical
Systems,* 184–200. *See* Basham 1976.
Berman, Peter. 1985. *Equity and Cost in the Organization of Primary Health Care in
Java, Indonesia.* Ithaca, N.Y.: Cornell University Press.
Bhardwaj, Surinder M. 1975. "Attitudes toward Different Systems of Medicine: A Sur-
vey of Four Villages in the Punjab—India." *Social Science and Medicine* 9:603–
12.
Burghart, Richard. 1984. "The Tisiyahi Klinik: A Nepalese Medical Center in an Intra-
cultural Field of Relations." *Social Science and Medicine* 18(17):589–98.
Colomy, Paul B. 1986. "Recent Developments in the Functionalist Approach to
Change." *Sociological Focus,* 19(2):139–158.
———. 1990. "Uneven Differentiation and Incomplete Institutionalization: Political
Change and Continuity in the Early American Nation." In *Differentiation Theory
and Social Change: Comparative and Historical Perspective,* ed. Jeffrey Alexander
and Paul Colomy, 119–62. New York: Columbia University Press.
Dunn, F. L. 1976. "Traditional Asian Medicine and Cosmopolitan Medicine as Adap-
tive Systems." In *Asian Medical Systems,* 133–58. *See* Basham 1976.
Durkin-Longley, M. S. 1982. *Ayurveda in Nepal: A Medical Belief in Action.* Ph.D.
diss., University of Wisconsin–Madison.
Feagin, J. R. 1989. *Social Problems: A Critical Power Conflict Perspective.* Englewood
Cliffs, N.J.: Prentice-Hall.
Foster, G. M., and B. G. Anderson. 1978. *Medical Anthropology.* New York: John Wiley
& Sons.
Fox, Renee. 1976. "Medical Evolution." In *Explorations in General Theory in Social
Science,* ed. Jan J. Loubser, Rainer C. Baum, Andrew Effrat, and Victor Meyer Lidz,
773–87. New York: Free Press.
Gesler, W. M. 1984. *Health Care in Developing Countries.* Washington, D. C.: Associa-
tion of American Geographers.
Grenholm, G. G. 1983. "The Paradigm of Health Care Delivery Systems: Implications
for the Third World." In *Third World Medicine and Social Change: A Reader in
Social Science and Medicine,* ed. John H. Morgan, 91–110. New York: University
Press of America.
Heggenhougen, H. K. 1980. "The Utilization of Traditional Medicine: A Malaysian
Example." *Social Science and Medicine* 14B:235–364.
Joseph, George, John Desrochers, and Mariamma Kalathil. 1983. *Health Care in India.*
Bangalore: Center for Social Action.
Justice, Judith. 1981. *International Planning and Health: An Anthropological Case
Study of Nepal.* Ph. D. diss., University of California, Berkeley.
Kleinman, Arthur. 1980. *Patients and Healers in the Context of Culture: An Explora-
tion of the Borderland between Anthropology, Medicine, and Psychiatry.* Berke-
ley: University of California Press.
Leslie, Charles M. 1976. "Introduction." In *Asian Medical Systems,* 1–15. *See* Basham
1976.
———. 1980. "Medical Pluralism in World Perspective." *Social Science and Medicine*
14B:191–95.

Lindsey, L. L. 1983. "Health Care in India: An Analysis of the Existing Models." In *Third World Medicine and Social Change*, 111–24. *See* Grenholm 1983.

Ministry of Health. 1979. *Midterm Health Review 2035: Research and Evaluation of Health and Health Services Mid Fifths Plan Period (2031–2036)*. Kathmandu: Ministry of Health, HMG of Nepal.

Nepal Janch Bujh Kendra. 1976. *Long Term Health Plan*. Kathmandu: Royal Palace, HMG of Nepal.

Polednak, Anthony P. 1989. *Racial and Ethnic Differences in Disease*. Oxford and New York: Oxford University Press.

Shah, Moin, P. Mathura Shrestha, and Robert Parker. 1978. *Rural Health Needs: Study No. 1. Report of a Study in the Primary Health Care Unit of Tanahu District, Nepal*. Kathmandu: Institute of Medicine.

Smelser, N. J. 1959. *Social Change in the Industrial Revolution*. Chicago: University of Chicago Press.

Starr, Paul. 1982. *The Social Transformation of American Medicine*. New York: Basic Books.

Statistical Pocket Book. 1984. Kathmandu: Center Bureau of Statistics, HMG of Nepal.

Streefland, Peter. 1985. "The Frontier of Modern Western Medicine in Nepal." *Social Science and Medicine* 20 (11):1151–59.

Subedi, Janardan. 1989a. *Factors Affecting the Use of Modern Medicine in a Pluralistic Health Care System: The Case of Nepal*. Ph.D. diss., University of Akron.

———. 1989b. "Modern Health Services and Health Care Behavior: A Survey in Kathmandu, Nepal." *Journal of Health and Social Behavior* 30 (December): 412–20.

Subedi, Janardan, and Sree Subedi. 1990. "Health Care System of Nepal: A Theory of Incomplete Differentiation." Paper presented at the annual meeting of the American Sociological Association, Washington, D.C.

Surace, S. J. 1992. "Incomplete Differentiation: New Forms." In *The Dynamics of Social Systems*, ed. Paul C. Colomy, 93–119. London: Sage International.

Susser, Mervyn, William Watson, and Kim Hopper. 1985. *Sociology in Medicine*. 3d ed. Oxford and New York: Oxford University Press.

Taylor, Carl E. 1976. "The Place of Indigenous Medical Practitioners in the Modernization of Health Services." In *Asian Medical Systems*, 285–99. *See* Basham 1976.

Tsai, Wen-Hui. 1988. "Industrialization and Health Care in Taiwan," In *Modern and Traditional Health Care in Developing Society: Conflict and Cooperation*, ed. Christiane I. Zeichner, 35–47. New York: University Press of America.

United Nations Fund for Population Activities (UNFPA). 1979. *Report of Mission of Needs Assessment for Population Assistance—Nepal*. Report no. 21. New York: UNFPA.

United Nations International Children's Emergency Fund (UNICEF). 1978. *Annual Report on Nepal*. Kathmandu: UNICEF.

USAID, World Health Organization (WHO), HMG of Nepal. 1975. *Report on the Evaluation of Basic Health Services in Nepal*. Kathmandu: USAID.

Wolinsky, Fredric D. 1988. *The Sociology of Health: Principles, Practitioners, and Issues*. Belmont, Calif.: Wadsworth.

World Bank, South Asia Regional Office. 1979. *Country Study: Nepal, Development Performance and Prospects*. Washington, D.C.: World Bank.

Zeichner, Ben. 1988. "Modern and Traditional Psychiatry in the People's Republic of China." In *Modern and Traditional Health Care in Developing Society*, 21–34. *See* Tsai 1988.

Chapter 6

Traditional Medicine in Africa:

Past, Present, and Future

COLLINS O. AIRHIHENBUWA *and*
IRA E. HARRISON

The use of traditional remedies to treat and cure illness in Africa dates back for centuries. In examining health services there, as well as in other parts of the world, the cultural framework must be carefully considered in order to gain an understanding of how the indigenous people view sickness, disease, and appropriate treatment methods (Harvey 1988; Airhihenbuwa 1990–91).

Researchers who study health practices and beliefs are now cognizant that patients and clients who seek the prevention or cure of an illness or disease do so in a variety of ways, and that they depend upon a variety of sources (Dennis 1985). Moreover, it is now well understood that the sources of prevention and cure for a given problem are determined to a great extent by the client's sociocultural and religious backgrounds (Holzer 1973; Airihenbuwa 1987). Because African cultural evolution has often been misunderstood and misrepresented, it is no surprise that its healing modalities have been victims of allopathic hegemony—that is, Western biomedical science. "In Africa, it has been argued that the harsh experience and upheavals of the slave trade, colonialism and neo-colonialism preclude the pattern of development experienced in the west" (Pearce 1989). Similarly, the evolution of traditional medicine in African countries is different from that of countries that were not colonized, such as China.

Reappraisal of Traditional Health Care Delivery

The existence of a large corpus of literature on a country's traditional medicine tends to depend on whether or not the country was colonized and the extent to which the colonizers directly outlawed the practice of traditional medicine and, indirectly, the documentation of it. In the nineteenth and most of the twentieth centuries, Europeans were concerned with colonization, exploitation, and commerce. J. M. Janzen, in a discussion of Belgian colonial policy in the Congo, notes that "indigenous therapeutic practices were never mentioned within colonial manuals or laws. These laws sought only to establish European-modelled institutions regardless of what may have pre- or co-existed in African society" (1974–75, 109). In Ralph Schram's *History of the Nigerian Health Services*, the author never mentions the traditional healers who were serving the people prior to British colonization (Harrison 1984).

During the early part of the twentieth century, there was a shift of emphasis from conquest of African, Asian, American, and Oceanic peoples to control and administration of these peoples. The major goal was the maintenance of law, order, and economic growth. Non-Western beliefs and values were ignored or dismissed as primitive, savage, or barbarian, being based upon magic, religion, or witchcraft (Seijas 1975). Laws were promulgated to criminalize the practice of traditional medicine.

A few decades later, Bronislaw Malinowski (1954) and A. R. Radcliffe-Brown (1952) formulated the basic concepts of cultural anthropology. They discovered that religious rites, beliefs, and practices serve to maintain order in society and to regulate individual and group sentiment and behavior. "Generally speaking, religious ceremonies take believers away from the mundane affairs of life, sometimes by presenting exhilarating experiences" (Harvey 1988, 103). Religion is critical in understanding the psychosocial dimension of health. Health care delivery systems do not exist in and of themselves, they exist as parts of larger sociocultural wholes. Health care systems are a set of resources that may serve nonmedical as well as medical goals.

A reassessment of the disease-focus approach to health care has led many social and behavioral scientists to think anew about health care delivery, particularly in developing countries. Medical and health beliefs and practices once deemed superstitions are being reassessed and given a fresh interpretation. These beliefs can be seen as symbolic representations of various realities—many of them non-Western. Maladies resulting from hot–cold imbalance, the dislocation of internal organs, impure blood, unclean air, moral transgression, interpersonal struggle, and the human relation to the spirit world are now seen as different manifestations of a more general reality. When indigenous people cope with physical or emotional symptoms, they are likely to classify them within a traditional taxonomy and to seek help in the traditional health system. Thus, Nigerian health education specialist Z. A. Ademuwagun indicates, Nigerians in the Ibarapa district of Oyo State go to traditional healers for excessive worry, sleeplessness, malaria, yellow fever, and snakebite (Ademuwagun 1974–75). T. A. Lambo, retired deputy director general of the World Health Organization (WHO), faults the Western medical practitioner as being "invariably preoccupied with immediate natural causes, almost to the exclusion of the causal relations between conflicts and irregularities in the field of social relations on the one hand and disease or misfortune on the other" (Lambo 1978). Traditional healers generally became a focus of research because they were thought to have herbal concoctions for dealing with hypertension, diabetes, and other chronic diseases that Western physicians found difficult or impossible to cure (Harrison 1974).

Traditional Healing Concepts

The belief that a state of balance exists within the individual on the one hand and between the individual and the environment on the other hand is a concept found in traditional healing modalities worldwide. How this concept is operationalized varies among cultures and hence among the different traditional healing systems.

African traditional medicine seeks to secure and maintain a balance between the individual, elements of nature, and the heavenly bodies. Within the individual, a balance is maintained between organic disorders, physiological disorders, and social conflicts. This balanced state is, in turn, balanced with elements of nature—earth, fire, water, air, and metal. Finally, balance is sought with the heavenly bodies—the sun, moon, and stars.

In the African healing context, an understanding of social conflict is pivotal in curing the person who has become ill. This is where the healer deals with the *ultimate* cause of an illness: who or what caused it, and why. The *proximate* cause, or specific etiology, deals with how it happened, not why it happened. For people who believe in this concept of disease nosology, allopathic knowledge of the germ theory is useful only in explaining the medium through which health problems manifest themselves.

Traditional medicine is a desirable part of a nation's formal health care system because it is widely available, particularly in rural areas. Seventy percent of the doctors in Nigeria live in six cities: Benin, Enugu, Ibadan, Ife, Lagos, and Zaria (Osuntokun 1975). Most of the rural population in Nigeria relies solely on traditional practitioners to care for health care needs (Oyebola 1986). Therefore, health professionals and planners should examine the strengths and weaknesses of traditional medicine, so that its strengths can be promoted and its weaknesses minimized for the benefit of the people who believe in and use it.

Traditional medicine has paralleled the practice of Western allopathic medicine in a number of ways. In 1879, Robert Felkin, a British medical missionary traveling in Baganda (modern-day Uganda), reported a high level there of medical and health practice. He observed the successful performance of cesarean section with antiseptic technique by a native surgical team. He also saw experiments devised to discover a cure for a local epidemic (Davis 1959). Although Felkin witnessed this two years after Joseph Lister advocated antisepsis use in surgery in London, it was clear to him that the team, surgical technique, and public health experiments were a part of the tradition of the Baganda.

Other contributions made by traditional healers to health care delivery include the discovery of *Rauwolfia serpentina* (medical plant known as snakeroot), whose active principle, reserpine, is used today as a tranquilizer and hypotensive agent (Basch 1990); *Erythropleum guineense* (identified from the bark of the sasswood tree), a powerful laxative substance (Foster 1963); and *Periwinkle vinca rosea*, an herb that contains insulin and is used for the treatment of diabetes mellitus (Teller 1968; Foster 1963). In addition to their contributions in the use of medicinal plants, traditional healers were very successful in treating psychosomatic disorders. Lambo (1961) illustrates the healer's (*babalawos*, in Nigeria) ingenuity in his or her treatment technique in this example: "A toad is tied to the penis of a bed wetter. If the child urinates, the heat from the urine wakes up the toad who then begins to croak. The croaking of the toad wakes up the child. The similarity of this device to the modern anuretic machine is evident. The modern anuretic machine delivers a shock to the bed wetter on urinating. Behaviorally speaking, the electric shock and the croaking of the toad function as negative reinforcers."

Another example was shared by a British-trained physician from Mauritius at a lecture in June 1991 that C. O. Airhihenbuwa gave on traditional medicine as part of the Boston University School of Public Health summer certificate program "Health Care in Developing Countries." The physician recounted the story of a soccer player in Nigeria in the seventies who had suffered a compound fracture and was healed by a traditional bonesetter. When the limb was healed, however, it was shorter than the uninjured limb so that the patient started to limp. The patient went back to the traditional healer to seek a solution for his shortened limb. In the allopathic system, the bone would have been rebroken in the hospital and reset. Fortunately, the traditional healer had a different approach. The patient was advised to ask a friend or relative to go to the river with him and tie him up in a part of the river with the heaviest waves. This patient was left in the river for one hour every day for six months. By the end of the six months, the patient's limb had returned to its normal length. The force of the waves had realigned the bone to its normal length. Though it would be naive to suggest that traditional medicine is a panacea for the health problems of Africans, it has selective potentials for improving health care delivery.

An understanding of traditional medicine in any society must acknowledge its culture and history. This is a challenge for those behavioral and social scientists who are interested in health problems and solutions for developing countries. As a result of the renewed interest in traditional medicine, partly due to the primary health care movement and more recently to the child-survival revolution, the concept of integration is now in vogue. Even given the problems that have been identified with integration (Pillsbury 1982), the renewed interest in traditional medicine falls under programmatic interests of international donor agencies concerned with primary health care, child survival, and safe motherhood. Often they view the contributions of traditional medicine as very limited. However, these agencies, on the strength of their economic resources, have dominated health policy and practices in the Third World since World War II (Justice 1987). Along with their influence and funding resources came policy guidelines and priorities that promote allopathic hegemony.

Integration

The Thirtieth World Health Assembly in 1977 adopted a resolution (WHA 30.49) urging governments to give "adequate importance to the utilization of their traditional systems of medicine, with appropriate regulations" (Akerele 1984). This became the spark that galvanized WHO's promotion of traditional medicine on a global scale. It has been estimated that 80 percent or more of the world's rural people rely mainly on traditional medicines for their health care needs (Bannerman, Burton, and Wen-Chieh 1983). Three major recommendations were made: (1) evaluation of traditional healing practices, (2) traditional medicine as part of a national health system, and (3) providing training for traditional healers. To accomplish this goal, attempts have been made in different countries to find a common ground for traditional medicine and allopathic medicine.

The struggle to locate a common ground between traditional health care and allopathic health services has led many to advocate the integration of the two systems of care. Integration has been promoted by many respected organizations such as WHO and the United Nation's Children's Fund (UNICEF) and by scholars such as Robert Bannerman, John Burton, and Ch'en Wen-Chieh (1983); Lambo (1978); Olayinola Akerele (1984); B. L. K. Pillsbury (1982); L. M. Maclean and Bannerman (1982),; and A. K. Newman and J. C. Bhatia (1973). Unfortunately, the implementation of integration has been based on a "donor–deficit model" for the traditional healers, even though this may not have been the intent of those who advocate integration. There is the belief that traditional healers can be trained to "modernize" their healing practices by having allopathic professionals teach them what they don't know (assessing healers from a deficit model). In the process, the allopathic expert finds out what traditional healers know so that their knowledge can be improved when applied to allopathic practice. This model assumes that the healer needs some training but has little or nothing to contribute to improving the knowledge and practice of the allopath. In discussions about integration of health services, seldom is the traditional healer pictured as a health provider with adequate or superior knowledge that will benefit to the allopathic provider (the physician) in certain aspects of training. The sources of the traditional healers' concoctions and pharmacopoeia, however, are eagerly, even exploitively, sought (Harrison and Cominsky 1976). Though deficient in some areas, traditional healers could be donors in other areas. They are expected to surrender their herbal knowledge without proper recognition of their skill and knowledge.

Mistakes in professional judgment do not end with allopathic physicians. Some social scientists who believe in aspirin, yet cannot explain how it relieves pain, demand that traditional healers explain their medications before the social scientists consider such medicine valid. This kind of inconsistent and one-sided judgment has led to reluctance and suspicion on the part of traditional health care providers. Instead of integration or cooperation based on mutual trust, respect, and collaboration, the result is antagonism.

As one further explores the concept of integration, three problems become evident. First, as stated above, the healer is seen as one who needs to be trained but has nothing to contribute to training the allopath. Second, a conflict exists between didactic learning, which is how allopaths are trained, and experiential learning, which is how traditional healers are trained. Third, there is a lack of systematic protection of ownership of orally transmitted information, which is a vital form of intellectual property in traditional medicine.

Integration seems to have be more successful with traditional birth attendants than with other types of traditional practitioners (Pillsbury 1982). This success has often been attributed to traditional birth attendants not posing any serious competition to physicians in terms of their professional status, their power, and their resources (Green 1988). In other cases of integration, governments have attempted to incorporate traditional healers into the "modern sector" projects or program (Pillsbury 1982). These attempts almost always involve some kind of training for the healers, to upgrade their knowledge. Unfortunately, the healers often receive training only in the most basic tasks, such as mixing oral rehydration solution, even though they would also like to learn how to give injections and read X rays (Green 1988).

A training session designed for integration should be one where allopathic providers (particularly physicians) and traditional healers participate both as trainers and trainees, because both have information to contribute and gain. I. E. Harrison's analogical model of traditional health–metropolitan health "mealth" relationships outlines professional areas of cooperation (Harrison 1984). Integration should involve the healers in planning, implementation, and evaluation, to foster cooperation and participation. This does not necessarily mean moving the traditional healer into a hospital practice setting any more than it should mean moving the physician to the healer's practice setting. Integration may mean referral from physician to a bonesetter for fracture, as well as referral from an herbalist to an internist for appendicitis.

The second problem with integration lies in the difference between allopaths and traditional healers in methods of knowledge acquisition, as applied to proposed training programs. It is a misapplication of formal, didactic modes of teaching to apply them in traditional healing practice, where learning in the apprenticeship mode (experiential learning) is more appropriate and culturally customary (Jordan 1989). This is particularly true in training programs developed to "upgrade" the knowledge and skills of traditional birth attendants (Maclean and Bannerman 1982, 1815).

The third problem with integration is that physicians have requested that traditional healers share their knowledge about their treatment and medicine without any systematic procedure for protecting the ownership of the information that is revealed. In Western culture such protection of information and medicine discovery is guaranteed under copyright and patent laws. In the United Nations debate over how developing nations are to be rewarded for contributions to plant species, Henry Shands, a U.S. delegate, argued that without a strong patent law there would be no incentive for people to create superior medicinal properties out of plant species (Simons 1989). Although patent and copyright laws are not customary in oral tradition, one should understand that revelation of information within this context has nevertheless been regularly protected, one method of such protection has been to reveal information only to one or two individuals who will be protégáes of the healer. Thus an open, widespread revelation is an allopathic phenomenon and should carry with it the protection and rewards that go with it or, alternatively a culturally appropriate modified version. When traditional healers possess the knowledge for discovering creating, and using medication of superior therapeutic properties, such information should not be shared with others in the absence of some system of guaranteeing that the original source of such information or medication is protected and appropriately rewarded for its revelation. Although the healers may not articulate such a right, it is a basic human desire to receive the comfort and protection of those fundamental principles regarding information-sharing and proprietorship, regardless of the pattern of knowledge acquisition. Information and medication protection and ownership is paramount in promoting open information-sharing and true reciprocity between and among health providers and policymakers. The resistance of physicians to sharing information with traditional healers can also be considered an example of such protectiveness.

Health professionals will have a better appreciation for international health problems if they understand that treatment modalities, like disease and disease patterns, are intricately tied to beliefs and values within cultures. As long as Africans successfully seek treatment from both allopathic and traditional healers, it is prudent to strive for collaboration based on respect and trust between the two health providers. Perhaps the term "cooperation" should be preferred to "integration." The latter term tends to conjure up resistance among those who interpret this process as an encroachment on their territory. This has been our experience during workshops and lectures on traditional medicine.

Implications for National Health Policy

Major difficulties with government policy are its perception and definition of traditional medicine. Murray Last observes that, "though within most nations there are usually a large number of medical sub-cultures, each with its own characteristics and structure, policy-makers often have in mind apparently a single, paradigmatic culture from which they generalize about 'traditional medicine.' Inevitably such stereotypes are likely to reflect political conditions—as of course happened under colonial rule when traditional healers were categorized as 'witches'" (Last 1986). An important factor in a successful national health policy in developing countries should be a clear definition for the healing modalities. Such a definition should involve people from both allopathic and traditional healing systems.

In *The Professionalization of African Medicine* (1986), Last and G. L. Chavunduka argue that traditional healers ought to organize themselves and seek professional status, not only to survive but also to get their share of governmental support. Integration, registration, and professional-

TABLE 6-1. Stages of Recognition of Traditional Healers

Form	Level	Context
1. Private Meeting	Personal	Informal Contact
2. Conference	Institutional	Sharing of Knowledge
3. Publication of Ideas	Institutional	Sharing of Knowledge
4. Registration	Institutional	Recording of Members and Expertise
5. Certification	Institutional	Monitoring of Members and Practice
6. Licensure	Societal	Practice: Limited/Full; Rural/Urban

ization, however, may be possible only after a period of official governmental recognition. Such recognition may take various forms, at various levels, in various contexts (Harrison 1984; see Table 6-1).

By recognition we mean an array of relationships between traditional healers, government officials, and medical personnel, which may range from informal private meetings to formal licensure. At the most basic level, healers, traditional or modern, may interact and exchange information as family, friends, and professionals. J. O. Lambo, president of the Nigerian Association of Medical Herbalists, is a chief, a traditional healer, and the older brother of Dr. T. A. Lambo. T. A. Lambo is black Africa's first Western-trained psychiatrist and is the retired deputy director-general of the WHO. The Lambos together employed traditional healers at Aro Psychiatric Hospital (1964). This is an example of stage-one recognition: there was an agreement at the personal level in an informal context to use the best traditional and Western procedures for patient care. Stage two might include the sharing of such information institutionally within clinics and hospital conferences and might evolve into stage three with the publication of results in a conference report (Lambo 1961).

In terms of conferences, the First International Symposium on Traditional Medical Therapy—A Critical Appraisal, sponsored by the University of Lagos, Nigeria, provided an excellent context for the exchange of ideas (Harrison 1974). The various papers presented at the 1973 symposium at the University of Lagos, were published in *Proceedings of the International Conference on Traditional Medical Therapy—A Critical Appraisal* (Akisanya 1973); this represents the form, level, and context for stage-three recognition (for a list of similar national and international conferences, see Harrison and Cominsky 1984).

Certification and licensure are the final stages in the formal recognition of traditional healers as an officially viable part of a society's health care delivery system. Nevertheless, the earlier stages of recognition identify these healers and illustrate their potential in health care.

Policymakers should decide on the unmet community health needs and then involve social and behavioral scientists, as well as the communities, in health program planning, implementation, and evaluation. The community thus helps to define a range of acceptable healing practices. Such definitions will be based on indigenous reasoning that may not be obvious in Western contexts. Cultural diversity among peoples of the nation and the impact of such diversity on program replicability cannot be overemphasized. Community involvement is one strategy for acknowledging the impact of culture on a national health system. This is often realized when individuals, families, and communities, for whom a program is intended, and service providers (traditional healers) all have the opportunity to be a part of the team that both states the health problem and formulates the solution as a particular health program. Sensitivity to traditional customs and social norms will be ensured by the community members; thus the program will be culturally representative.

Allopathic health providers can learn from traditional healers, just as traditional healers can learn from allopaths. Understanding the components of a healing system is critical in influencing the health behavior of those who subscribe to the modality in question. Consequently, one should learn to be more humble about one's profession and programs and become more understanding of others (Torrey 1972). Some allopathic physicians have already started to utilize lessons learned from traditional healers. For instance, some allopaths now place an amulet around a child's neck so that the child will return for a follow-up visit. Reciprocally, some healers now send their fracture patients to have their bones x-rayed in the hospital. In child-survival programs, the traditional wearing of beads around a child's wrist is being used for growth monitoring. Thus there is already some level of cooperation.

Conclusion

One of the key primary health care providers in most developing countries is the traditional healer. Because traditional medicine is based on cultural and traditional values, ignoring this treatment modality is tantamount to ignoring the cultural impact of health and disease in these societies. In Africa, one cannot begin to address health care delivery without acknowledging the role of traditional medicine. It behooves social and behavioral scientists who are interested in health care delivery in developing countries to devote some time to exploring the past, present, and future contributions of traditional healers to health care delivery in these countries. This was done, for example, when the WHO's Global Programme on AIDS and Traditional Medicine Programme convened an informal consultation in Geneva in February 1989 to review the status of research and services in traditional medicine as applied to human immunodeficiency virus (HIV) infection and acquired immunodeficiency syndrome (AIDS) (WHO 1989). Social and behavioral scientists must be willing to experiment with various forms, at different levels, and with definitive contexts in order to establish and to promote proper communication between traditional and allopathic health providers. Communication and cooperation must prevail for an optimal working relationship to exist between these forms of health service.

Social and behavioral scientists have a vital role to play in formulating health care policies and in working with traditional healers to ensure the provision of an adequate health care system in developing countries. Such a system would assure that Africans will have available, accessible, acceptable, and affordable health services. Thus they can benefit from "the best of both worlds" (Akerele 1986).

REFERENCES

Ademuwagun, Z. A. 1974–75. "The Meeting Point of Orthodox Health Personnel and Traditional Healers/Midwives in Nigeria: The Pattern of Utilization of Health Services in Ibarapa Division." *Rural Africana* 26 (Winter):57–78.
Airhihenbuwa, C. O. 1987. "Nigerian Heads of Households' Attitude toward Modern and Traditional Medicines." *Journal of Rural Health* 3(11):21–30.
———. 1990–91. "A Conceptual Model for Culturally Appropriate Health Education Programs in Developing Countries." *International Quarterly of Community Health Education* 11(1):53–62.
Akerele, Olayinola. 1984. "WHO's Traditional Medicine Programme: Progress and Perspectives." *WHO Chronicle* 38(2):76–81.
———. 1986. "The Best of Both Worlds." *Social Science and Medicine* 21(2):177–81.
Akisanya, Akiasola. 1973. "Traditional Medical Therapy—A Critical Appraisal." *Proceedings of the International Conference on Traditional Medical Therapy—A Critical Appraisal* (December 10–16). Lagos: University of Lagos.
Bannerman, R. H., John Burton, and Ch'en Wen-Chieh. 1983. *Traditional Medicine and Health Care Coverage: A Reader for Health Administrators and Practitioners.* Geneva: World Health Organization.
Basch, P. F. 1990. *International Health.* New York: Oxford University Press.
Davis, J. N. P. 1959. "The Development of Scientific Medicine in the African Kingdom of Bunga-kitara." *Medical History* 3(49):47.
Dennis, R. E. 1985. "Health Beliefs and Practices of Ethnic and Religious Groups." In *Removing Cultural and Ethnic Barriers to Health Care,* ed. Elizabeth L. Watkins and Audrey E. Johnson, Chapel Hill: University of North Carolina Press.
Foster, E. V. 1963. "Treatment of African Mental Patients." In *First Pan African Psychiatric Conference Report,* ed. T. A. Lambo, 267–79. Ibadan, Nigeria: Western State Government.
Green, E. C. 1988. "Can Collaborative Programs between Biomedical and African Indigenous Health Practitioners Succeed?" *Social Science and Medicine* 27(11):1125–30.
Harrison, I. E. 1974. "First International Symposium on Traditional Medical Therapy." *Medical Anthropology Newsletter* 6(1):10–13.
———. 1984. *Colonialism, Mealth (Metropolitan Health Care) Care Systems, and Traditional Healers.* Occasional Papers no. 5. Urbana, Ill.: Association of Black Anthropologists.

———. 1986. "Colonialism, Health Care Systems, Traditional Medicine and WHO: Health Care for All by the Year 2000." Paper presented at the Second International Conference on Traditional Healing Systems of the African Diaspora, University of California at Berkeley, February 8–9.

Harrison, I. E., and Sheila Cominsky. 1976. *Traditional Medicine.* Vol. 1, *Implications for Ethnomedicine, Ethnopharmacology, Maternal and Child Health, Mental Health and Public Health—An Annotated Bibliography of Africa, Latin America, and the Caribbean.* New York: Garland.

———. 1984. *Traditional Medicine.* Vol. 2, 1976–1981: *Current Research with Implications for Ethnomedicine, Ethnopharmacology, Maternal and Child Health, Mental Health and Public Health—An Annotated Bibliography of Africa, Latin America, and the Caribbean.* New York: Garland.

Harvey, W. B. 1988. "Voodoo and Santeria: Traditional Healing Techniques in Haiti and Cuba." In *Modern and Traditional Health Care in Developing Societies: Conflict and Cooperation,* ed. C. I. Zeichner, 101–14. New York: University Press of America.

Holzer, Hans. 1973. *Beyond Medicine.* Chicago: Henry Regnery.

Janzen, J. M. 1974–75. "Pluralistic Legitimization of Therapy Systems in Contemporary Zaire." *Rural Africana* 26:105–22.

Jordan, Brigette. 1989. "Cosmopolitan Obstetrics: Some Insights from the Training of Traditional Midwives." *Social Science and Medicine* 28(9):925–44.

Justice, Judith. 1987. "The Bureaucratic Context of International Health: A Social Scientist's View." *Social Science and Medicine* 25(12):1301–5.

Kegley, C. F., and A. N. Saviers. 1983. "Working with Others Who Are Not Like Me." *Journal of School Health* 53 (February): 81–85.

Lambo, T. A. 1961. "Mental Health in Nigeria: Research and Technical Problems." Reprinted in *World Mental Health* 13.

———. 1964. "The Village of Aro." *Lancet* 2:513–14.

———. 1978. "Psychotherapy in Africa." *Human Nature* 1(3):32–39.

Last, Murray. (1986). "The Professionalization of African Medicine: Ambiguities and Definitions." In *The Professionalization of African Medicine,* ed. Murray Last and G. L. Chavunduka, 1–19. Manchester: Manchester University Press, International African Institute.

Maclean, C. U., and R. H. Bannerman. 1982. "Utilization of Indigenous Healers in National Health Delivery Systems." *Social Science and Medicine* 16:1815–16.

Malinowski, Branislaw. 1954. "The Rationalization of Anthropology and Administration." *Africa* 3:405–29.

Newman, A. K., and J. C. Bhatia. 1973. "Family Planning and Indigenous Medicine Practitioners." *Social Science and Medicine* 14A:23–29.

Osuntokun, B. O. 1975. "The Traditional Basis of Neuropsychiatric Practice among the Yorubas of Nigeria." *Tropical Geographical Medicine* 27:422–30.

Oyebola, D. D. O. 1986. "National Medical Policies in Nigeria." In *The Professionalization of Traditional Medicine,* 221–36. See Last 1986.

Pearce, T. O. 1989. "The Assessment of Diviners and Their Knowledge by Civil Servants in Southwestern Nigeria." *Social Science and Medicine* 28(9):917–24.

Pillsbury, B. L. K. 1982. "Policy and Evaluation Perspectives on Traditional Health Practitioners in National Health Care Systems." *Social Science and Medicine* 16: 1825–34.

Radcliffe-Brown, A. R. 1952. *Structure and Function in Primitive Society: Essays and Addresses.* Glencoe, Ill.: Free Press.

Schram, Ralph. 1971. *A History of Nigerian Health Services.* Ibadan: Ibadan University Press.

Seijas, Heijas. 1975. "An Approach to the Study of Medical Aspects of Culture." *Current Anthropology* 14(5):344–45.

Simons, Marlise. 1989. "Poor Nations Seeking Rewards for Contributions to Plant Species." *New York Times* (May 16):138.

Teller, Ayo. 1968. "Studies on Aspects of Traditional Medicine." *Lagos Notes and Records* 2(1):18.

Torrey, E. F. 1972. "What Western Psychotherapists Can Learn from Witch Doctors." *American Journal of Orthopsychiatry* 42(1):69–76.

World Health Organization (WHO). 1989. "Memoranda: In Vitro Screening of Traditional Medicines for Anti-HIV Activity: Memorandum for a WHO Meeting." *Bulletin of the World Health Organization* 67(6):613–18.

Chapter 7

Curricular Goals and

Student Aspirations in a

New Arab Medical College

EUGENE B. GALLAGHER

It is as difficult to envision a modern society without doctors as it is to envision a modern society without motor vehicles or telephones. The doctor has become a culture hero who wields the complex, often dramatic, endlessly advancing paraphernalia of health care—Nuclear Magnetic Resonance (NMR) devices, computerized axial tomography (CAT) scanners, transplants, intricate neurosurgery, emergency medical services, and precisely targeted drugs—and who is the promulgator of hopes for still better techniques to come. Health care is an important vector of modernity in two senses: directly, for its powerful practical effects in curing or alleviating illness; and symbolically, for its representation of a society's capacity to mobilize the agents and institutional structures that can implement biomedical science to human benefit. With physicians leading the charge, so to speak, against illness, medical education is a particularly strategic component of a society's health effort and index of its modernization.

Except for a few schools dating back to medieval times, most medical schools in Western industrialized societies were founded in the latter part of the nineteenth and the early twentieth centuries. These schools were in a comfortable position to absorb the great discoveries of early biomedicine and to evolve ways of transmitting that knowledge to students, both in preclinical or theoretical forms and in clinical form, that is, as applied to the diagnosis and treatment of illness in patients. From one school to another, medical curriculums came into a remarkable degree of similarity, in methods of instruction and evaluation as well as in content.

As in many other aspects of development, the developing societies got a late start in creating their own modalities of medical education. Although several medical schools were established by colonial powers during the nineteenth century (in Brazil in 1808, in Egypt in 1827, and in India in 1835), and more in the first half of the twentieth century, the great surge came after the Second World War (*Directory of Medical Schools* 1987). In the two decades between 1955 and 1974, the number of medical schools in developing societies substantially more than doubled, and many more have been established since 1974 (Kindig and Taylor 1985).

This rapid move into medical education has the appearance of a straightforward catching-up with the industrialized societies—the acquisition by the developing societies of the capacity to produce their own physicians from their own resources. This, however, is too simple a characterization of what is occurring, because the Third World societies are making their current progress under historical conditions that differ markedly from those prevailing when medical education began in the industrialized societies.

Two differences stand out as especially important. First, the immediate utility of medical intervention is far greater now than it was one hundred years ago. Consider the life-saving benefit of these few examples: antibiotics, insulin, blood transfusion, cesarean section for difficult birth presentations of the fetus, and hemodialysis. Even in developing societies with low literacy rates, people learn about the "miracles" of modern medicine; public expectations for health care rise accordingly.

Second, in response to rising public expectations, Third World governments play a more active oversight role in medical education than did governments in the initial phases of medical education in Western societies. It is also true in many Third World societies that, given the generally low economic level of the populace and the laissez-faire orientation of the government toward the practicing medical profession, the urban elites benefit most from the services of physicians. The ratio of physicians to population is very low, and the quantum of available medical services is far from evenly distributed. Nevertheless, whatever the actual distribution of medical care and the career paths of Third World physicians once they graduate from medical school, an ideology of national service figures importantly in planning the medical curriculum, as well as in the motivation and aspirations of many medical students.

Research Objectives and Setting

The foregoing statement identifies the two focuses of research that I report in this chapter. This research was carried out in the Faculty of Medicine and Health Sciences of United Arab Emirates (UAE) University. This is the only medical school in the nation and the newest of the eight faculties that now comprise the United Arab Emirates' only university.

I traced out above the ways in which medical education is an important avenue for modernization on the national or societal level. Medical education leads to the production of physicians, who taken together are centrally important in directly providing medical care and, more broadly, for guiding most of the health care effort of the nation.

This formulation leads to the two questions I answer in this report.

1. What importance is attached to the meeting of national health care needs—compared with other goals—in the curriculum of the new medical college?
2. Are the medical students oriented, in their career thinking and aspirations, toward social objectives in the practice of medicine?

I carried out this research in the course of my academic appointment on the medical faculty. I explained to faculty, students, and staff that I wanted to obtain a rounded sociological picture of teaching and learning in the medical school; many individuals went out of their way to supply me with information and interpretation. My data collection thus stemmed broadly from participant observation—conversations, informal interviews, observation of student response to my lectures and tutorials. In addition to these varied encounters, I was given access to invaluable written materials—official documents, administrative surveys, student notes and reports, admission applications for students, faculty recruitment applications, and minutes of several faculty committees. In short, my position as a faculty member gave me wide-ranging exposure to student, faculty, and staff perspectives and information on many aspects of the educational process.

In addition to carrying out teaching duties, I served as a consultant on library development and instructional resources to the administration of the newly founded medical library. This responsibility gave me further insight into attitudes about teaching and related matters, such as student preparation for exams and faculty utilization of library resources.

During my tenure as a visiting professor in 1990, the faculty size was thirty-five. Three of the thirty-five were physicians native to the United Arab Emirates; the other thirty-two (both physicians and Ph.D. basic scientists) were recruited diversely from the United Kingdom, United States, Germany, Australia, the Netherlands, Sweden, Yugoslavia, Ghana, Nigeria, Egypt, the Sudan, Turkey, Jordan, India, Pakistan, and Sri Lanka. Faculty size is expanding rapidly: by June 1991 it had reached seventy-five.

The first class, consisting of twenty-two women and eleven men, was admitted in 1986 and scheduled to graduate in 1993. No students were admitted in 1987. In 1988, twenty-five women and nine men were admitted. In 1989, twenty-seven women and three men were admitted. At the time of my study, there were altogether eighty-four female students and twenty-three male students.

The curriculum consists of two years of premedical study followed by five years of medical courses. The latter, medical phase is divided into two years of preclinical or basic science study, followed by three years of clinical clerkships.

Students are admitted to the university at an average age of eighteen, upon completion of secondary school. Only UAE nationals are admitted. The language of instruction is English, with the exception of two courses in Islamic studies and one course called Emirates Society, all of which are taught in Arabic.

The United Arab Emirates: A Brief Sketch

Although my research was carried out within the confines of the medical school, it dealt with questions of health care delivery at the national level. In that sense, the research looks outward. It becomes important to understand the sociopolitical environment of the medical school for two reasons: because the United Arab Emirates is the society wherein the medical graduates will practice, and because it is the society from which the students (and a few of the faculty) are recruited.

The United Arab Emirates was established as a loose confederation of seven separate emirates in 1971, following British withdrawal from political and naval suzerainty in the gulf region. Prior to that, the emirates had engaged in acrimonious boundary disputes. With the discovery and production of oil starting in the 1960s, the nation that became the United Arab Emirates moved rapidly from being a poor nation to one of the world's richest nations, with per capita income in 1987 standing at $15,770—compared with $660 for Egypt, $1,760 for Mexico, and $19,840 for the United States (World Bank 1990, 178–179).

The past two decades have seen tremendous expansion of the physical infrastructure of the United Arab Emirates. The seven emirates are linked by good roads; automobile ownership is widespread, and there is an extensive network of public bus transportation. Four of the seven emirates have international airports; two, the airports in Abu Dhabi and Dubai, have substantial traffic.

Although illiteracy is common among men over fifty years old and almost universal in older women, virtually all children now receive at least primary school education. All education is free; university students, including medical students, also receive a monthly stipend from the government.

The population of the United Arab Emirates is about 1.8 million, of which only 25 percent are UAE nationals. The other 75 percent consist of expatriate workers and their dependents. The expatriate workers carry out many vital functions, from unskilled construction workers, who are essential in the many building projects, to skilled professionals such as petroleum geologists, architects, physicians, and nurses. Although most of the expatriate workers are male, there is also a sizable cadre of women brought to the United Arab Emirates, mainly from Thailand and the Philippines, to serve as domestic workers—cooks, nannies, maids—for UAE families.

Islam is the state religion of the United Arab Emirates. Arabic is the official language, although English is also widely used.

The United Arab Emirates have until the recent past been a strongly tribal society, with many tribal groups following a nomadic desert life and others engaged in fishing and pearling activities in the gulf. It is now a heavily urbanized society and the role of the tribe as an economic and political force has diminished considerably. Nevertheless, tribal ties retain social and emotional force. I heard, for example, that certain students keep their distance from each other because they belong to tribal groups that have been traditional enemies.

The position of women in UAE society is of particular interest for my research because of their potential for contributing substantially to UAE medical care. As their contribution crystallizes in coming decades, it will mark a radical departure from the traditional activities of women in the United Arab Emirates. As in most Arab–Muslim societies, UAE women have traditionally played a dominant role in domestic and family affairs, as wives, mothers, household managers, marriage arrangers, and counselors, but their public role is very limited. Currently, very few UAE women are employed outside the household; the main occupations open to them are teacher, physician, and social worker—all dealing entirely with female clients. Education at all levels, including the university, maintains strict sex segregation.

Planning the UAE Curriculum: The Principal Actors

The UAE ministries of health and higher education had in mind the establishment of a medical faculty from the time of UAE University's founding in 1977. Sustained planning did not start, however, until 1983. The three principals in the planning process were Sheikh Abdul Ahmed Al-Naimi, Dr. Lamont Fisher, and Dr. Murbarak Fouad Al-Khameri. (I use fictitious names here.)

Shaikh Al-Naimi was at the time the chancellor of the university, reporting directly to the UAE minister of higher education (in 1990, Al-Naimi became minister of higher education). As chief administrator of the university, with its diverse faculties, the Sheikh had little familiarity with medical education. Indeed, his main occupational post was not the position of chancellor but rather the chairmanship of a large UAE commercial bank. To familiarize himself with contemporary medical education, he visited several medical schools in the United States and Canada. Then he engaged Fisher, a renowned Canadian internist and "medical educationist," to advise him on policies and procedures in setting up the school. He also appointed Al-Khameri, an Egyptian public health specialist, to be the founding dean of the medical faculty. Al-Khameri had previously founded a medical school in the Sudan, in which the curriculum was heavily weighted to provide students with knowledge and practice opportunity in community medicine.

The dynamics of curriculum development and educational policy can, without undue simplification, be understood in terms of what these three figures stood for and sought in planning the medical school. Their positions and interactions also constitute a representative picture of what has happened in many other Third World medical schools.

To understand what happened—the planning process and the provisional outcome—in the UAE faculty, it is useful first to look more generally at contemporary issues in the training of doctors and the ambiguity of the medical role within the totality of health care.

Issues in the Training of Physicians for a Medically
Relevant Contribution in Third World Health Care

There is a remarkable similarity worldwide in the curriculums of medical schools—in the subjects taught and information conveyed and in the teaching methods, moving from lecture–lab theoretical training into later clinical contact with patients in range of specialties and primary care or family medicine. This similarity is matched by a similarity in statements about the goals of medical education—the attributes of the "product" of the curriculum, and how he or she, as a medically educated and qualified individual, will function as a professional in society. These attributes include, at a minimum, the physician as a person dedicated to the patient's health; competent to diagnose and treat illness; caring in his or her orientation toward the patient; conscientious and responsible in his or her conduct with the patient and other health professionals.

Though this listing is in one sense a full roster of the attributes of "physicianhood," it exists in an empty social space, saying nothing about the role of the doctor in addressing the health problems of society, the resources at his or her disposal, the composition of his or her clientele, patterns of access to medical care, and a host of parameters vital to the actual conduct of medicine. This detached conception of the physician's role—leaving entirely unresolved the question of medical priorities in society—has implications for medical education. In a social vacuum, medical education usually comes, by default, to emphasize academic excellence and clinical responsibility—but not concern with health problems of the society.

The World Health Organization's (WHO) program Health for All by the Year 2000 (HFA/2000) (WHO 1981) is a well-known statement of how societies should organize personnel and technology to meet health care needs with both preventive and curative modalities. The general thrust of HFA/2000, however, is more strongly preventive than curative. It advocates the training of community health workers who can, under medical and public health supervision, carry out the tasks of immunization and environmental health protection. The implications of this are to place the physician in a managerial rather than a clinical role. Its implications for medical education are not clear-cut, beyond emphasizing training in primary care for meeting the health needs of society.

Producing a competent generalist physician, well grounded in the basic medical sciences and the major fields of medicine (especially internal medicine, pediatrics, and obstetrics), is the proclaimed goal of many medical schools in both industrialized and developing societies. In the course of medical education, however, and at sharp variance with the publicly proclaimed goal, medical students receive strong encouragement to become specialists. That many students should actually move in this direction is due to their receiving almost all of their clinical training at the hands of specialist faculty and their having virtually no exposure to physicians carrying out primary care in communities. It should also be noted that there is nothing in the content or setting of their preclinical studies, taught by biomedical scientists devoted to research rather than to medical practice, that would incline the students toward primary care. The implicit message of preclinical studies is: "Do not end up as a generalist physician but continue on to specialize in a field of medicine that functions from a sophisticated knowledge base."

When medical schools in developing societies espouse the goals of HFA/2000 and the training of primary care, generalist physicians, they must still face the influence of the specialists on their faculties, most of whom have been trained in Western medical schools. The stance of these key medical teachers is aptly described by Ronald Frankenberg and Joyce Leeson as follows:

> The medical school in a developing country . . . has to recruit expatriate medical teachers who are chosen for their specific skills. The required anatomists, physiologists, biochemists, neurologists, surgeons, and physicians of various specialties come from a wide variety of backgrounds and countries, but they have been trained mostly in advanced industrial countries, in modern

teaching hospitals. . . . such teachers usually consider their own education to have been ideal and seek benevolently to allow others hitherto less fortunate to share in it. (Frankenberg and Leeson 1974, 270)

The pro-specialization influence to which students are exposed has a particular aspect and a general aspect. In its particular aspect, the student is expected to learn the rudiments of diagnosis and treatment in each specialty. That expectation is an open, formal requirement of the curriculum. On a more subtle level, the clinical teachers in that specialty will try to engage the student's interest in it—to encourage him or her to think about going beyond the basics and to become a specialist like themselves. Faculty will try to entice the brightest and most strongly motivated students to follow in their footsteps.

The general aspect of pro-specialty influence transcends each of the specialties and stresses clinical excellence, that is, creation of the physician who is capable, by intellectual mastery, experience, and technical know-how, to deal with disease expertly in the light of the latest information within the specialty. Whether blatantly or subtly, this canon disparages generalist practice and forms of medical care carried out under technologically rudimentary conditions. The latter are seen as second-rate medicine, stultifyingly routine, and work that paramedicals can carry out—or work that is superfluous, because most patients most of the time seek care for minor, self-limiting conditions.

Medical schools in developing countries are especially susceptible to the mandate for clinical excellence. The push in this direction comes from the administration as well as the faculty. The administration, through its contacts with the national Ministry of Health and other political entities, is aware of social priorities in medical care and medical training and is in some measure sympathetic with the implied objective. When the diverse goals and pressures that administrations must accommodate are resolved, however, social priorities in medical training as a rule come up short. In matters of faculty recruitment, curriculum design, and teaching ambience, there is little more than a courtesy nod toward a social role for medicine.

Academic Excellence versus Health Care Orientation in the UAE Curriculum

From documentary evidence of the planning history, the foregoing issues were evidently much on the minds of Al-Naimi, Fisher, and Al-Khameri as goals and priorities to be variously sought or avoided, according to one's vision of the role of medicine in health care and society. These three people felt the tensions between the objective of educating to meet health needs of the nation and the objective of educating for academic excellence. The various planning documents, letters, and memos that I surveyed suggested a keen consciousness of choice between these goals, experienced as disjunctive rather than complementary alternatives. In the end, as will be seen, the choice came down heavily on the side of academic excellence.

In addition to the two competing aims already discussed, Al-Naimi had a third idea in mind, namely, that the medical school be created to provide the means for young UAE nationals to obtain training in a prestigious, demanding modern profession. One of the Sheikh's most frequent and cogent statements was "We are not bedouins," by which he meant that he and his fellow citizens were an able, ambitious, sophisticated people who were fully capable of mastering complex modern science. The bedouins to whom he referred were his own ancestors, who lived in the desert some fifty years ago; bedouins occupy a wholly honorable place in UAE history and legend, but they were not known for self-discipline and methodical devotion to a long-term task such as learning medicine.

Al-Naimi was also concerned, of course, with the fruits that the medical school would produce in the form of UAE Arab–Muslim doctors who would eventually be able to displace the many foreign doctors there. However, the notion of proving to the world that UAE citizens could make good doctors seemed even more important in his thinking. On the whole, this notion resonated more strongly to the goal of academic excellence than to that of providing health care to meet the needs of the nation.

Partly from his own convictions and partly from his sensing of the Sheikh's priorities, Fisher fashioned a "comprehensive planning memorandum" that nodded strongly in the sheikh's direction (UAE University 1986). Thus, under "immediate" objectives, it states that the goal of the medical school should be "to provide for citizens of the U.A.E. an opportunity to qualify for the M.D. degree of international standards of quality, so that the M.D. graduates of U.A.E. University would be able to compete successfully in any of the clinical specialties in Canada, the U.S. or the U.K." (In examining similar documents from U.S. and British medical schools, I have not found any goal statements to the effect that the medical school exists to give students the opportunity to become physicians; instead, the goals include statements about educational standards of the school and its value to society by providing society with well-qualified physicians).

The long-term objective (in contrast with the immediate objective) that Fisher's memorandum proposes is "to develop . . . a center of scholarship in medicine and medical sciences which can provide intellectual leadership to the Islamic world, and beyond it." This second objective extends the first one: once the medical school has demonstrated its ability to transform UAE students into doctors of international caliber, it can then establish itself as a center of advanced medical learning.

Fisher's memorandum is notable for the absence of any reference in its eighteen densely packed pages to what the graduates will do once they have completed their education, nor does it contain a statement about medical needs or priorities in the nation that the medical school will help to solve or alleviate. Other parts of the memorandum show clearly that the failure to specify health care goals was not a mere oversight or an idea lying outside the framework of consideration. Rather, the document displays an explicit antipathy to any emphasis on community health or social goals in medicine.

In arguing against a socially oriented curriculum, Fisher noted that the United Arab Emirates was now a highly urban society and that several modern, well-equipped hospitals had already been built and staffed with expatriate physicians. He used this fact as the basis for his conjecture that, once graduated, the UAE doctors would not be content to work in primary care clinics or rural outposts while foreign doctors continued to work in the hospitals.

In other statements, Fisher expressed doubts about the ability of Al-Khameri to provide broad academic leadership to the medical faculty. He referred negatively to the dean's earlier experience in founding the Sudanese medical school; this marked him, he said, as an educator with a shallow commitment to clinical excellence and the advance of biomedical knowledge. He predicted that, with these limitations, the dean would find it impossible to attract top-notch faculty from North America and the United Kingdom.

By the time the first class was admitted, a well-qualified core faculty had been recruited, composed predominantly of North American, British, and European medical specialists and basic scientists who had been selected from many hundreds of applicants. Contrary to Fisher's predictions, Al-Khameri was able to launch the enterprise. After two years, however, the dean resigned to take a post with an international health organization dedicated to promoting primary care in developing nations. He was replaced by an Irish anesthesiologist who, along with stress on high academic standards, wanted to build up emergency medicine in the medical school's two teaching hospitals.

Priorities in faculty recruitment and the thrust of decisions in key committees, such as the curriculum committee, strongly favored "biomedical excellence" over a more innovative social–community orientation for the new school. The interviewing of faculty prospects and subsequent recruitment proceeded slowly for the "social" fields of community medicine, family practice, behavioral science, and primary care, by comparison with "hard science" fields such as pharmacology, physiology, surgery, and nuclear medicine. This meant that the socially oriented fields of medicine lacked representatives to articulate their mission in the medical faculty during the school's formative years.

The Faculty–Student Gap

The vulnerable position of the social–community side of medical education at UAE University was due, I felt, to lack of support for it in the medical faculty leadership, especially after the departure of the founding dean. Another factor even more basic, however, leads to the same result: the fact that the faculty was over 90 percent expatriate. Many of the faculty members had taught in many different countries. They were employed on two-year renewable contracts and did not expect to settle indefinitely in the United Arab Emirates; further, the government makes it virtually impossible for any expatriate worker ever to obtain citizenship.

As cosmopolitans, many of the faculty were at home everywhere and yet nowhere. They did not know the culture and health situation of the UAE citizens. They were brought into the nation strictly for their biomedical expertise, not on the basis of their knowledge or concern for UAE people. Very few faculty members could speak Arabic.

The "faculty strangeness" factor, repeated many times over in Third World medical schools, introduces into the teaching–learning situation a cultural dimension that has been understandably absent in sociological studies of medical education in the United States. Whatever the survival anxieties of students and the expectations of faculty for student performance, students and faculty in the United States are cushioned by a common environing culture. In the United Arab Emirates there was, instead of a cushion, an uncomfortable gap. I had found a similar gap in two earlier studies of student–faculty relationships in a Saudi medical school (Gallagher 1985, 1988).

The logic of curriculum planning cannot deal with factors such as this. The curriculum planners set the general standards for student performance; they count, implicitly, on admitting students who are bright enough and eager enough to invest themselves successfully in the prescribed learning tasks. The students have a great stake but no say in laying out the curriculum. Their voice is silent because they do not know much about what a person should learn in order to qualify as a physician. Nevertheless, even at an early learning stage of their career, they have impressions of what will be expected of them in medical education and, beyond that, aspirations and ambitions for their own careers.

I decided to probe the thinking of the students in these directions. I was particularly interested in the question of how they perceived the issue of academic excellence vis-à-vis socially oriented medical education. As I indicated above, the drive for academic excellence arises partly from the situation of the faculty being expatriate, with no grasp of the culture or health care needs of the United Arab Emirates. The students, as UAE nationals, might have a stronger drive toward a socially oriented curriculum, as well as practical ideas about how to implement it. Further, although there is no direct mechanism by means of which students' aspirations can affect the learning requirements of the curriculum, there might be channels for this in the long run, as I explain below.

I gathered data relevant to students' aspirations through the medium of students' responses to the question "Why do I want to be doctor," which I put to them as an exercise in English writing. This question was far from new to them; they had earlier, in applying for admission, dealt with it. In varying degrees of conscious preoccupation, their concern with it remained as they moved through the curriculum.

The reason I believe the students' attitudes toward their prospective careers in medicine are relevant to the future functioning of the medical school lies in the following considerations. The first generation of UAE medical students—the first four or five classes—were destined to provide a major component of the faculty ranks once their medical training, including specialty training, was complete. The virtual inevitability of their recruitment into teaching lay in the widely proclaimed goal of "emirization" of the UAE work force—replacing the expatriates with qualified UAE nationals (*Emirati*). This goal was particularly critical for high-prestige occupations such as airline pilot, petroleum geologist, practicing physician, and medical school faculty member.

In analyzing the students' responses, I found that four themes occurred frequently. I present them below with illustrative quotations (I have allowed the sometimes awkward English phrasing to remain intact). These responses show what was in the minds and feelings of the UAE students about their medical futures; they illuminate the issues my research dealt with.

Learning Medicine to Help an Ill Family Member

It is by no means unknown for medical students in West to offer this as an impelling reason to study medicine. Given the strength of the family system throughout the Arab world, however, this reason probably crops up more frequently among Arab students than those in the West.

(STUDENT A, MALE): All my family tried to prevent me when I was choosing this college. But I was doing what I want. . . . The biggest reason is to help my brother who has mental disease. I'll help my brother when I graduate. Something's wrong with his behavior, for example, he don't like to contact his wife or other ladies. A lot of people, his wife, secretary, friends, hope to understand what he want or mean, but they can't.

(STUDENT B, FEMALE): Medicine was a dream of my childhood. As I grown up my dream grew with me. I insisted more and more to be a doctor when my father needed a kidney transplantation and did it twice, which makes me take a decision to be a surgeon especially a nephrologist. [Note: This student is not yet aware that nephrology is a branch of internal medicine rather than surgery.] Nobody in my family ever encourage me to study this field because they thought and some of them still thinking that it is difficult and long for a woman to study medicine. In addition that she is probably not going to marry—if she wants to be a doctor, she has to choose between a husband and a career. Now I think that some of . . . my family begin to accept that I will be a good doctor in the future because my level was A in the previous semester, and some of them already begin to call me Dr. Zainab. But I'm still the only person who is responsible about her own decision, and it is a real challenge between my community and my family on one side and me on the other side.

In view of the vicissitudes of medical careers, it may be that relatively few of the students who start out with the "family-helping" motive will actually move into a position that enables them to fulfill this ambition. That does not, however, diminish its importance as an initial attractor.

It is interesting to compare this motivation with the educational philosophy that places primary care and social objectives at the center of health service provision and education. If we take the aspirations of the foregoing students literally, it would appear that they wanted specialized care rather than primary care for their relatives, who were notably ill or disabled. I mention this not to discredit the primary care-oriented philosophy education but to indicate that it is not much on the minds of students who have a personal, family-based motivation for studying medicine. This suggests the difficulty of promoting primary care and socially oriented medicine: patients and relatives of patients (including medical students) want "the best" treatment—the most focused, intensive, and specialized attention. The rationale for primary care can, however, be found elsewhere, as is shown below.

Demonstrating Female Ability

This theme applies only to female students. Whatever their intrinsic interest in medicine, many female students wanted to prove that they were as capable as male students and as other women who were already doctors. The following excerpts make the point.

(STUDENT C, FEMALE): I want to become a doctor because four of my sisters are doctors, and I am not less than them.

(STUDENT D, FEMALE): I want to be a doctor, I want to be something special in my family. . . . I don't forget forever my cousin looking askance at me when I told him I want to be a doctor.

(STUDENT E, FEMALE): When I complete 17 years old I promised myself to work hard to be a doctor. I'm always think about that day when I will wear a white dress and cure people. I will of course happy when I will change their sadness to happiness. I want people to know how can woman realization her hopes.

(STUDENT F, FEMALE): I want to be a good doctor to confirm that woman can learn with high efficiency like a man. Some time in our community people think that woman cannot treat people like a man so when they see a lot of clever woman who practice medicine they will change their mind.

Interpretation of the foregoing responses must be tempered by the realization that medicine is one of the few occupations open to women in conservative Arab societies. This narrowness of choice may mean that some of the female students were more concerned with proving themselves academically than they were specifically interested in medicine.

This motivation on the part of the female students can be viewed as a refinement on the earlier discussion of goals for the medical school. As I said, an important goal was to prove that a developing society such as the United Arab Emirates or Saudi Arabia can produce doctors of international caliber from their indigenous population—an "I'll prove I can do it" compulsion that exists in virtual independence of the fact that medicine is a socially useful vocation. The female students were offering a gender-specific version of this compulsion that put their gender first, but I suspect that they also harbored the sentiment that "we as UAE nationals will prove we can do it."

The fierce, openly expressed determination of the female students to meet the challenges of medical education had a strong implication for the administration and operation of the medical school, namely, that the women accepted full equality with the male students in the demands of the curriculum and examinations and expected to receive fully equal learning opportunities. The female students were quick to complain to the dean about any shortcomings in their domain, for example, books and journals that they had learned were available in the men's library but not in their own.

Female Doctors for Female Patients

Like the preceding, this theme is expressed only in the statements of the female students. The issue of whether women are capable of becoming doctors is not at stake here; instead, the issue here is the need or preference of female patients for female doctors.

(STUDENT G, FEMALE): Another point is I feel that as I am a Muslim lady my responsibility to become a doctor is much greater because in our country ladies need a lady doctor to examine them due to our cultural and religious instructions.

(STUDENT H, FEMALE): In Islam it is not allowed for women to be examined by male doctor except in serious cases. I like to help those ladies who has to be examine by male physicians because there are not female doctors in the same specialty.

(STUDENT I, FEMALE): I will treat those women who refuse to be treated with a man doctor, where they cannot talk with him freely as if they are talking to a woman like them.

The precepts of Islam concerning female patients seeing male physicians are far less definitive than, for example, the injunctions against pork and alcohol. It is common, however, in Islamic countries to hear conservative interpretations advanced as if they were universally accepted dogma.

Whatever the predilections and inhibitions of individual female patients, there can be no doubt that the availability of female physicians will transform the medical care situation in the United Arab Emirates. Those female students who stressed their desire to treat female patients are at the leading edge of this transformation. It goes beyond the simple replacement of male by female physicians for female patients; it also points to the probability that, in times past, some women shied away from treatment because they did not want to see a male physician—or because no physicians of either sex were available. Within a larger picture, this transformation in medical care is related to the fact that the more abundant provision of medical care is part of the general transformation of the society. Yet in certain areas, such as the availability of female doctors for female patients, the transformation will recognize and reinforce traditional preferences and values.

Emirization of Health Care

This theme showed up very frequently in the array of student responses. Here are four expressions of it.

(STUDENT J, MALE): Our country needs doctors in every specialist because there is not too many citizen doctors in it, so that the least things that we can introduce it to our country is medicine. . . . I will treat all the people without differentiating between them. . . Also I will try as I can to help our community by the health education.

(STUDENT K, MALE): My country trying to develop itself in order to reach a good level in which it can be compared with highly progressed countries. I think that medicine is a good field which may push my country forward.

(STUDENT L, FEMALE): What influenced me to enter this school? It was because I wanted to be that human being that could help a lot of people. I thought that I can understand and help our local people more than unlocal doctors.

(STUDENT M, FEMALE): Maybe we have good doctors in the hospitals but this is not going to last forever. One day will come and all of them or some of them will go back to their home country. No matter they are loyal to the host country but it is an accepted fact that nobody can be as loyal as the sons and daughters of the country.

It is notable that many of the student responses, including those above, referred to communication gaps between physicians in UAE health centers, hospitals, and private practice offices, and the UAE patients. Probably not more than 2 to 3 percent of the practicing physicians currently in the United Arab Emirates (I am not referring here to those on the medical faculty) are UAE nationals. Of the other 97 to 98 percent, some are from Arabic-speaking regions—the Sudan, Egypt, Jordan, and the West Bank. They can understand the patients, though even then there are important Arabic dialect differences. Most of the expatriate physicians, however, come from India and Pakistan, and a few from Europe and North America. None of the expatriate doctors understands enough Arabic to deal with UAE patients without the mediation of institutional interpreters. Reports abound—and there have been some complaints—about the distortions introduced into diagnosis and treatment by these mediators.

It is this situation that the students have in mind: by becoming doctors, they will improve the communicative access to medical care of their fellow citizens. This theme clearly goes beyond the "let's prove we can do it" motivation for studying medicine, for here the students are intent on being useful to patients through being culturally similar to them—in addition, of course, to the overt activity of providing medical treatment.

Some of the "emirization" responses hold a broader idea: that improved health status of the populace is part of national development or of becoming "modern." Their responses also suggest a quasi-political role for the citizen doctor: he or she will be better able than an expatriate doctor to educate and motivate citizen patients toward a higher level of health awareness and health behavior (several of the male students mentioned to me that they wanted to eradicate the widespread use of tobacco, and they deplored that several members of the UAE national football team were heavy cigarette smokers). In other words, indigenous medical leadership can contribute to the health progress of the society.

Earlier I noted that the students, in their career aspiration of treating ill members of their own family, were looking toward specialized medical care. These "emirization" responses show a revealing contrast to that. In their thinking about a role for themselves in relation to their compatriots, the students are strongly oriented toward health education, health promotion, the prevention of illness and dysfunction—close indeed to the aspirations of the WHO HFA/2000 program.

Conclusion

In many developing countries, both medical education and biomedically based health care are, on a broad scale, relatively new phenomena. Both accelerate the collective definition and consciousness of a society as "modern." They signal new, nontraditional ways of meeting health care needs and of training practitioners for this function.

Thus students who undergo medical training, like students in other fields of higher education, are personal carriers of knowledge and technique that kindle the expectations of the populace for effective, sophisticated treatment of their ills. The actual burden of illness in developing societies, however, lies heavily on the side of infectious disease and conditions that are largely preventable or—short of prevention—manageable with relatively simple, community-based medical resources. This realization is incorporated into the thinking of WHO in its promulgation of HFA/2000. HFA/2000 rationally attempts to produce health resources attuned to population needs. Therefore, however, a tension arises within the sphere of medical education (and health professional education more generally) between the heavily science-oriented curriculum that has become the norm in industrialized societies and a curriculum that would have greater immediacy for the health problems of developing countries.

Another element that places pressure upon medical education in developing societies is the fact that new medical graduates can be immediately absorbed into the typically understaffed, slender base of national health personnel. Indeed, there is the need, and the opportunity, for the whole apparatus of medical education—teaching hospitals, ambulatory clinics, laboratories—to become a major component in the totality of health care delivery, to a greater extent than it is in industrialized societies.

A further, strategically significant nuance is given to this study in the fact that the medical school examined was located in a wealthy Arab country that has chosen to invest a goodly portion of its oil revenues into medical education. The United Arab Emirates at present employs many foreign physicians. If health care were seen as purely a rational activity driven by utilitarian needs, as in HFA/2000, then it might be difficult to attract young UAE nationals into the long course of medical studies. Under that mandate, the United Arab Emirates would be content to continue its exclusive reliance upon expatriate physicians. In contrast with that view, my data suggest that the students are drawn to medical study by the prospect of being in the vanguard of national doctors trained to international standards by a cosmopolitan, expatriate faculty.

At the same time, the students are motivated by the prospect of being of service in assuring the good health status of their fellow citizens; they are probably ambivalent about providing medical services for the many foreigners present in the United Arab Emirates. These foreigners are more needed than wanted; yet there is at present ample provision for their health care as part of their total employment contract.

Sociologists who have studied medical education in the United States have been alert to the many-sidedness of students' aspirations and expectations (Bloom 1971). Students anticipate that high prestige and a good income will be theirs one day, but they know it will take effort. They relish the monetary and status rewards that go with medicine, but they also value the appreciation that patients can give them, and they do want to help patients as much as possible, not simply to make masterful diagnoses. Medical students in developing societies also have diverse, sometimes competing motivations such as these. In addition, the students are caught up in the cultural complexity of development, which has an impact on medical education as well as many other aspects of society.

NOTE

Acknowledgments: I thank Nabil Banna, Peter Grantham, Bashir Hamad, Iain Ledingham, Khalil Qayed, and John Wales for their engaging discussions and interpretations of events in the Faculty of Medicine and Health Sciences at United Arab Emirates University. I thank the medical students there for their youthful wisdom and their gracious tolerance of me and other faculty in the growing pains of a new institution. I thank Jack Bryant for his energetic vision of health care futures in developing societies. I thank Peter Conrad, Joan Ferrante, Fred Hafferty, and Phil Moody for their astute, thorough critiques of earlier drafts of this manuscript.

REFERENCES

Bloom, Samuel W. 1971."The Medical School as a Social System." *Milbank Memorial Fund Quarterly* 49, Part 2 (April).
Directory of Medical Schools Worldwide, 4th ed. 1987. Miami: U.S. Directory Service.
Frankenberg, Ronald, and Joyce Leeson. 1974. "The Sociology of Health Dilemmas in the Post-colonial World: Intermediate Technology and Medical Care in Zambia, Zaire, and China." In *Sociology and Development*, ed. Emanuel De Kadt and Gavin Williams, 255–78. London: Tavistock.
Gallagher, Eugene B. 1985. "Medical Education in Saudi Arabia: A Sociological Perspective on Modernization and Language." *Journal of Asian and African Studies* 20(1/2):1–12.

————. 1988. "Convergence or Divergence in Third World Medical Education? An Arab Study." *Journal of Health and Social Behavior* 29(4): 385–400.

Kindig, David A., and Charles M. Taylor. 1985. "Growth in the International Physician Supply." *Journal of the American Medical Association* 253(21): 3129–32.

Rathgeber, Eva M. 1985. "Cultural Production in Kenyan Medical Education." *Comparative Education Review* 29(3): 299–316.

United Emirates University. 1986. "An Analysis of and Recommendations for the Current Planning of the Faculty of Medicine." Unpublished memorandum. Al-Ain, U.A.E.

World Bank. 1990. *World Development Report 1990—Poverty.* New York: Oxford University Press.

World Health Organization (WHO). 1981. *Global Strategy for Health for All by the Year 2000.* "Health for All" Series, no. 3. Geneva: WHO.

Chapter 8

Family Care Work and Duty in a "Modern" Chinese Hospital

JOSEPH W. SCHNEIDER

From December 1986 through early April 1987, I did fieldwork at a hospital in a north China city where I lived and taught sociology. I proposed to the Chinese authorities that I examine how Chinese family members and friends contribute to the work of caring for patients in the hospital (see Strauss et al. 1985). My own experience as a son whose father recently had died after a long illness, my research on the experience of people with chronic illness (Schneider and Conrad 1983; Schneider 1988), and the stories I had heard in China about how much care work Chinese family members do in the hospital made the question both personally and professionally interesting.[1]

Although I thought my research was politically "safe," that is, it did not seem to touch topics sensitive that the government might consider I nevertheless anticipated difficulty in gaining access (cf. Wolf 1985). After all, I was a foreigner wanting to observe and write something about modern Chinese life. I told officials that I wanted to describe sociologically (scientifically) and not to criticize Chinese practices or people, and that perhaps we Westerners could see our own high-technology, highly professionalized, and often impersonal system of health care delivery in a critically helpful light as a result of my research; that "the Chinese" may indeed have something to teach "us" in these matters.

As I began to see the officials endorse and repeat the characterizations of my work as "scientific," I appreciated as never before the legitimating power of this discourse in the face of skepticism about motives and ends. Although subsequently I would applaud the deconstruction of scientific realism and epistemology back home, I saw that I was again using it uncritically to get what I wanted—access—and to assure my audience of my "objective" methods and "progressive" ends. Yet I knew how easy it would be to critique what I might see; how what I would write as nonevaluative description easily could be read as (that is, could be) highly critical. Moreover, because I had decided to privilege the perspective of family members, it would be easy to sympathize with them— to "take sides"—and thus no doubt run afoul of various official or policy perspectives in the hospital and elsewhere. Although I could perhaps use the current renewed Chinese faith in science (see Goldman and Simon 1989; Anderson 1990) and "facts" to get in, questions of the authority and power of my own voice would have to be managed each time I began to write (Schneider 1991; Fabian 1990; Clifford 1983a). And I could enter only with the endorsement of those in positions of power—hospital leaders and doctors—yet I would try to tell a story about the work and care that family members give. What posture would I effect (then and now)?

Obviously, these dilemmas have not kept me from writing; and since they are so fundamental to the practice of modern social science and, I think, unsolvable within its confines, it seems better to make them explicit in this writing, critiquing and perhaps abandoning some of these conventions rather than abandoning the writing itself. Accordingly, in what follows I use conventional practices of ethnographic reportage to create realist scenes ("I/eye was there and I/eye am reporting the facts"; and note the opening sentence of this chapter; see also Kondo 1990, 7–9) about care work in the hospital, along with self-reflexive commentary that seeks to point to my own presence both in the story the text tells as well as in the construction of the text as vehicle for that (still quite modern) story.

First, I describe the hospital I visited—invoking "the field"—and the kinds of work family members and hospital staff did around their patients. I proceed then to organize segments of conversations (interviews) and observations I made—data—into a story about how, in doing the work of giving care, these family members took up positions in a complex web of often contradictory and always power-saturated discourses that characterize urban China in the late twentieth century.[2] Sometimes I saw these family members as victims of power; at other times they seemed to be skillful wielders of power, yet usually to defend themselves and their patients against what they saw to be much greater forces inclined not to operate in their interests.

At the Hospital

Over the course of four and a half months I visited three hospitals, but I went most often to the critical care unit (CCU) of one five-hundred-bed general hospital. Officials told me this CCU was "one of the best" of its kind in all of north China and that it had received many foreign visitors. Because only Western medicine was practiced in this unit, I took this to mean it was offered to foreigners, and to me, as an example of China's progress in "modern medical care" (see Henderson 1989).

My first visit was in the company of a doctor–official from the public health bureau, who introduced me to the unit's leaders and displayed the necessary certified papers showing who was responsible for the decision to give me this access. After I explained my interests and research procedures, the leaders invited me to "come any time" and "see whatever you like." I quoted them to myself several times during the course of my visits, when I was unsure about whether or not to move into certain spaces.

In my proposal, I had offered to provide an interpreter to accompany me. Bureau leaders were hesitant to allow an "outsider" whom I would choose, and they found it difficult to secure a bureau person who had the time and English skills. After two visits with a bureau-supplied interpreter, I began to go to the unit by myself.[3] As a result, I suffered not understanding most of the conversations overheard and was unable to converse with most of the patients and their *peiban*[4]—people, mostly family members, who accompany the patient, most of whom could not speak English. Yet, because such an interpreter–official likely would have further constrained the conversations I hoped to have, I felt the loss was also a gain of sorts. I would rely on my own observation and those conversations I could have in English, supplemented by any information I could gain by asking simple questions in Chinese. I also spoke to many English-speaking Chinese not connected to the hospital but whose experience of their own hospital caregiving was informative. (In short, I'm not making this up. Am I?)

Posted visiting hours in the unit were from 4:00 to 7:30 P.M., Monday, Wednesday, Friday, and Saturday. Doctors told me that family members and friends who wished to visit at other times were required to obtain a *peiban zheng* or visitor's card from the head nurse, who would write on the card the reason for the visit, such as to bring the patient "delicious food" or to "serve the patient." This discourse of modern medical administration to the contrary, it seemed that at almost any time of the day or night there were some *peiban* on the unit. This was perhaps the first of several contradictions between what I was told and what I thought I could see.

The CCU consisted of the first floor of a two-story wing at the hospital, a building probably dating from the early 1950s. Patient and staff rooms of various sizes opened from either side of a single, long corridor. The largest ward was called the "monitor room." It had nine beds reserved for the most critically ill patients. Moveable fabric screens separated the beds, and one end of the room had storage cabinets and several wooden desks pushed together as a place for doctors and nurses to sit and write. Two smaller rooms, one ten-bed unit for women and a six-bed unit for men, were called "convalescent wards" and often received patients from the monitor room, as well as from outside the unit. Two additional rooms housing various machines and equipment were reserved for treatment. The doctors' room, nurses' station, unit director's office, and washroom and toilet were on the facing side of the corridor. Often two or three additional patient beds were placed against one wall in the corridor, along with cabinets, equipment, oxygen tanks, and carts.

I spent most of my time in the monitor room, standing along the wall near the door or sitting at the desk. There I could strike up quiet conversations with doctors as they sat and wrote in charts or chatted. I also had a full view of the room, the patients, and the *peiban*. I recall fancying that I was somehow less visible in those spots (the "fly on the wall" fantasy of the powerful, unnoticed gaze), although in fact, such practices located me quite visibly "with" the doctors in that space. I was thankful for my conjured sense of the "witness" of those moments at a time when I felt quite alone (the "heroic" white man holding forth under difficult conditions in the exotic place? I/eye *was* there!).

I made a few visits to an obstetrics ward and an internal medicine ward at two other hospitals, always in the company of a public health bureau or hospital official. One of these hospitals was new and both were larger than the one containing the CCU. In neither case did I have the same freedom to move and look around as I did on the CCU.

Caregiving Labor: Something *Peiban* "Like to Do"
because "Doctors and Nurses are Few"

As a bourgeois Western sociologist familiar with the complex specialization and control of work common to U.S. hospitals, I was immediately struck by all of the physical labor family members were doing in the CCU. This was notable in contrast to the considerably more constrained repertoire of activities for their U.S. counterparts in similar circumstances. I noticed a lot of washing and cleaning, bringing and taking— work that seemed, for its ordinariness, largely unnoticed by most Chinese eyes, but that I wanted to see as a display of deeply felt duty.

Washing and Cleaning

Emblematic of this physical work was a young woman I noted, perhaps a daughter, who, having served supper to an older woman in the convalescent ward, went out into the hall, returned with a large steaming mop, and began cleaning the floor around the woman's bed. None of the *peiban* or patients took much notice of her, but I did. As she finished the floor near her patient's bed, she proceeded to mop under and around the bed of the patient nearby, with *peiban* for that woman helpfully moving stools and shoes out of the way. Before finishing, she had mopped all of the central floor space in the ward. I saw similar mopping by both men and women *peiban* in this ward and in the monitor room. In the two specific cases where I could take note, there seemed to have been nothing spilled on the floor to occasion the mopping. Nurses and doctors were regularly in and out of the room, and they seemed to take no note of this work. Rather, it was simply another project in the evening round of bringing food, serving it, conversing, washing the supper cups and bowls, packing these away to be taken home, changing the sheets, and ministering to the patient—all proper practice for *peiban*.

Bringing and Taking

Some of what was brought and taken included the patient's "favorite food" from home; soiled bedpans and urinals; thermoses of boiled water; supplies of medicine and materials from outside the hospital; large and heavy oxygen tanks, put next to a patient's bed; doctor-written orders for lab tests on the *peiban*'s particular patient, delivered to the appropriate offices; and even patients themselves, taken to other departments in the hospital. An immense amount of work was done by people who were not part of the official hospital work force, on tasks that in the United States usually were done by employees.[5] I was deeply impressed by what I read as "the Chinese sense of family duty." Being part of and contributing to my own family and being able to care for my father had been so important to me (and no doubt still was/is).

After noticing a patient's wife bring an X-ray film into the ward for a doctor to examine, I asked the doctor why she, rather than a hospital worker, had brought it. He said that she had gone to another department and gotten it. "Is this something that *peiban* often do?" I asked. He said, "Yes, family members like to do this kind of thing, and sometimes the doctor and nurse are too few and cannot take time to get these things."[6]

Peiban sometimes carried doctor-written requests for lab work to another part of the hospital. One night I watched as one doctor filled out such a form and gave it to a man whose young sister had just been admitted. After the man left, I asked this doctor and another sitting nearby, whose English was a bit better, "These forms. You gave that man three of them. What are they and where is he taking them?" Together they offered the following:

> Maybe observe this at night. Two labs, one outpatient and one inpatient. All doctors use outpatient lab at night because inpatient lab closed. *Peiban* take to outpatient department and this

would probably cause technician to come to patient and get samples and take back to laboratory. Sometimes *peiban* go to lab to get result back. Or, doctor may call. If doctor and *peiban* do nothing, maybe tomorrow lab will send.

Although one senior doctor told me that *peiban* were definitely not allowed to get lab reports and bring them back to the ward—according to "modern" hospital administrative procedures—there seemed to be a good deal of energy given over to this kind of expediting work. As the doctors quoted above implied, it was not so much that the lab would not come to do the tests or would fail to send the results. Rather, *peiban*, doctors, and nurses alike saw this kind of taking and bringing work as expeditious and sensible—as normal—for family members to do. What otherwise might take three days could be accomplished in one or two. Besides, "They like to do this kind of thing," said the doctor, something I willingly heard as confirming my sense of "the Chinese sense of duty," as well as "good sense."

Similarly, if a patient was to be taken to another hospital for a special test, the work of contacting that hospital, making an appointment, and arranging transportation by means of some work unit's car all might be taken over by a family member. I spoke to one man who had done this for his father:

> The doctor here suggest to us that you should have an exam for your patient . . . CT—do you know? (Yes.) But if you want to have, you must contact with that other hospital by yourself. (How?) My brother-in-law have a classmate who work at CT department there . . . so my father went very soon. Otherwise, you wait a long time because there are so many people need and so few hospitals—only two—that have that equipment. It is often broke down and the technicians can't repair it. Perhaps some of that machines are imported from America. ((We share a laugh.))

Although not officially responsible for making these arrangements, neither this son nor the doctors could be sure just how long it otherwise might take. To rely on much slower institutional channels and the people whose job it was to activate them would be considered, I think by all parties (even by me), both foolish and lazy—falling short both of common sense and proper filial duty. Besides, "Family members like to do this kind of thing, and sometimes the doctor and nurse are too few and cannot take time" to do it, the doctor said. Yes, yes, I thought. This is precisely what it means to be a "good" family member. (I liked to think of myself as a good family member.)

One man in his early thirties described how he got the peritoneal dialysis fluid used in his father's care. We had been discussing the intravenous (IV) drip going into his father's stomach as we stood near the bed. Because I had heard other *peiban* describe how they went outside the hospital to get scarce medicines, I asked him how he got this fluid. Our conversation went on like this:

HE: Yes, I go to medicine box . . .

I: What do you mean, "medicine box," what is that?

HE: At the factory, not far from here . . .

I: Wait. You mean you go to a factory to get this medicine yourself?

HE: Yes, it is not far from here. This kind of medicine all people here go get themselves. The other kind of medicine the doctor has to give.

I: How much do you get at one time?

HE: Three yuan, two jiao a bag. Each time [father] must use two bags. One day, four times. He uses eight bags a day.

I: How many bags do you buy at one time?

HE: There are ten bags in a box. At one time I buy twenty boxes.

I: You buy twenty boxes?! Do you have to take a bicycle?

HE: ((Smiling)) No, my father's factory provides a vehicle . . . what shall I say, a simple truck.

I: And a driver?

HE: Yes, a driver, and he helps me bring the medicine here to the hospital.

I: Where do you put the medicine when you bring it here?

HE: Outside. . . . I am going to use a long sentence now. When there is a flat and it is second or third floor, outside there is sometimes a place ((makes motions with his hands)) . . . what is it called?

I: Balcony? A balcony?

HE: Balcony, yes. There is in the third building a balcony and I put the medicine there. Other people put their medicine there too.

I: So, each time you need the medicine you go there, four times a day?

HE: Oh, no. I put some boxes under the bed, three boxes under the bed here. When it is time for the medicine, I give it to the nurse.

Each time I read this dialogue, I am tempted to modify it so that I don't appear so naive, so impressed by his explanation, such a "straight man" for his account. This underlines for me both the distance between and the closeness of their and my experiences and, more generally, of the Western bourgeois social scientist in the "exotic" place. It also points to my (our) presence "there" as an occasion for such accounts and performances (cf. Clifford 1983b) and thus confounds simple notions of social scientists gaining entrée and "trust" as vehicles toward making "valid" characterizations of "the setting." And, as is now widely appreciated, this passage helps us see how such data are jointly produced.

Ministering and Monitoring

Another kind of work seemed to demand greater judgment and decision-making, such as in watching the patient, noting his or her condition, and reporting same to hospital staff. It revolved mostly around (IV) drops, routine reports of fluids taken in and passed, temperature readings, foods eaten, frequency and volume of bowel movements, and the operation of various machines attached to patients.

Late one cold January afternoon as I sat in the monitor room, a sixty-five to seventy-year-old man was brought from surgery, where he had been operated on that morning for pancreatic cancer. After a few minutes I asked a doctor about his condition. He said, "He is jaundiced, in shock, has lost a lot of blood, and has respiratory failure." Over the next hour, *peiban* did a good deal of ministering and monitoring work around this patient. Here are some notes—again, here set off as data—that I made as I watched:

A middle-aged woman, not a nurse, comes in, slightly breathless, and unlatches the other swinging door and props both doors open. Slowly, a bed is wheeled to the center of the room—there is very little space here—pushed and surrounded by eight or nine people. I assume they are family members. They are accompanied by two doctors in blue surgical clothes. Two of the *peiban* are carrying, and holding high, IV bottles, one with blood and another with a clear solution. As doctors and nurses begin to attach the patient to machines and put the IV bottles on stands, the relatives cluster around the bed, their attention focused on the man and the doctors and nurses. I am standing a foot or two below the end of the bed when a nurse comes in and seems to ask most of the *peiban* to go back out into the hallway, leaving three people beside the bed. I'm still there too. The middle-aged woman and a man are on either side, crouched on the floor, each with one hand on the patient's knee and the other holding down a hand. As the patient tries to move his legs, these family members—children?—push the legs back down straight. They look haggard and worried. The man lets go of the knee and hand to check the blood drip going into the patient's wrist. He flicks the IV line with his fingers. Another *peiban* comes in from the hallway and they both examine the bottle and tube. One adjusts the valve and looks closely at it. Apparently not satisfied, he says something to the nurse, who has calmly noticed him doing this.

She turns, examines the valve, adjusts it and goes back to her work. I can see the other drip is connected to the man's right ankle as the woman moves the blankets to examine the place where the needle is placed. Every few minutes one or two of the other *peiban* in the hallway come in, stand for a moment at the foot of the bed, say something to the woman or man there, and then go out.

Another patient in the monitor room, a young man in his late twenties or early thirties who had suffered brain damage in a truck accident, was in a coma and tended to regularly by his sister. She seemed to be in the ward every time I visited, over the course of one month. The doctors told me her brother had been in the hospital three months, all together. He had had a tracheotomy and was fed through a tube inserted in his nose. Another quote from my detailed notes (these really are data):

Patient 9's sister comes in and goes to the bed. She pulls the covers back, lifts the man's left and then right arm up, and pushes the blanket up under his armpits. She touches the back of her hand against the man's cheek and looks down at him, steps away from the bed to a small stand at the head of the bed, and appears to be pouring something that looks like honey into a cup, followed by some white liquid, mixing the two. Then dry powder goes in; more mixing. She puts this down and takes the thermos out into the hall, returning moments later. She pours some of this water into a basin, testing it with her hand and on her own face, puts in a cloth, squeezes it out and proceeds to wipe the man's face, hands, forehead, neck, holding the tube that goes into his stomach through his nose carefully to one side. She resticks the tape against his upper lip, rearranges the gauze pad covering the opening, and then takes a large syringe from the stand and draws some of the mixture into it. She connects the end of the syringe to the tube and pushes the plunger to empty the syringe. She repeats this two to three times until the mixture is gone.

Finally, I watched one evening as a middle-aged son repeatedly re-attached a ventilator connection taped over his father's mouth. Each time the son would have the tube in place, the father would pull it out. This went on for twenty minutes before I left. The son looked very tired. I, too, felt tired and wondered how long it could continue, imagining his anguish out of my own from past care enforced against a father's will.

The Burden of Duty and the Opportunities of Care

Family members were often called upon by doctors to sign permission forms for emergency procedures, tests, or surgery—to be, in short, the "person responsible." When I asked three doctors on the unit, "What is the most important thing *peiban* do for their family members?" they all said, "To sign permission forms," especially for patients who were seriously ill.

I observed such a permission form-signing by a middle-aged man whose father had suffered a cerebral hemorrhage (I thought of my favorite uncle, who died from that) and was having trouble breathing. The doctors decided the patient needed a tracheotomy. I stood at this man's shoulder, outside the closed doors of the monitor room, and watched several doctors and nurses bent over his father. Suddenly, a doctor and nurse turned toward the door and motioned for the man (us?) to come into the room. (Did they want me, too? Oh, no. Of course not.) The nine doctors and nurses who had been around his father's bed gathered around him as one doctor spoke, making a downward thrusting motion with his hands. This talk at the center of the huddle of white coats went on for a few minutes, with the man and doctors talking in turn. They moved to the desk and the son was given a permission form, which, after some hesitation, he signed. He came back out into the hallway and stood near the wall, looking away from the door. He had behaved like a good son, at least in the doctor's script. It perhaps wasn't that clearly so in his own.

But family members' sense of duty was considerably more diffuse than this form-signing coerced by doctors. It seems captured succinctly by a proverb one man cited when I said he was working very hard to care for his father, who suffered from a cardiopulmonary problem. He replied: "There is a saying, if a father lay in bed for a long time, his son not care well for father" (*jiu bing chaung gian wu xiao zi*). I was immediately struck by how unreasonably demanding this seemed; what, after all, was a son expected to be able to do? Quite a great deal, apparently. I couldn't avoid thinking of my own father's long illness and time in bed and the care I gave him. He was, so often, such a long time in bed; but I felt this Chinese wisdom was unreasonable. How could *we* be held responsible?

Another, older man, when discussing the routine practice of *peiban* spending the night beside a patient's bed and the importance of being vigilant, told me the following story passed on to him by another family member on the ward:

> Some *peiban* told me there were two *peiban* here with a patient who was very serious and couldn't breathe. The . . . [he points to his throat] sput . . . (Sputum? Yes, I know) . . . and the *peiban* were sound asleep. The patient died and *the doctor said that if the* peiban *paid more attention, the patient would not die so soon.* If the patient is so serious, like in bed 4, the *peiban* never go to sleep. [my emphasis]

Here are complex moral instructions indeed. They draw on the *peiban*–son's sense of duty and responsibility (felt by him and fully understood by the doctors) and the authority of the doctor in the modern hospital, and they shore up the political and economic conditions of contemporary Chinese urban life. The unasked question seems to be: Who is really responsible for the proper in-hospital care of the patient? Children—perhaps especially sons—are quite familiar with the discourse of filial duty; the proverb offered by the other son specifies the scope of this work. The "doctors" indexed in the story reaffirm the nature of this duty while eliding their own and that of the nurses. The family member's task seems impossible to fulfill; yet acceptable options seem not to exist ("*meiyou banfa*—I have no choice"). Arguing that it is, rather, the doctors, nurses, and hospital who failed the patient would have to be a private discourse, which would be foolish and shortsighted to offer publicly. To ignore the duty would seem an even less available option. Family members thus reaffirmed the traditional discourse, paradoxically shoring up a system of care delivery that they often privately criticized.

Even when a patient was not "so serious," a family member might not sleep. The man who told me this story said his father suffered a gastric ulcer but was "not so serious." A few moments later he said that he routinely spent the night awake at his father's bedside, reading English books. Having heard the prophetic and chilling tale from his fellow *peiban*, I felt I could understand why.

Moreover, there was both cultural and institutional support for sons' and daughters' in-hospital care work. *Danwei*[7]—work units in China—as a matter of policy released sons, daughters, and spouses from their duties at work, usually with full pay for a specified period of time (such as one month), so that they could be at the hospital doing various caregiving tasks. If family caregivers were few, work units also might send fellow workers to the hospital to help care for a patient. Although this could provide needed extra hands, *danwei*-supplied caregivers could bring new burdens. One middle-aged man said he was glad he and his only sister had not accepted the offer from his father's work unit to send "a person to assist us." When I asked him why they had not, he said, "Because that person is not as . . . serious as a family member in care." He added, "Even if some unit person come here, it's that person's job to look after the patient. But also that person feels he does something for the family and so he thinks we should do something [for him or her. . .like] . . . like take him out to eat . . . in a restaurant. So, we don't like that idea."

This reflects an intersection of traditional conceptions of proper family responsibility and good everyday politics; and, from the *danwei*'s side, such policy might be cheaper than paying the additional fees for special nurses. But that these conceptions do not always fit together well is indexed by the family's refusal of help from the father's *danwei*. Here the son invokes the traditional discourse of reciprocal exchange to block what might be seen as good socialist practice. The official discourse and the policy, however, remain relatively intact.

Caregiving needs, quite in contrast to being a burden, could provide a fine opportunity to demonstrate oneself as a suitable candidate for traditional family relationships while, paradoxically, serving the official discourse of "revolutionary humanitarianism" (*geming rendao zhuyi*; see Wang 1986) in the hospital in the face of "too few doctors and nurses." One man and I had the following conversation:

> I: Last night when I left I noticed that there was another man sitting here [by the bed] after you had gone. Who was that?
> HE: That was the boyfriend of my sister.
> I: Oh, really? Why did he come?
> HE: In our society, if a young man see a young girl, if father or mother is ill, that boy or girl must take much care. It is a good chance to express kindness ((chuckles and smiles broadly)).

Moreover, not only was this care work a "good chance" to show oneself as a proper candidate for husband, it was a good chance for anyone to do what might be called "the good person."

As I watched and was impressed by all this effort, I found myself recalling scenes from hospital waiting rooms and corridors back home, scenes that I had come to read as sometimes "contests of character," in which various degrees of sacrifice and selfless work could be displayed among relatives in what seemed almost a competition to display oneself as the son or daughter or grandchild *"closest* to," "caring *most* for," "loving and loved *best* by" the patient. I myself felt ever-so-virtuous in the various caregiving tasks I did for and around my father.

The concern for "face" and the proper display of traditional duties and responsibilities in today's urban China, coupled with the official discourse of scarcity and collective responsibility for "modernization" and the still quite alive remnants of what Gail Henderson (1989) has called the "Maoist model of health care," would seem to render this work a terrain to be sought out and, perhaps, even contested. This might be one way to see, to read, all the extraordinary work these *peiban* did.

Connections and Care

As Mayfair Mei-Hui Yang (1986) has pointed out in her study of *guanxi* in Beijing, establishing, nurturing, and using relationships or connections to solve life's routine but important problems is a kind of work that today is ubiquitous in China. Similarly, problems of allocating and obtaining "scarce resources"—a theme in both official and common discourses— often bring forth discussion of "back doors," *hou men(r)*, as the best way to get whatever is desired.[8] One of the most desired "objects" a family member might obtain for a sick relative is to find a back door that would open into the critical care unit I visited. It could, on the one hand, literally mean the difference between life or death. On the other hand, it could mean the difference between more and less comfortable care. In either case, opening such back doors was an important way to do one's duty as a good son, daughter, or spouse. Standing in those shoes, it seemed to me a very reasonable pursuit; one I could lament, for the effort and groveling it sometimes required, but one I sensed it would be most difficult to ignore (*"meiyou banfa!"*).

Early in my visits to the CCU, I began to understand that many, if not most, of the patients had gained admission in this way. Of course, some patients were admitted because they suffered from the critical care conditions the unit was designed to serve. *Guanxi* and backdoor admissions, however, seemed easily as common. The best—and luckiest— patient was perhaps one who both fit the protocol and had good connections, providing everyone a chance to behave properly: the official discourse of modern medical administration could be invoked, pointing to this patient as exactly the sort of case the unit could serve (good, i.e., "modern" administration and delivery); the doctors could work hard for this (special) patient, invoking the discourse of selfless, perhaps even socialist, medicine (good doctors); the family members could hope, with varying degrees of certainty, that their patient would be given good care by doctors and nurses, at the same time that they could see their own activities as successful and themselves as properly responsible family members (good son/daughter/spouse).

One way *guanxi* operated was when the patient or *peiban* and one of the doctors or nurses had some personal relationship (*pengyou guanxi*). Speaking one afternoon about a newly arrived patient, one doctor said, "He has stroke and myocardial infarction. That patient's relative knows some doctor who work in our ward, so we receive this patient. The patient's relative wants the patient to have better care, so he came here from . . . [another] hospital." Later, when I asked whether all unit doctors and nurses could provide such an avenue into the unit, this doctor said:

> I will say yes, because *we help each other. We have to work together.* We have a rule in the CCU. The doctors' and nurses' direct relatives—father, mother, child, brother, sister—if they are ill, we receive the patient immediately, even though the patient suffers from things like advanced cancer and chronic renal failure. We accept them immediately. Why do we have this rule? *We want to make our doctors and nurses happy. We want to let them feel warm to work here.* [my emphasis]

The connection to a doctor did not have to be quite so direct as family or *gingi guanxi*. One man I spoke to explained his father's access to the unit by saying that his sister was going to marry a young doctor who worked in another department in the hospital. When I asked him if he thought it would have been difficult to gain admission without this contact, he said, "Yes, very difficult. I think many patients are more serious than my father . . . [but] have to stay at the emergency room . . . or not even there. Just give some medicine and told to go home." And, as the prospective husband noted earlier, this doctor could demonstrate his own goodness in this way.

When I heard these stories, I thought how important it would be to make friends with a doctor in China, even to put him or her in your debt, as a kind of insurance. Speaking about one patient, a doctor said:

> This patient was introduced by some of our doctors [as a candidate for admission] because the patient give our doctors some help. Two doctors ask me, two or three times a day, urge me to receive this patient. I thought about it. *This patient helps these doctors* get new houses. If I not receive, these doctors may not be happy. . . . *I want to keep things peaceful and quiet,* so I admit this patient. [my emphasis]

Doctors often explained to me that the unit's scarce renal dialysis resources, for instance, were more wisely used for patients suffering acute renal failure. But, like other displays of the medical administrative discourse, this could be juxtaposed, in a very matter of fact way, with an explanation that this patient, having suffered a cerebral vascular accident (CVA)—what one doctor called patients "waiting to die"—had connections, and the patient was therefore admitted.[9]

Another kind of back door, publicly criticized of late, opens to allow officials—"important people"—entry. A man in his early forties had suffered cardiac arrest that produced brain damage. One doctor told me, "The father of patient is the head of . . . [a city] district. If his father not this kind of man, this patient we not receive in our ward." Another man about sixty-five, who suffered from liver cirrhosis linked to an earlier hepatitis infection, was described to me by another doctor as a "police official" to account for why he was on the ward.

Such connections also could exist between other work units and the critical care facility (cf. Yang 1986, 136–90). Because, for cadres and workers, the *danwei* will inevitably bear some or all of the costs of hospitalization and care,[10] work unit leaders can become rather directly involved in negotiating not only admission to the unit but also continued treatment. If one were an important leader, a loyal and valued worker, or if the unit were somehow liable for the injury or illness, such connection could be invaluable both to the *danwei* and the patient.

One afternoon I sat in the director's office and watched the head of a prospective patient's factory urge the director to admit a man in his thirties with chronic renal failure—a condition not officially treated in the CCU. Not surprisingly, however, work units were interested in striking a balance between proper care and cost. Family members and patients in such situations are often happy to stay in the hospital as long as possible. As one man said, "Because the cost is supported by my father's unit, we are in no hurry to go back home. Here my father get good care and good look after."[11]

If a work unit were responsible for a worker's injury, the expectation seemed to be that they would pay all expenses, including hotel room costs for out-of-own family members and fellow workers who came to give care. One young man had been seriously injured in his work at a factory in another town. His *danwei* leaders seemed to assume responsibility: they came to the unit to encourage the doctors to "save this patient"; otherwise, as one doctor told me, "They would be seriously criticized. They have many accidents there." Not only was the work unit paying for all the care of this patient, who had been there for more than one month, but they also continued to pay his salary; they paid for all his brother's expenses to come to the city where the hospital is located; and they paid the expenses of seven fellow workers who came to share the care work. When I asked this brother how the patient came to the unit, he said, "The . . . [*danwei*] has a connection to this hospital." And in the work unit leaders' view, that this young man's father was the party secretary of the *danwei* could only strengthen their case before the hospital's leaders.

At another hospital I visited, a man had suffered chemical poisoning at work and would never regain consciousness. His unit paid for a private room, for one shift of a private nurse, and for two eight-hour shifts of fellow workers' care at the hospital. He had been a patient there for three years. I asked if his family members—a wife and two children—came to see him often. The nurse said, "Not so much anymore."

Such situations involving work units and costs can put doctors and the hospital in a difficult position relative to the patient and family members. Two doctors said that one of the reasons there is so much trouble between doctors and nurses on the one hand and family members on the other is that whereas work units want to keep care costs down, family members and patients want as much care as they can get. After invoking the supply-and-demand discourse—too few nurses and resources—one doctor said, "The doctor have trouble with patient and with patient work unit director. For example, if patient suffer from some disease, this patient need many money. The patient unit director don't hope do, so this is controversy. If patient spend money, unit must pay this money." Here, the family members may draw fully on both the *danwei*'s responsibility—using the socialist discourse—and on strongly held notions of harmony—the traditional discourse—to try to keep the patient in the hospital. The harmonious image produced by the official discourse that the doctor, nurse, *peiban*, and *danwei* all "work toward the same goal," as one senior doctor said, seemed hard to sustain in the face of these diverse efforts and interests. I doubted that any of the *peiban* I had spoken to would take it seriously as a description of the circumstances of care.

Peiban and Medical Staff: Strains in Managing Care

Contrary to handing over responsibility for care to the specialist or expert, a position that family members in the West might find more familiar, these Chinese sons and daughters were likely to see their relationships to medical staff as requiring complex and crucial management work. I came to see that one should not merely assume that doctors and nurses will do their jobs well and give good care. The assumption in Chinese families seemed to be that if it indeed were a "job," one could count on it not being done well. The outcome of caregiving had to be managed by a range of interactions, offers, and deferences directed toward positively influencing people with authority—doctors, nurses, unit or even hospital leaders.

This, however, is not to say that the doctors whom I met or whom these *peiban* knew had behaved badly or irresponsibly. It is rather to say that the operative assumption—under the circumstances of "scarce resources," the power-infused system of "back doors," and the importance of filial duty—was that without the requisite display of appreciation or "help" to those in power, without very concerted attempts to marshal resources to control the course of events, one's patient's care likely would go badly. This then could weigh very heavily indeed on those who had ignored or failed in this kind of work.

Next to these efforts, my assumption, nurtured in the United States, that such care work is primarily a question of professional training and responsibility, requiring little "intervention" and "connections," has since come to appear more than a little naive. Indeed, it now seems to me ideological, pressing me to think more critically about the discourses that bring that naive subject who still trusts modernism—"me"—into being (Althusser 1971). But I recall that at the time, in that hospital, thinking about those strange assumptions, I stood firmly and uncritically on my Western, bourgeois, modernist "truth," quietly thankful to be "an American" consumer of medical care (even after more than a little experience at seeing it up close and writing about it).

For "them," however, to ingratiate oneself to doctors and nurses was an abiding and serious question. This was explained by a doctor who himself had received such help. I had asked him to translate a question to one *peiban*, asking how he knew when he would be permitted to come into the monitor room after posted visiting hours. The doctor, answering the question himself, said:

You must understand the psychology of the *peiban*. In this ward, *peiban* are forbidden but in other wards they are more. Strictly not allowed in this ward; must stay in hall [outside the unit]. Many *peiban* try many times [to come in]. *If the nurse is kind-hearted*, easy to talk to, *peiban* will try and maybe nurse will criticize or let go in or pretend not to see *peiban* come in. (So, the *peiban* should be sensitive to the nurse's and doctor's idea?) Yes, to clean the floor, to ask if this or that is easy for you, can I buy something for you—if you need movie tickets? There are *many ways maybe to make a doctor happy. There are many things that can help with*, and different things from different people and different occupations. For example, if I want to have heat in my house, they may help with the tube . . . and this kind of thing. Everything. *I am the person here who can help him.* [my emphasis]

With so much emphasis on calculated help-giving and receiving, it was not surprising to hear that "some" doctors and nurses received gifts from patients—although this seemed to be a sensitive subject. It was mentioned in anger by one *peiban*, who criticized one doctor whom he and his family did not like. After saying the doctor was "cold," he added, "And he receives gifts from his patients."[12]

For their part, although doctors and nurses usually acknowledged the importance of *peiban* labor in Chinese hospitals and agreed that they themselves would want their own family members' care in the hospital (the traditional discourse), they felt *peiban* could be a nuisance to their work and even troublesome to the patient (the discourse of modern hospital administration; see Henderson 1989). If a patient were seriously ill and required constant attention, they reasoned, then perhaps it was important to have a family member available most of the time. There simply were not enough nurses and "conditions were poor" (the discourse of a developing country, struggling to "modernize").

One senior doctor at another hospital said, bluntly, "We doctors don't like *peiban* because they interfere with . . . work and some treatment. But patient very like to have family member stay with him." One young nurse said, "Most of the *peiban* do not understand the treatment and care in the hospital and are very worried sometimes and angry when nurse uses treatments. They think that if we use a machine on the patient, the patient be die . . . do not want us to use the machine." Although nurses acknowledged *peiban* labor, they usually were quick to point out that today nurses themselves were able to do all the necessary care work. I asked one young nurse about this. She said that even when she was very busy, she did not like having *peiban* on the ward "because the relative ask the nurse many questions and this take time. Sometimes this kind of condition has a bad influence on the patient." This administrative discourse casts family members as not behaving in the best interests of the patient, necessitating the intervention by the medical staff (whose interests are, of course, with the patient) to curb these negative effects, that is, to restrict and coerce the presence of *peiban* in the hospital. This sounded quite familiar to me.

By considering a hypothetical but, I think, telling account of how doctors might effect this coercion, we can appreciate how the tensions between doctors and *peiban* easily could build. The following comes from a longer conversation about permission form-signing:

DR: The most important thing a relative can do is to sign the paper!

I: What if the relative says no, won't let you do it?

DR: We continue to work until . . .

I: What if the patient says yes and the son says no?

DR: We ask the son, why do you not agree? Is it because of money? We tell him it is not important to worry about the money. We may try to *bring public opinion or family opinion against him*. We may go to other members of the family to try to force him to agree, or, even tell him I will tell his father in the bed that his son won't agree to pay for the treatment we want to do. This public opinion and the opinion of other family members is very important in China. *We don't want criticism*. We might even *go to the unit where the son or daughter works* and say, "*How do you educate your workers?* This son does not want to pay money for a treatment his father needs. You should do better!" This way we try to force the son.

I: What if the patient or the father says no and the son says yes?

DR: That is no problem. We do it. [my emphasis]

"Harmony" can thus be achieved coercively, using diverse discourses in quite artful ways.

Given the above, it is not surprising that doctors and nurses sometimes saw *peiban* as people who might "make trouble" for them of a more consequential kind.[13] They did seem to consider the external resources a controlled, chastened, or disappointed *peiban* could draw on in possible retaliation. For instance, the truck driver–patient who had been injured in an accident in the countryside and suffered brain damage had become a problem for the unit. His condition was medically stable and there were no treatments available, save routine maintenance care. The doctors wanted the patient to leave, but the patient's sister and family members would not agree to a transfer. One of the doctors said:

This patient is give me a headache. He is a driver and there was a car accident . . . in the countryside. . . . During his stay there [in a small county hospital] the patient's condition became worse and worse. He had ARDS syndrome [Acute Respiratory Distress Syndrome], so we received this patient here . . . three months! I would like this patient to go away. He was discharged [once] . . . and went to . . . [another hospital in town] but that hospital refused to accept the patient because they have no special treatment for such a condition. He stayed only at emergency room for three days, then nowhere to go so the relative came back and met me and the head nurse. My opinion was we should receive. The head nurse said we should refuse. *I was afraid the relative would have some quarrel with us if the patient died.* The patient's relative has a lot of trouble with us. The trouble is the accident occurred in the countryside and the patient stayed at [the small hospital]. Came here from there, so [that hospital] refused to receive this patient too. The other side is the [city hospital in patient's hometown]. We want to transfer [patient] to [that] hospital, but *the relative doesn't believe in that hospital. . . . She refuses to transfer.* (Could you just send the patient there, to that city hospital even if the sister says no?) No. *The patient relative must agree with the opinion.* [my emphasis]

I asked this doctor what sort of trouble this sister might be able to cause. He said, "She maybe go to the health bureau or find the hospital president and say that the patient is severely ill but Dr. [his name] refuse to receive the patient. Patient die. I will be criticized." While this doctor here considers his own and the hospital's liability—something familiar in the West—he also gives great attention to *peiban* opinion and refuses to override directly their position (a posture less familiar in the United States).

I heard stories about family members beating doctors when something "went wrong" in their patient's care. Asking direct questions about this usually brought chuckles and asides in Chinese from doctors. During a conversation with three doctors, in which I explained something about malpractice suits and insurance in the United States, one middle-aged doctor quipped, "In our country, relatives always beat the doctor, not sue the doctor." Two doctors I spoke to actually had experienced physical assaults by relatives and patients: one was attacked when a patient died unexpectedly during a delicate cerebral vascular procedure; the other, by a patient and his wife when he worked in the emergency room. Writing in the English-language *China Daily* about a possible shortage of doctors in China, a journalist reported that one reason for a "lack of enthusiasm" for the job was the "lack of necessary legislation to protect medical workers from harassment and even physical assaults by family members all too ready to accuse them of medical malpractice" (Chen 1987).

Nurses, because they were largely responsible for managing *peiban* in the hospital, often were criticized by both *peiban* and doctors. While praising "these nurses here," critics typically connected the presence of *peiban* to "too few nurses." Some family members added that nurses didn't do their work well, that they were "lazy," and that they treated relatives and *peiban* badly. In the strongest explicit condemnation of hospital care and, especially, nurses that I heard, one *peiban* said (the following is a translation):

> The trouble is they play with you in the hospital. They do not provide adequate service, not to say good service, but they play on your anxiety for the comfort of your sick family member by telling you the patient needs a companion and giving you the I.D. card, as if they were bestowing a great favor. In the intensive care unit you're told to go home and take a rest by the head nurse because there are three nurses on duty day and night for eight or six patients, but the minute you're out of the room the nurses demand to know where the family is or tell some other companion to call you because the patient wants to urinate or something. In fact, they're always right and you're always wrong. The nurses never tell you that a seriously ill patient can do without a companion. They won't do the work! What I can't understand is why they can't do their jobs by themselves like everybody else. I believe that if the hospitals provided something like normally decent service, *nobody is such a sucker as to want to stay by a sick bed day and night, going without proper meals and sleep.* There may be such suckers but they certainly are not in the majority. [my emphasis]

Nurses and medical officials were sensitive to such criticism and usually countered it with the modern medical discourse that separated nurses' and *peiban*'s interests on the grounds of the former's expert knowledge and training and the latter's ignorance and emotion.

One head nurse in another hospital, whom I spoke to through an interpreter, early in the project clearly invoked this discourse. When I asked her, a woman in her fifties who said she had been a nurse for thirty years, about *peiban* on her floor and in the hospital, she said:

> There has been a directive from the public health bureau that the *hospitals had to be managed according to correct managing principles. This means not so many* peiban. (In the past, what did these *peiban* do in the hospital?) They would feed the patients, clean the wards, carry urine and blood samples to the laboratory, get food from dining hall, wash patient's hands and face, help them eliminate urine and go to the toilet. Sometimes they were

also responsible for watching the solution for injection [IV] because they would tell the nurse when the bottle was empty. If patient had a high fever, they could wash the patient with alcohol to bring the fever down. *This is now forbidden because this work belongs to the nurses and nurse assistants. Before there was disorder, during the Cultural Revolution, and now there are new standards for the management of the hospital.* We have the responsibility system. Everybody has his or her work to do and even if you want to, you can't ask the patient's family members to do this work. *This is the work of the staff.* [my emphasis]

This is the "modern" Chinese hospital. It leaves little room for the more traditional discourse on caregiving that is typically invoked by family members and patients. In fact, family members appear here only at visiting hours. Moreover, it assumes adequate numbers of well-trained ("modern") medical personnel in the hospital. That all of what she described as part of a disordered past was precisely what I would soon witness in such great variety and detail helped me understand the power of the official view and the resentment of those who actually did such a great part of this work.

Modernization and *Peiban* Care

It is wonderfully convenient that, as one doctor put it, "family members 'like' to do this kind of thing"—this caregiving work—because, as another said, "If all the *peiban* in the hospitals in China were removed, that would be a social problem." That this contradiction of "modernization" in China—relying on a traditional discourse to shore up a considerably less established, "modern" one—is in some sense recognized by the Chinese health bureaucracy is indexed in a brief article titled "View on Visiting Patients in the Hospital" which appeared in a 1986 issue of the *Chinese Journal of Hospital Administration* (see also Zhong 1985). The author, arguing that it is, of course, necessary to place certain limits on "companionship" in the hospital, writes that without more resources, such tight controls on *peiban* will "only create difficulties for the patient":

Generally speaking, the patients tend to be in low spirits, particularly the severely ill ones. Some are depressed and worried, some anxious, some in dark moods, some lonely. Most of them wish to have someone from their families at their sides. *This not only assures them of better care*, it also reduces the patients' tenseness. It has the effect of providing them with solace and contributes to their sense of security and *is helpful to medical*

treatment and the patients' recoveries. . . . Many patients feel
unaccustomed to nursing care from anyone who is not a family
member. Some feel embarrassed or uneasy. . . . Clearing the hospitals of companions often gives rise to arguments that affect the
relationship between the patients and the medical staff. . . . In
order to be at the patient's bedside, family members sometimes
force their way into the ward, which causes rows and fights. . .
the hospitals have made great efforts toward reducing the number of companions and controlling visiting hours. A large number
of people have been employed to guard the entrances. In addition,
measures have been taken, such as sudden inspections, which
involve a large amount of manpower and resources. . . . [All of]
this means there perhaps is not such a great advantage in exercising a tight control on companions and visitors. [Wang 1986, 192;
my emphasis]

Indeed, from this description one might ask what the benefits of such
controls are, apart from greater consistency with the "modern hospital"
discourse.

What this characterization doesn't begin to acknowledge is the complex and endless *guanxi* work the family members I met performed to get
their patients into the hospital, not to mention efforts toward helping
ensure what they hoped would be good care once their patients were in.
The deeper tensions that define the complex relationships between hospital staff and *peiban* are also ignored. In the hospital, doctors, nurses, and
officials have authority in the official discourse that they use to try to
gain *peiban* conformity with stated "modern" hospital rules. At the same
time, they draw on traditional discourses of filial duty and harmony to
coerce cooperation and care work by *peiban*, work that then goes largely
unnoticed and, most recently, has even been repudiated by official regulations. Yet the doctors themselves are subject to traditional discourses of
proper conduct, as well as a kind of "negative control" that keeps them
mindful of their own debts to and transgressions against both traditional
and socialist codes of behavior. While invoking discourses of bureaucratic
authority and "modern medicine," these doctors and nurses cannot afford
to forget that not only are they "Chinese" but also their official political
line is a communist one—a line that, as has so often been the case in the
past, can be invoked effectively by those below and beside them against
all manner of "counterrevolutionary," bourgeois, individualist, and even
"feudal" conduct. The possibilities of "making trouble" for others seem
to proliferate both on these official grounds and from what could be
called more traditional Chinese ways of being. Finally, to complicate the
picture further, family members themselves use the traditional discourses of filial responsibility in the hospital, perhaps sometimes in spite

of themselves, as a way to create and recreate themselves as proper and dutiful Chinese sons, daughters, and spouses.

You will have noticed, however, that I here have moved into a totalizing, analytic voice, one common to narratives' endings, where authors are hard put to slip off the stage unnoticed and leave a pleasurable feeling of order and understanding in the audience about the object of study—in this case, "how family members care for their relatives in urban Chinese hospitals." Yet even as I began this ending I wanted to step away from it, to leave the story open, uncertain; not a story that claims to tell you what was "really there."

Although in the beginning I justified the project using my status as an experienced U.S. social scientist, from the earliest days on the CCU my own personal experiences as an American and recollections of virtue and guilt connected to my family and to my father's long illness and death strongly influenced what I saw. After initial drafts of this paper sat quietly for some time, a colleague, Min-Zhan Lu, helped me see in the paper a sentimentality and nostalgia for duty properly done, personal sacrifices made, and a sense of family and connectedness in social relationships that, to me, often feels quite absent in the "(post)modernized" life of the United States. Readily available to help me fall into this trap were other, dog-eared, totalizing notions of "the Chinese" and of "Chinese duty." The real risk, one greater than being critical of things Chinese, was nostalgically to valorize the dutiful and seemingly never-ending care work family members in China did, while neglecting the contexts of power and coercion in which this work was done; in effect, to affirm the doctor's assessment that the way to understand this work was to see it as the product of what "[Chinese] family members 'like' to do." It was to make them out as fools, "suckers" (shan yao dan), as the one peiban put it so shatteringly. The Western bourgeois social scientist going to urban China in the late twentieth century to find parts of a cherished but gone past at home is not a picture we should abide. It affirms, at the expense of the difficult and coerced lives of the natives, imaginary selves and lives seemingly lost by privileged outsiders not subject to these complexities.

But mine is only one small instance of the endless dilemma of speaking from a centered place, from a discourse that is not simultaneously subjected to criticism and destabilization. There is no Truth there to be "brought back" (cf. Geertz 1988; Rorty 1983); and perhaps not even a "there." A sense that the ground in "modern(izing) China" is itself full of contradictions and complexities, even as I try to make it cohere in a "scientific story," provides the nonsolution on which I might end.

NOTES

Acknowledgments: An earlier version of this paper was delivered at the annual meeting of the American Sociological Association, San Antonio, Texas. 1988. Thanks to William Liu, Min-Zhan Lu, Richard Madsen, Mark Selden, Anselm Strauss, and

Hong Zhu for helpful comments on earlier drafts of the paper. Particular appreciation goes to those Chinese officials, doctors, and common people in Tianjin who helped me gain access to the hospital and to develop an understanding of what I saw.

1. I have been influenced by the symbolic interactionist ideas of Everett Hughes (1971) and Herbert Blumer (1969) in their arguments that sociologists should provide detailed descriptions of how people do things together in natural settings (see also Becker 1986). Recent critical work in anthropology (e.g., Marcus and Fischer 1986; Clifford and Marcus 1986) and feminist deconstructive criticism (e.g., Clough 1992; Penley 1989) have begun to undermine this position and my own faith in it, as is reflected in this paper.

2. I use "discourse" here in a quite casual way but influenced most by some of Michel Foucault's (1972) writing and especially by the rereadings of his ideas by feminist poststructuralist writers Chris Weedon (1987) and Bronwyn Davies (1989).

3. My sense of how this unaccompanied access came about is that it was too difficult to find someone to come along each time. Also, those responsible had agreed to higher officials' requests to help me; and I would be supervised by the English-speaking doctors and nurses on the unit. I feel quite sure no formal decision was made to allow this.

4. The Chinese *peizhu*, literally translated as "accompany stay"—people who come with the patient and stay in the hospital—is also used to refer to family members and perhaps speaks more accurately to what I here describe. It was only later in the project that I discovered this other usage, and so I decided to retain the somewhat less specific term, *peiban*.

5. While this sort of unpaid labor might be attributed to socialist or party ways of conduct, sociologists of work in the United States have noted how various private and public organizations and institutions alike seem to rely on large amounts of unpaid and unrecognized labor for their continued operation (see Bucher and Stelling 1977).

6. Throughout this paper I have tried to quote the Chinese I spoke to in English as closely as possible. Some early readers objected to this "pidgin English," suggesting it demeans the Chinese speakers. I believe it to be quite the opposite. To edit their English into smooth and standard form would seem to dismiss their efforts to learn and speak English. Moreover, from the beginning of the project I was quite surprised at how much I, then having only rudimentary skills in Chinese, was able to learn from these people who, without exception, told me they "could not speak English." Finally, to the extent that these "data" are taken to be informative, they are testimony that one need not have mastered Chinese language to pursue a project such as this. Perhaps this latter point is no surprise to Sinologists. To those from other lines of work who are approaching China, it may be an encouragement.

7. My introduction to the *danwei* system came with reading Gail Henderson and Myron Cohen's 1984 book, *The Chinese Hospital: A Socialist Work Unit*, before I went to China. Although their book helped me understand the hospital I visited, my concerns were considerably narrower than theirs. Henderson and Cohen do note the presence of family members in the hospital, but they do not discuss in detail their work or their relationships to medical staff.

8. Mayfair Mei-Hui Yang describes several kinds of relationships that can obtain between people based on "the degree of personal emotional and moral commitment" on the one hand and "the degree of gain-and-loss calculation and interest at stake" on the other (1986, 128–35). So-called *hou men(r)* contacts thus might easily be set off from the more general *guanxi*, which can include ties of intimacy and deep commitment. I believe such distinctions go beyond the limited scope of this paper and therefore have not made them here.

9. This is not to suggest that these decisions were made easily. The director of the unit expressed his frustration at being asked to treat a thirty-year-old man, then in the emergency room, suffering from chronic renal failure, who had come from a county

hospital thirty miles away. He said to me, "What am I to do? Maybe sociologists have an answer to this. What am I to do?" Later he told me he had allowed the treatment, "at least for a few days."

10. The circumstances for peasants are less supportive in that, because they have no *danwei* to support them, they have to bear the costs of medical care themselves. For rich peasants, however, this might not represent the burden it at first seems to be. Obviously, for poor peasants circumstances are quite the opposite.

11. Gail Henderson's (1989, 206–10) recent paper on modernization in Chinese medical care helps us put this remark in the context of general trends of the rising cost of hospital stays, contributed to especially by those—such as this man's father—whose *danwei* pay most or all of the costs of care. At the same time, she reports, part of the Western and modernizing model, especially found in cities, is an attempt to increase turnover of patients, reducing the average length of stay. This pressure exerted by doctors and hospital officials is especially strong for those who lack some form of subsidy.

12. Given the gift-exchange calculus that Yang (1986) has described and the present context, it was not surprising to have heard stories of surgeons receiving rather large gifts of money (*hong bao*) from family members in advance of surgeries performed. Although I did not hear any firsthand accounts of this, it was brought up often in discussions with other foreigners about medical care in China. Chinese who commented on this said that "it was more common" in the recent past but that crackdowns on corruption in the hospital had reduced occurrences of the practice. That it has disappeared seems unlikely.

13. This concern that others might try to bring "trouble" seemed a fundamental adjunct to all relationships, possibly with the exception of the most intimate family ties. I felt such concern worked like a wedge to prevent or reduce the cultivation of what we in the West, perhaps especially in the United States, call "openness" in such relationships. Of course, such openness in the United States is located in a quite different context of resource availability and management and of social exchange, not to mention the presence of differences in larger cultural themes, such as individualism and privacy.

REFERENCES

Althusser, Louis. 1971. *Lenin and Philosophy and Other Essays*. London: New Left Books.
Anderson, Marston. 1909. *The Limits of Realism: Chinese Fiction in the Revolutionary Period*. Berkeley: University of California Press.
Becker, Howard S. 1986. "Telling about Society." In idem, *Doing Things Together*. 121–35. Evanston, Ill.: Northwestern University Press.
Blumer, Herbert. 1969. *Symbolic Interactionism*. Englewood Cliffs, N.J.: Prentice-Hall.
Bucher, Rue, and Joan G. Stelling. 1977. *Becoming Professional*. Beverly Hills: Sage.
Chen, Guanfeng. 1987. "Top Expert Warns of Shortage of Doctors." *China Daily* (March 31):1.
Clifford, James. 1983a. "On Ethnographic Authority." *Representations* 1:118–46.
———. 1983b. "Power and Dialogue in Ethnography: Marcel Griaule's Initiation." In *Observers Observed: Essays on Ethnographic Fieldwork*, ed. George W. Stocking, Jr., 121–56. Madison: University of Wisconsin Press.
Clifford, James, and George E. Marcus, eds. 1986. *Writing Culture: The Poetics and Politics of Ethnography*. Berkeley: University of California Press.
Clough, Patricia Ticineto. 1992. *The End(s) of Ethnography: From Realism to Social Criticism*. Newbury Park, Calif.: Sage.
Davies, Bronwyn. 1989. *Frogs and Snails and Feminist Tales*. Sydney: Allen & Unwin.

Fabian, Johannes. 1990. "Presence and Representation: The Other and Anthropological Writing." *Critical Inquiry* 16:753–72.

Foucault, Michel. 1972. *The Archaeology of Knowledge and the Discourse on Language*. Translated by A. M. Sheridan Smith. New York: Pantheon.

Geertz, Clifford. 1988. *Works and Lives: The Anthropologist as Author*. Stanford, Calif.: Stanford University Press.

Goldman, Merle, and Denis Fred Simon. 1989. "The Onset of China's New Technological Revolution." In *Science and Technology in Post-Mao China*, Denis Fred Simon and Merle Goldman, 1–22. Cambridge: Harvard University Press.

Henderson, Gail. 1989. "Issues in the Modernization of Medicine in China." In *Science and Technology in Post-Mao China*, 199–222. *See* Goldman and Simon 1989.

Henderson, Gail, and Myron Cohen. 1984. *The Chinese Hospital: A Socialist Work Unit*. New Haven: Yale University Press.

Hughes, Everett C. 1971. *The Sociological Eye*. Chicago: Aldine-Atherton.

Kondo, Dorinne K. 1990. *Crafting Selves: Power, Gender, and Discourses of Identity in a Japanese Workplace*. Chicago: University of Chicago Press.

Marcus, George E. and Michael M. J. Fischer 1986. *Anthropology as Cultural Critique*. Chicago: University of Chicago Press.

Penley, Constance. 1989. *The Future of an Illusion: Film, Feminism, and Psychoanalysis*. Minneapolis: University of Minnesota Press.

Rorty, Richard. 1983. "Method and Morality." In *Social Science as Moral Inquiry*, ed. Norma Haan, Robert N. Bellah, Paul Rabinow, and William M. Sullivan, 155–76. New York: Columbia University Press.

Schneider, Joseph W. 1988. "Disability as Moral Experience: Epilepsy and Self in Routine Relationships." *Journal of Social Issues* 44:63–78.

———. 1991. "Troubles with Textual Authority in Sociology." *Symbolic Interaction* 14:295–319.

Schneider, Joseph W., and Peter Conrad. 1983. *Having Epilepsy: The Experience and Control of Illness*. Philadelphia: Temple University Press.

Strauss, Anselm L., Shizuko Fagerhaugh, Barbara Suczek, and Carolyn Wiener. 1985. *Social Organization of Medical Work*. Chicago: University of Chicago Press.

Weedon, Chris. 1987. *Feminist Practice and Poststructuralist Theory*. Oxford: Basil Blackwell.

Wang, Lin Ren. 1986. "Dui yiyuan peizhu tanshi wenti zhi guanjian." ("View on Visiting Patients in the Hospital.") *Zhongguo Yiyuan Guanli Zazhi* 23:192.

Wolf, Margery. 1985. *Revolution Postponed: Women in Contemporary China*. Stanford, Calif.: Stanford University Press.

Yang, Mayfair Mei-Hui. 1986. "The Art of Social Relationships and Exchange in China." Ph.D. diss., Department of Anthropology, University of California, Berkeley.

Zhong, Shi. 1985. "An Investigation into Irregularities in Hospitals." *Chinese Sociology and Anthropology* 27:36–48.

Chapter 9

A Comparative Analysis of the
Culture of Biomedicine:
Disclosure and Consequences for
Treatment in the Practice of
Oncology

MARY-JO DELVECCHIO GOOD, LINDA HUNT,
TSUNETSUGU MUNAKATA, *and*
YASUKI KOBAYASHI

Modern biomedicine of the late twentieth century is frequently considered to be "international" and cosmopolitan, based on "universal" scientific knowledge and standards of practice. Yet when we examine the practice of biomedicine, we find variations that cannot be explained solely by differences in the political organization of health care delivery systems or in levels of a society's wealth and investment in health care expenditures (as critically important as these may be to shaping practice). This chapter addresses selected cross-national differences in the practice of oncology; we focus in particular on how culture influences ideologies of "disclosure" and on the conveying of information about diagnoses and prognoses of cancer from physicians to their patients. In this chapter we explore the hypothesis that the cultural foundations of medicine, the way culture shapes the physician–patient relationship, the definition of how and with whom communication takes place, and professional standards and ethics all have critical consequences for how treatment processes are structured and biomedical interventions availed. Practices of disclosure in turn influence and are influenced by the availability of treatment choices and investment in anticancer therapies and research.

In this chapter we compare ideologies about the disclosure of information in the practice of oncology and the care of cancer patients in the United States, Japan, and Mexico (see Good 1990; Good et al. 1990; Good 1991, for additional comparative analyses).[1] The American case provides the foil against which we examine the highly distinctive practices of disclosure of diagnoses and communication about prognoses in Japan (tacit nondisclosure) and Mexico (assertive and frank disclosure).

Cancer, the "dread disease" (Patterson 1987), universally poses grave challenges to physicians, patients, and their families. Discussions about diagnosis, prognosis, and anticancer therapies are seldom unproblematic, regardless of cultural context or the availability of therapeutic resources. Yet we find vastly different professional and lay ideologies about the purpose, content, extent, and mode of disclosure considered appropriate in the three cultures under our consideration. Although the type of source material and data available vary for each of the cases (published literature for Japan; interviews and yearlong field observations for Mexico; and interviews, clinical observations, and published literature for the United States), our analysis of practices (reported or observed) and professional ideologies of disclosure reveals three dimensions of distinctively cultural medical practice. The implications of this analysis for studying biomedicine internationally, in cosmopolitan and local contexts, is addressed in our concluding discussion.

The American Perspective

The influence of American biomedicine, and American oncology in particular, in the creation and promotion of medical knowledge, education, and therapeutics extends worldwide. Not only are oncologists and general physicians in Europe, Asia, and Latin America aware of American practices, but in local debates about medical standards and ethics (as well as about levels of expenditure and cost) the American case is frequently used as an ideological foil, both positive and negative. Biomedicine in the recently industrializing world, and the practice of oncology in particular, is also in part shaped and influenced by practices and ideologies of cosmopolitan medicine of postindustrial societies, such as the United States and Japan. The exportation of anticancer therapies, including radiation technology, chemotherapy, and surgical protocols, proceeds not only through economic channels but through vehicles for conveying medical knowledge, including pharmaceutical company publications and medical texts. The exportation of styles of practice is more highly contested. American practices regarding disclosure are critiqued not only by Japanese physicians but by others in Asian, European, and Middle Eastern countries.[2]

American oncology has its own cultural foundations, its own "local" culture—core symbols, constellations of meanings, and forms of discourse that organize and reflect practice and experience (Geertz 1983). The dominant symbol "hope" and popular American notions about the relationship of psyche to soma—the deeply felt cultural conviction that individualized *will* can influence bodily processes—play a powerful role in shaping physicians' communication with patients about disease and treatments. In the popular domain, the American Cancer Society introduced and promoted "the message of hope" in the "war on cancer," beginning with political activities in the 1930s (Patterson 1987). This American social movement provided popular support for the expansion of research and investment in anticancer therapies and the development of the National Cancer Institute. The "message of hope" also encouraged greater frankness in acknowledging cancer in American society, with profound effects on clinical practice and the profession's ethics of disclosure.

In the United States, disclosure of cancer diagnoses by physicians to patients is now the norm, although communication of the seriousness of the disease usually occurs over several clinical encounters, as physicians construct partnerships with patients (see Good, Good, et al. 1990; Good 1991; Novack et al. 1979; Oken 1961; Taylor 1988). Remarkably, it was only three decades ago that American physicians' fear of direct disclosure of cancer diagnoses to patients and worries about patient and family response to the "dread disease" led to a consensus against disclosure. A comparison of three groups of university physicians documented the change in practice since then: 90 percent of those surveyed in 1961 reported that they generally did not inform patients of diagnoses of cancer (Oken 1961); 91 percent surveyed in 1971 reported they frequently or always informed patients; 98 percent surveyed in 1971 reported that disclosure was their usual policy, and all surveyed felt it was the patient's right to know the diagnosis (Novack et al. 1979).

American physicians and patients have come to an agreement that there should be full disclosure regarding diagnosis of cancer and options for treatment. Discussions about prognosis continue to be problematic for both, however, in part because of the clinical mandate to instill hope (Good, Good, et al. 1990; Good 1991; Lind et al. 1989; Holland 1989; Buchholz 1990). Table 9-1 illustrates the responses of oncologists practicing at Harvard Medical School to questions on optimism and hope; these fifty-one physicians participated in a study on the culture of oncological practice in cosmopolitan medical centers, which we conducted in 1988. Although the oncologists in our study expressed skepticism about the impact of hopeful attitudes on the longevity of cancer patients, heated debates within oncology (Cassileth et al. 1985; Cassileth, Walsh, and

TABLE 9-1. American Oncologists' Efforts to Encourage Patient Optimism[1]

A. Do you usually make an effort to change your patient's attitude to a more optimistic view?

Specialty Affiliation	Responses	
	No	Yes
All physicians	12%	88%
Radiation	7	93
Surgery	14	86
Medicine	13	87

B. Reasons noted for encouraging patient optimism (percent of yes responses).

Reasons	Specialty Affiliation			
	Radiation	Surgery	Medicine	All
Tolerate Adversity	71%	50%	65%	63%
Live Longer	14	21	0	10
Live Better	71	79	74	75
Easier to Manage	29	7	30	24
Enhance M.D. Relationship with Patient	29	21	39	31

1. Sample: N = 51: 14 radiation oncologists, 14 surgeons, 23 medical oncologists.

Lusk 1988; Angell 1985; Cousins 1985, 1989) have intensified discussions about the management of information and the effects of promoting patients' hopefulness and optimism. Information about cancer and its treatment was viewed by many oncologists in our study as knowledge essential for marshaling the "will" to engage in toxic treatments and to fight disease. Nevertheless, oncologists voice the tension experienced over how much and what to tell. Full disclosure is seldom considered possible or therapeutic, especially for cancers with poor prognoses. Thus, although American oncologists recognize that aggressive treatment requires disclosure, total frankness about prognosis is still a contested domain.

In a small study of fifty-five radiation oncology patients, we found that most wished their physicians would be more forthcoming in discussions of prognoses (Lind et al. 1989). By contrast, physicians interviewed expressed concern about the confusing effects of too much information. One medical oncologist spoke of the threat of "overdisclosure" when referring to American patients' quest, even outside of the physician–patient relationship, for ever-greater details about treatment options. A radiation oncologist, expressing dismay at "our national mania for numbers," questioned the value of excessive explicitness in discussing prognoses with patients. These apprehensions may reflect physicians' concern with preserving control over medical information, a control that enables physicians to pace and structure the experience of treatment and the illness course for patients (see Mattingly 1989, on therapeutic narratives; and Good 1990, on narrative time and therapeutic emplotment in the practice of oncology).

The communication of information about diagnosis, prognosis, and treatment is part of the persuasive and relational tasks of the physician, part of the effort to "get patients into treatment," to accept the toxicity of cure or palliation, to invest in the therapeutic endeavor. Therefore information is tailored to the clinical task, to perceived capabilities of patients, to the maintenance of the hierarchy of the physician–patient partnership, to the efficacy of biomedical treatments, and to the goals of instilling hope. American oncologists, like their counterparts in other parts of the world, are concerned with encouraging patient morale and maintaining optimism throughout their clinical partnership. The dynamics of clinical interaction and the shaping of the physician–patient relationship, however, take this explicitly American form of mutuality and "truth-telling." Thus patients are regarded as partners to be educated; knowledge, although medically managed, is to be conveyed; and patient will, in ideal clinical work, ought to be enhanced through clinical communication. It is through such efforts that American physicians believe their patients will be able to "fight" the disease, invest in treatment, and make the most of what biomedicine has to offer in prolonging life or curing cancer.[3]

The Japanese Perspective

In contrast to the United States, Japan and other countries of the Pacific Rim have followed quite a different ethic and culture of disclosure in medical practice (*Scope* 1987; Holland et al. 1987). Diagnoses of cancer and other serious illnesses are generally masked for patients, and often for families as well (see Long and Long 1982; Feldman 1985; Munakata 1986, 1989; Ohnuki-Tierney 1984; Swinbanks 1989a; *Wall Street Journal* 1990). Clinical communications are modeled after an idealized relationship between physicians and patients, one that should be "protective," positively paternalistic, and emotionally deep. Frankness in clinical communication with patients is not only not the norm but is considered unthinkable and professionally inappropriate. Ambiguity is highly prized. Some Japanese physicians regard the American practice of disclosing diagnoses of serious illness, particularly cancer, as overly frank, cruel, legalistic, and protective only of the physician or shaped by legal concerns over patients' right to know (Feldman 1985).

The Japanese, however, are beginning to scrutinize and reconsider their tradition of nondisclosure and ambiguity in communicating with patients (Reynolds 1989; Hattori et al. 1991). In the late 1980s, an "event set" stimulated this reconsideration. During Emperor Hirohito's terminal illness, the Japanese press was admonished not to use the term "cancer" in referring to his illness (*Wall Street Journal* 1988), and his radiation treatments were carried out at the palace with great circumspection. Yet the press broke the traditional taboos on using the term "cancer" in print. The emperor's illness intensified a developing discussion within Japanese medical, health psychology, and media circles about the appropriateness of masking the diagnosis of cancer.

The international dimensions of biomedicine, as well as Japanese participation in anticancer protocols and recent research on quality of life of cancer patients, encouraged by the World Health Organization, also heightened the health professions' awareness of diverse practices and ethics in the treatment of cancer patients. (One of the authors of this chapter, Tsunetsugu Munakata, is carrying out a longitudinal study of "Quality of Life" for cancer patients.) The Japanese, ever astute observers of American and worldwide medical practice and ethics, began to reevaluate their own traditions in comparison to these diverse international practices and to question what the implications and consequences of those traditions are for the care of patients and the utilization and choice of anticancer therapies. This concern is evident in both professional medical and popular lay literature.

We draw on three types of Japanese data to document the reevaluation of professional ideologies about disclosure and medical practice: popular media publications, stories of clinical experiences, and surveys on "telling the truth" to cancer patients published by pharmaceutical firms in medical journals and academic and government literature. The themes recurrent in this literature suggest that the Japanese are framing new directions for medical practice and medical ethics concerned with physician–patient communication and disclosure.

The popular media has focused on the question of "truth-telling" in the physician–patient relationship throughout the past decade. The prominent newspaper *Asahi* published a weekly series on "Living with Cancer" by Atsuko Chiba, a well-known *Asahi* journalist (the equivalent of a *New York Times* journalist). She wrote about her experiences with breast cancer and contrasted the medical treatment and style of communication of her American and Japanese physicians. Her articles were followed by a best-selling book, *Living with Cancer in New York* (1986). During the late 1980s, Chiba became one of Japan's noted intellectual commentators who articulated concern over traditional Japanese medical practices of nondisclosure and who urged that Japanese physicians "tell the truth" to cancer patients. Remarkably, her American physician was not only a noted breast surgeon but also a Japanese American, perhaps suggesting to her audience that being Japanese and informing patients about their diseases were not essentially incompatible (Chiba 1986).[4]

A similar account of personal experiences with cancer was published by Hiroshi Agatsuma, a Japanese anthropologist who had lived in the United States for nineteen years. He too contrasted the American and Japanese practices of disclosure and nondisclosure and called for the patient's right to be informed of diagnosis, prognosis, and the effects and outcome of treatment (Agatsuma 1985).

Recent events indicate that, despite this ongoing debate in the popular media, traditional forms of physician–patient relationships and ethics of disclosure remain deeply embedded in the practice of modern oncology in Japan (Hattori et al. 1991). In a "precedent-setting" court case, the family of a nurse who died of liver cancer brought a malpractice suit against the treating hospital for failure to inform the patient of "the true nature of her illness," leading her to reject recommended surgery "for gallstones," which she knew was not a life-threatening disease (Swinbanks 1989a, 409). Lawyers for the family argued that had the patient been told the true diagnosis, she would have sought aggressive and possibly effective treatment and would not have unknowingly succumbed to the disease. The court rejected the suit, ruling that, although it is the physician's duty to "explain accurately and concretely about the sickness," the extent of disclosure is at the discretion of the physician (Swinbanks 1989a, 409). This case and other legal suits noted below suggest that not only are patients not informed of their diagnoses but that nondisclosure may extend to family members.[5] A series of similar court cases arguing for the patient and family's right to be informed about diagnoses and treatments indicate that the Japanese public is accelerating its challenge of the medical profession's ethics regarding disclosure and nondisclosure (*Wall Street Journal* 1990).[6]

Japanese Medical Literature

Japanese sensitivity to and concern with the problem of disclosure is also evident in the literature designed for physicians in clinical practice, as well as in the more formal academic professional literature. *Scope*, a popular medical journal published by the pharmaceutical company Upjohn and circulated to the majority of Japan's private physicians, devoted its September 1987 issue to cancer and problems of disclosure. The issue began with an interview with one of Japan's noted "classic" clinicians, Suboi Eniko, who had spent ten years at the National Cancer Center prior to turning to private practice in a Tokyo suburb. The interview with Eniko was titled "Again We Think about the Diagnosis of Cancer." It was followed by the article "Again We Think about Disclosure and Cancer," which reviewed survey data from almost two thousand physicians.

The journal also reported on a survey of Upjohn employees, 613 from Japan and 268 from Pacific Rim countries, the United States, and Belgium. A series of brief case accounts volunteered by the surveyed physicians were also presented. These cases provided a "model" for when telling the diagnosis to patients worked well and when it did not. The range of comments favoring greater disclosure, as well as those warning of the potential dire consequences of revealing diagnoses, were also presented.

The Upjohn studies highlight the ethical dilemmas about disclosure that Japanese physicians experience, and they illustrate the nature of the current debate within the Japanese medical profession.

The Surveys

The 1987 Upjohn readers' survey elicited responses from 1,839 physicians, indicating high interest among clinicians from both hospital and clinical practices in the dilemmas posed by disclosure of diagnoses to cancer patients. The Japanese term *kokuchi*, which was used in the *Scope* survey for "disclosure" or "notification," conveys clarity and seriousness, an almost sacred sense of "revelation" and of "truth-telling."[7]

Table 9-2 summarizes the physician survey findings (*Scope* 1987, 10–14). Respondents were almost equally divided between hospital-based (52.3 percent) and private-practice physicians (47.7 percent); one-half were surgeons (50.2 percent) and one-half were in medicine (49.8 percent). Seventy percent of respondents were age fifty or older.

Clearly, great variety characterizes the opinions of the practicing physicians who responded to the survey. No clear pattern emerged either by generation or by specialty, although younger physicians appear to be more attuned to possible changes in the ethics of disclosure. Given that one-half of the respondents viewed disclosure of cancer diagnoses as continuing to be problematic, it is not surprising that 47 percent felt that physicians should not reveal a diagnosis of cancer to patients except in unusual cases. Physicians were clearer about what they wished for themselves if they should suffer from cancer; yet, although the majority would wish to be told the diagnosis clearly and correctly, the state of ethical flux is evidenced by those who prefer the traditional mode of informing with "ambiguity" or who prefer not to be informed. Physicians in the younger age groups (thirty to fifty years old) were somewhat more likely to want to be explicitly informed. In a similar reader survey conducted by Upjohn and *Scope* in 1981, 31 percent of physician respondents stated that they would not want to be informed of their diagnosis if they had cancer. The change in attitude is evident across all age groups, suggesting that regardless of generation, individuals are beginning to rethink the meaning and practice of nondisclosure.

Reports about actual experiences in revealing diagnoses of cancer are

TABLE 9-2. Japanese Physicians' Responses to Questions Regarding "Revelation/Notification" of the Diagnoses of Cancer

Comments	Percent
Notification will become popular	43.1
Notification will still be difficult	49.7
Uncertain	7.2
Favor move toward notification	52.8
percent of surgeons who favor	58.4
percent of medicine (internists, general practitioners) who favor	54.2
If you get cancer, would you want	
to be informed correctly	61.0
to be informed ambiguously	22.0
not to be informed	17.0
Have you notified family members who have cancer of their diagnosis? (46.8% had family members with cancer)	
informed family member	25.0
did not inform family member	75.0
If you did inform, was it the right thing to do?	
yes	81.2
If you did not inform, was it the right thing to do?	
yes	80.9

Note: N = 1,839. Revelation or notification is comparable to "disclosure"—telling the diagnosis.
Source: Scope 26(9):11–12, September 1987 (in Japanese); an Upjohn Pharmaceuticals, Japan, publication.

perhaps most revealing of the state of flux in the Japanese ethics of disclosure. Curiously, of physicians who reported having family members with cancer, an equal proportion felt they had erred whether they had told or not told the diagnosis.

In a second survey, 613 Japanese Upjohn employees responded to comparable questions (see Table 9-3). Like the physician readers of Scope, Upjohn's Japanese employees were not likely to inform a family member of their diagnosis. Twenty-nine percent had family members who suffered from cancer, and most neither had told the diagnosis nor felt that they had erred in not telling. The experience of telling family members appears to have been frightening but generally positive for the majority of the Japanese employees who did tell. Remarkably, the vast majority of employees interviewed also wished to be informed of a diagnosis of cancer if they should become ill with the disease. Thus personal preference for knowing and family experience at revealing diagnoses are at odds with current traditional practices for these Japanese.

Upjohn employees from the United States, Belgium, South Korea, Taiwan, and Thailand were asked about Japanese and local practices of disclosure of diagnoses of cancer in a third survey (see Table 9-4). The sampling and method are unclear for this survey, but the findings are suggestive and represent Japanese sensitivity to international variety in

TABLE 9-3. Japanese Upjohn Employees' Attitudes on Revealing the
Diagnosis of Cancer

Comments	Percent
Will notification or disclosure be accepted in Japan? (yes)	71.3
Will revealing the diagnosis be common in the near future? (yes)	60.0
If you had cancer, would you want to be informed?	
let me know	79.4
don't let me know	20.6
Have you notified family members who have cancer of their diagnosis? (29.2% had family members with cancer)	
informed family member	17.8
did not inform family member	82.2
If you did inform, was it the right thing to do?	
yes	74.2
If you did not inform, was it the right thing to do?	
yes	86.7

Note: N = 613.
Source: Scope 26(9):14, September 1987 (in Japanese); an Upjohn Pharmaceuticals, Japan, publication.

medical ethics. American attitudes regarding disclosure stand out as extreme when compared with the responses of employees from the Pacific Rim countries. Notably, respondents from the Upjohn Belgium office appear to hold attitudes about disclosure that have greater resemblance to those of their Asian colleagues than to those of the Americans.[8]

Physicians' Experiences

Physician respondents to the Upjohn survey volunteered experiences associated with informing patients that they had cancer. The journal published both accounts of experiences of failure and accounts of experiences of success. These case accounts were coded and categorized into 117 experiences of failure and 66 experiences of success. Experiences of failure, from the physicians' perspectives, included patients who suffered an obvious deterioration in physical condition or mental status after being informed. Physicians attributed depression and rapid physical decline to patients' knowledge of their disease. The responses included comments that patients "died of psychological shock"; "of apoplexy, perhaps caused by shock"; "of bleeding from a stress-induced ulcer"; and of suicide. Loss of interest in living was associated with knowledge of cancer, corroborated by "unexpected" or "more rapid" physical decline and psychological deterioration such as depression and "ceasing to speak." Physicians also felt that disclosing the diagnosis could endanger the physician–patient and physician–family relationship and gave accounts of patients leaving their care, doctor-shopping, and following irrational treatment processes or rejecting rational medical treatment altogether.

TABLE 9-4. A Comparative Study of Upjohn International Employee Comments Regarding the Disclosure of Cancer Diagnoses in Their Countries

Comments	Percent
Revealing is common	
United States	91.7
Belgium	13.8
South Korea	12.0
Taiwan	27.5
Thailand	6.0
Have you revealed diagnosis to family member? (yes)	
United States	92.1
Belgium	40.0
South Korea	50.0
Taiwan	29.4
Thailand	25.0
If you were afflicted with cancer, would you wish to be informed of the diagnosis? (yes)	
United States	97.9
Belgium	82.8
South Korea	92.0
Taiwan	93.4
Thailand	80.0
Do you find the Japanese practice surprising?	
United States	41.7
Belgium	3.5
South Korea	12.0
Taiwan	7.7
Thailand	8.0
Do you find the Japanese practice is because "people do not want to face reality"?	
United States	0.0
Belgium	6.9
South Korea	20.0
Taiwan	13.2
Thailand	8.0
The patient may be happy not to be notified	
United States	43.8
Belgium	48.3
South Korea	66.0
Taiwan	37.4
Thailand	16.0
It may be prudent not to tell	
United States	2.1
Belgium	13.8
South Korea	0.0
Taiwan	47.3
Thailand	18.0
Japanese practices are understandable because of cultural differences between countries	
United States	58.3
Belgium	10.3
South Korea	62.0
Taiwan	49.5
Thailand	42.0

Note: N = 268; U.S. = 48, Belgium = 29, South Korea = 50, Taiwan = 91, Thailand = 50.

Source: Scope 26(9):15–16, September 1987 (in Japanese); an Upjohn Pharmaceuticals, Japan, publication.

But physicians also identified positive experiences with disclosure of the diagnosis of cancer. Many physicians mentioned that many patients, once they learned the diagnosis, became positively involved in the therapeutic process, accepting recommended treatments and investing in fighting the disease. Positive psychological and social consequences were also mentioned; patients were able to "put their affairs in order," to "express tenderness to family members," to become "frank," to "live longer," and to "smile at death" and "die in peace." These changes in attitude were seen as beneficial for the patient–physician relationship, as well as for the patient's psychological and social health. Remarkably, from these physicians' comments it would appear that the disclosure of a diagnosis of cancer was generally equated with informing a patient that he or she had a terminal disease.

Physicians remained divided over whether or not it was ethical to inform patients of their diagnoses. Written comments gleaned from the survey included those that implied that patients had the right to know the truth, that "the Japanese should be tougher and confront their destiny," that "it is unnatural to conceal the truth," and that relationships with physicians and family members would be improved by disclosure. As with the case examples noted above, those physicians in favor of informing patients also felt that it would be easier to gain patient acceptance of treatment recommendations; and one commented that "to tell a cancer patient that he has tuberculosis is almost a crime" (*Scope* 1987, 17–29.

Physicians opposed to informing patients of their diagnosis argued nondisclosure better suited the Japanese, "who prefer a tacit understanding" and "indirectly [to] know the truth." Several physicians remarked that because cancer is still considered a fatal disease, informing a patient "means a sentence of death," and several commented that patients are at risk for suicide. Another noted, "I believe that living with the hope that [a disease] is not cancer, even with a bit of doubt that it might be cancer, is much better than being informed that one has cancer and encouraged to fight against it." Others felt that patients can undergo painful treatment because they have hope of recovery; clarifying their diagnosis would take that hope of recovery away. Finally, one physician volunteered that although Americans inform cancer patients of their diagnoses, they only do it to avoid lawsuits. Several others remarked that because Japan is a different culture, physicians should continue practicing medicine in the Japanese way (*Scope* 1987, 17–29).

Academic Publications

The concern over disclosure of cancer diagnoses expressed in the Upjohn studies was evident in academic articles in the professional medical journals. Two contrasting cases of young married women with children—

one in which the patient was informed of her diagnosis of cancer early in her care, and one in which the patient was not informed until four days prior to her death—were presented as model "telling" cases in the *Japanese Journal of Clinical Research on Death and Dying* in 1988 (Ochiai 1988; Inbe and Kato 1988). In both cases, the conflicts felt by physicians, nurses, and the patient's family were recounted. Both model cases emphasize how telling patients their diagnoses and prognoses can resolve psychological distress for all involved. Dependency on health care providers, and on nursing staff in particular, can be reduced and care rationalized.

Research on quality of life and psycho-oncology concerns also is beginning to be published in Japan. In 1989, the recently formed Japanese Psycho-Oncology Society published its first journal issue (JPOS 1989). Quality-of-life articles, discussions of pain management, and psychological support for cancer patients were featured.[9]

Perhaps the most significant indicator of a shift in Japanese considerations regarding disclosure of information to cancer patients was the publication of a manual titled *Terminal Care: Its Examination and Report* (1989), produced by the Ministry of Health and the Japanese Medical Society. The manual devotes an entire chapter to "Telling the Truth" to patients who are afflicted with cancer. As with other professional publications, case examples provide lessons for modeling new behavior, that is, how physicians and nursing staff can inform patients yet give and maintain hope. Criteria are proposed for when patients should be told their diagnosis (again disclosure has the force of a prognosis of terminal illness), when family members should be told, and when physicians should withhold information. The ministry has come out in favor of informing patients of their diagnoses for most cases.

The Political Economy of Hope

The Japanese case illustrates how the power of a cultural norm shapes investment and utilization of anticancer therapies. Several anticancer therapies marketed only in Japan are extremely popular with Japanese physicians (Fukushima 1989; Swinbanks 1989a, 1989b). Several prominent Japanese oncologists have suggested that one of these, the anticancer drug Krestin or PS-K, which holds 25 percent of the market share of all anticancer therapies, is particularly attractive because it has no noticeable side effects and therefore requires neither the patient's knowledge of the diagnosis nor participation in toxic anticancer therapies (Swinbanks 1989a, 1989b; Fukushima 1989). Krestin is an extract of a tree fungus and has annual sales of approximately U.S. $400 million. The manufacturer admits that it has not studied the drug's effects on mortality rates, and there are serious doubts about its efficacy. The drug has

recently been reevaluated by the government and recommended therapeutic uses of Krestin have been revised; physicians are urged to use it
only in combination with other chemotherapies (Swinbanks 1989b).

Masanori Fukushima of the Department of Internal Medicine and
Laboratory of Chemotherapy, Aichi Cancer Center, proposes that the utilization of Krestin and other Japanese-produced anticancer drugs without
proven efficacy appeals to Japanese physicians for three reasons: first, the
drugs have limited "tell-tale side effects," allowing physicians to avoid
informing patients about their diagnoses; second, "most Japanese doctors
are unfamiliar with the discipline of medical oncology" and thus are limited in their ability to assess the efficacy of anticancer chemotherapies;
and third, there exists what Fukushima defines as an "unhealthily close
relationship" between doctors, pharmaceutical companies, and the Ministry of Health and Welfare, leading to a less-than-critical assessment of
chemotherapies and the marketing of "dubious" drugs (Fukushima 1989,
851). Physicians acquire part of their income from the sale of medications, due to the unduly low fees for service and procedures that are set
by the government; and, perhaps as a consequence, "the Japanese are the
world's highest spenders on prescription drugs" (Fukushima 1989, 850–
51). Makoto Kondo, a noted radiologist at Keio, one of Tokyo's foremost
university hospitals, has concerns similar to those of Fukushima and
"gives provocative speeches calling on doctors to give patients information" (Wall Street Journal 1990). He was quoted in the Wall Street Journal as saying: "Our technology is at the level of the U.S., but our patients
aren't informed . . . [because] in Japan, doctors are all gods" (Wall Street
Journal 1990).

The Mexican Perspective

The Mexican perspective stands in stark contrast to the ethics and ideologies of disclosure expressed by Japanese physicians. The Mexican oncologists who were observed by Linda Hunt over a period of fifteen
months of anthropological field research practiced in a provincial capital
city in one of the poorest states in Mexico. These physicians cared for
patients over a range from the educated middle class to the rural poor, in
hospitals funded by the Mexican national health programs and in private
hospitals and clinics. Although oncological surgery and chemotherapy
were available in the city under study, patients were required to seek
radiation treatments and advanced radiography in metropolitan medical
centers in other cities. Most surgery and radiation treatments within the
publicly funded Mexican hospital system are of minimal cost or are covered by insurance. For uninsured patients, however, chemotherapy was
only available at market price, costing as much as U.S. $200 per month.

Uninsured patients also had to pay living expenses in the metropolitan centers where they received radiation treatments. Such stays could last from one to two months.

The oncologists in this study were consistently candid with patients; all were frank and assertive in informing patients of their diagnoses. For the most part, three modes of disclosure were employed; we have categorized these as commanding, disengaged, and consoling. The threefold purpose of all of these modes of communication appeared to be to force patients to understand the gravity of their illness, to ensure compliance with toxic therapies that often were only available in metropolitan medical centers in distant cities, and to encourage patients to commit to the "fight" that lay ahead. The goal of providing the "best treatment," as reflected in disclosure practices, takes on a distinctively assertive and blunt flavor within the cultural and political–economic context of Mexican medicine.

Styles of Disclosure in Mexico

When these Mexican oncologists were asked what they felt they should tell patients and why, they replied that patients should be told their diagnosis and what to expect from treatment: "What the doctor should always do is not lie." One physician explained the process of disclosure: "I tell them that they have a bad tumor. I inform them that it has to be studied and verified. Later I explain what the treatment consists of and the risks that can be with it, with the treatment. Then, depending on this, they decide if they're in agreement or not, in what to do."

A surgical oncologist, noting that the fundamental problem was to get patients to understand the gravity of their disease and the necessity of treatment, remarked:

> You have to explain things to patients so they can understand it. But the word "cancer" is usually not mentioned. We use the word "neoplasm," "malignant tumor," because the word "cancer" is usually associated with pain, suffering, death, and very costly treatment, and this depresses the patient and the family. . . .
> Well, sometimes you have to mention that without treatment they're going to die. If you come to this, there are patients too stubborn to understand it and accept it, right? Well, then as resources you can use these . . . these terms.

The manner in which information was shared with patients was closely associated with the stage of the disease, the point in the treatment process, how well the doctor knew the patient, and the daily routines of consultation.

Commanding

The stage of treatment was often the single most important determinant of the style of disclosure. When talking to newly diagnosed patients about to begin cancer treatment, the oncologists often employed a commanding or directive tone. They would state bluntly and forcefully that the diagnosis was "cancer" or a "malignant tumor," that the treatment would be difficult, and that the only alternative to treatment was imminent death. The goal of this style was to establish the physician's authority and to communicate a sense of urgency. Although physicians employed this style with most new patients, with lower-class and rural patients they often used a strident, even aggressive tone. As discussed above, the doctors believed it necessary to force uneducated patients to confront the gravity of the disease. The following case example illustrates the use of the commanding style by a surgical oncologist in treating a rural, poor patient.

THE CASE OF SEÑORA GUADALUPE. Señora Guadalupe, sixty years old, came from a farming village about fifty miles south of Santo Domingo and was dressed in the braids and apron typical of rural women in southern Mexico. She had had a positive Pap test, followed by a biopsy, and had returned to the hospital for the results. This was the first time she had been to see the oncologist. When she first came into the consultation room, she seemed unaccustomed to the situation, smiling, moving slowly, and hesitating at the door until shown where to sit. The doctor reviewed her chart and speaking emphatically, in a voice a little louder than seemed necessary, said:

> Your reports show a very advanced problem. The problem is not something for an operation; we'll send you to Mexico City. . . . I can't operate, it's very advanced. I'm going to send you to Mexico City for treatment with special equipment that they have there. Without treatment it will advance and kill you, this is your last chance, this is the fastest way. Be prepared to stay there four to six weeks. You've had this eight or nine years. Every year a woman should have a Pap test to catch it early, when it's early you can operate and cure it. Your daughters should do it. If it's caught early you can operate, but with you we can't operate now.

Señora Guadalupe said, "I went to a doctor in private practice, he was going to operate." The doctor responded, "If he wants to operate at this stage he is wrong, he's just trying to get money. With this treatment in Mexico City you can live years, but always with the chance that the illness will return. You could live well six to eight years but you're never going to be completely healthy again."

Señora Guadalupe, with a sly smile, said, "You know, I can still go to the doctor in private practice to get the operation." The doctor replied dryly, "If you want to go for the operation, that's your business." He turned his attention back to typing her referral forms. When he had finished, he called her son into the consultation room. The son was a very humble-looking farmer, approximately forty years old, unkempt and apparently confused, holding his hat in his hand in a classic gesture of servitude. Speaking slowly, in a measured tone, the doctor said to the son:

> Your mother has a cancer of the neck of the womb, very advanced. It's not for surgery, to operate would be a mistake because it will return and kill her right away. She needs special treatment in Mexico City called radiation. She's going to Mexico City to the General Hospital. They won't charge you. Go to the City. Now go and talk to the social worker, she'll give you the details. Your mother will have to be there about four weeks. With this treatment she can live several years.

The son answered in one word: "Yes." Señora Guadalupe was silent, chewing her nails. The doctor concluded, "Without treatment it will kill her soon, maybe this year." The doctor then left the room, and the nurse took the Señora and her son out to look for the social worker to complete the referral process to Mexico City.

This example illustrates the commanding style of disclosure. By using this tone, the doctor in this case attempted to establish his authority as a specialist against that of the private practitioner, who the patient says is willing to perform surgery on her.

The oncologists often stated their belief that educated middle-class patients are better able to grasp the implication of the diagnosis and the necessity of aggressive treatment than are rural, poor patients. They therefore addressed the former group of patients in a less exaggerated but equally decisive style. An example of a medical oncologist treating a middle-class woman illustrates this.

THE CASE OF SEÑORA MARTA. Señora Marta was a shy, twenty-year-old woman, recently married to a college student. The doctor looked over her chart and in a mechanical, almost icy tone of voice informed her: "You have no lung problem, but the womb problem is a cancer. Its from the incomplete abortion that you had, it's changed to cancer, it's very small. We will begin medicine to try to take care of it."

Señora Marta was visibly shaken, batting back tears, wringing her hands, and sighing continually. The doctor plugged on: "The treatment is hard. If you come and take it, it can cure you. If you don't come, the illness will get worse and you'll die. Do you understand?"

She answered, "Yes." The doctor then leaned back in his chair, looked at her silently for a moment, apparently for effect, then asked her if she knew the meaning of the word he had used for "die" (*fallecer*). She said, "Death" (*muerte*), and they both laughed nervously. He told her she wouldn't be able to get pregnant again for three years because of the medicine. He said she must not have sexual relations for several months, at least not while she is on the medicine. She agreed to this as well. He then sent her out with the nurse to get instructions regarding her chemotherapy. In this case, the oncologist employed a commanding style, forcefully laying out the diagnosis and lack of options, thereby creating an atmosphere in which the patient's compliance seemed virtually assured.

Disengagement

A disengaged style of disclosure was commonly employed during routine phases of treatment of long-time patients, especially in the context of instructing medical students. In this mode, oncologists discussed technical details of the diagnosis, the treatment, and the prognosis with students and the anthropologist (Hunt) in front of patients, although they did not directly engage patients or acknowledge that they were disclosing information. Physicians used this style when the details of a case were of particular instructional interest.

A CASE OF SURGICAL ONCOLOGY. A surgical oncologist was consulting with a lower-class patient who had surgery for cervical cancer eighteen months before in the same hospital. In the presence of the patient, he turned in disgust and said to the students, resident, and anthropologist, "This patient had incomplete surgery incorrectly done by Dr. Fuentes. The cancer came back, now I'm sending her to Mexico City for radiation. To the General Hospital there."

The patient then interrupted to ask the doctor, "How long will it take?" The doctor, addressing the patient directly for the first time, said indifferently, "It's a slow treatment—it will take about eight weeks." Then, turning back to the students, he said:

> The diagnosis is adenocarcinoma of the cervix—well differentiated, invasive. Fuentes operated July 8. '88. This type of cancer is the most aggressive type and she really should have had radiation after the surgery. There were two errors, one was incomplete surgery, the other was not giving radiation. Dr. Fuentes should have done a more extensive hysterectomy. . . . It's only just starting to come back, it's not yet a recurrence. But we can stop it with radiation.

He then turned to the patient and told her in a level tone, "Go to Mexico City, or it will grow; after that, come in here and bring the reports from Mexico City and we'll start seeing you every month."

The disengaged style of informing and communicating with patients was also used when patients were well known to the physician, when the clinical encounters were routine, and when informing patients of metastasis requiring further treatment. It was not unusual for physicians to be disengaged even though the information being conveyed may have been novel and distressing to patients.

A ROUTINE CASE. Señora Flor, a rural woman of forty-two years of age, had had a vaginal hysterectomy for cervical dysplasia five months before. She had been sent to talk to the surgical oncologist after having a positive Pap smear with another doctor in the I.M.S.S. Hospital. The surgeon performed a pelvic exam, took her medical history, then asked her if she had brought her husband with her. No, she said, she had only a teenage son with her. The doctor sent her to fetch her son, a boy about fifteen. Then, it seemed rather abruptly, he dropped the bomb: "You must go to Puebla as soon as possible or you'll die—there is no other choice."

Señora Flor laughed a little and said, "I'm not well?" The doctor replied in an emphatic tone, "No. Bring your husband for the next appointment so I can explain this to him. You have to go to Puebla for radiation treatment." He asked if she had any family in Puebla. Señora Flor, in a strained voice, answered, "No, no one." The doctor said, matter-of-factly, "Well, you'll have to find someone you know to stay with, near the hospital—you'll have to stay there one and a half or two months."

She seemed quite shocked at the whole idea, saying little but watching the doctor with a fixed stare, her mouth slightly open. The doctor took no notice and went on following his very standardized procedures: he completed the paperwork and sent her for X rays and blood work. As she was about to leave, she turned to him and said, "What do I have?" He answered, "A little tumor in the womb. Bad. Your treatment is not yet complete." She asked, "Can't I get it here?" He replied, "No, it's not here, it's only in Puebla. Bring your husband to the next appointment." Señora Flor and her son left.

This was not an unusual clinical encounter. Physicians would frequently give instructions about treatment requirements without leading patients through staged explanations. When patients had exhausted all treatment options, however, these same doctors often shifted to a consoling style in communicating prognosis to patients.

Consoling

All the oncologists employed a frank but consoling style with patients from time to time. Most commonly they used this with patients they had treated for a long time, after the prognosis had turned grim. The consoling approach was also common in breaking the news to parents that a child's treatment had failed and the child was terminally ill. Doctors would speak in low, soothing tones, sometimes making little jokes to lighten the atmosphere. They would explain that there were no more treatments and that they would now do all that was possible to assure the comfort of the patient. Terminal or severely metastasized patients were most commonly the object of this approach, as in the following case.

A CASE OF TERMINAL CANCER. Señora Cristina was a sixty-three-year-old woman, impeccably dressed in the style of the urban middle class with high heels, a tailored dress, and neatly arranged hair. She came to the hospital to consult with the medical oncologist, accompanied by her nineteen-year-old adoptive daughter. Señora Cristina had had a mastectomy eleven years before, and since then had been battling recurrences and metastasis in a series of surgeries, radiation treatments, and chemotherapies. Two weeks earlier the oncologist had told her that she was beyond curative measures. Upon entering the room, the patient began crying softly, through a brave smile. The doctor, in a half-teasing, half-consoling tone, asked the daughter if her mother was not "like the turtle now, crying all day long?" "Yes," the daughter said.

The Señora seemed desperate. She complained of pains everywhere in her body; her eyes continued to tear as she spoke. She cried as she talked about what an awful thing cancer is, about not wanting to leave her daughter alone. The doctor tried to soothe her by pointing out that her daughter was old enough to be on her own. The Señora continued crying about how few days she had left, how she knew she had to live day to day. The doctor spoke to the anthropologist in English: "There is nothing to be done, this is the end."

When the doctor marked the contours of a large tumor on the patient's belly, he joked about her having to bathe now. After the exam, he told her that he was going to give her a new medication. He remarked to the intern and anthropologist in Spanish, "There is no more chemotherapy. She knows the problem."

Then the oncologist spoke directly to the patient in a warm voice: "We've had success for eleven years, you've had lots of drugs. I don't want to give you more chemotherapy. We have to give your body a rest. So for now I'm just giving you hormones. We're only buying a little more time, we can't cure it."

The daughter responded, "My mother has bought a grave plot, she says she's resigned. All my family knows." The doctor replied, "Don't worry, a bad bug never dies." Everyone laughed. At the conclusion of the visit, Señora Cristina tearfully made a little speech about having a lot of faith in God and the importance of having faith.

Generally, for terminal cases, a frank and consoling mode of disclosure was used. A surgical oncologist's remarks regarding his thinking about sharing information with terminal patients are useful for understanding this practice.

Clearly, in terminal cases where you see the patient is dying, and he's going to die tomorrow, the day after tomorrow, in these cases then you talk to the patient frankly: "Look, there's nothing that can be done, we are going to take away the pain, we are going to make it so you don't suffer, but now there is nothing to do." In these terminal cases, yes, we have to tell the truth. What good is hope? They know because they are seeing the situation for themselves, right? Or when the treatments have already failed, then we speak frankly: "Now there is nothing to do, only to control the pain, control the bleeding, control the infection." They are spoken to frankly, right? But to this point he already has struggled a lot . . . with the hope that he could have been saved.

Masking

From time to time, the Mexican oncologists would withhold information from patients and speak frankly only with family members. This mode was employed principally at the family's request. Only middle-class families were observed to make requests of this sort, perhaps because they felt more confident to ask for special consideration than rural and lower-class families. Occasionally, in terminal cases, doctors decided on their own to mask information, usually when the patient was very old. Discussion in the presence of patients would be kept nonspecific, and physicians would speak frankly with families only when patients were not present.

Physicians reported they would sometimes actively participate in deceiving the patient, using phrases like "chronic infection" or "preventive treatment" at the family's request. Yet, having agreed to masking, physicians would let the diagnosis slip out unintentionally during a consultation, such as asking patients if any other family members had had cancer or if they had previously been diagnosed with cancer. Perhaps these routine indiscretions were due to a general detachment on the part of the medical profession regarding issues of disclosure.[10]

Professional Authority Contested

The physicians of Mexico, as in many other developing countries, primarily come from the urban middle class (Callado-Ardon et al. 1976; Rubel 1990). Most have little or no exposure to the urban and rural poor outside of their hospital practices,[11] and many physicians view uneducated patients as having limited capacities to understand their diseases and to comply with recommended treatments. What is perceived by physicians as resistance to accepting treatment or diagnoses is attributed to ignorance. Therefore physicians conceptualized their paramount clinical task as one not of building the physician–patient relationship but rather of aggressive persuasion. Their perception of the need to struggle to convince patients of the seriousness of illness and the necessity of treatment may be due only in part to class differences. It may also be an aspect of the contested authority of physicians in the Mexican context.

In contrast to much of the world (in particular, to Japan and the United States), the cultural authority of Mexican physicians does not go unchallenged, and the social status of physicians is not especially elevated. Mexican medical schools have experienced a massive expansion since 1967, resulting in a glut of unemployed and underemployed doctors (Frenk 1987; Frenk et al. 1991; Martuscelli 1986; ANUIES 1984).[12] Furthermore, under Mexican law physicians do not monopolize access to most drugs or to most diagnostic and treatment procedures: anyone has the right to buy and use most biomedical treatments and technologies. Finally, patients own and possess their medical records, X rays, and test results.[13]

The lack of assumed professional authority results in a recurrent need for the oncologists to establish authority with each patient, especially with lower-class and rural people who may not embrace the ideology of the innate veracity of "scientific" medicine. A remark by a surgical oncologist reflects his perception of this problem:

> You have to make them understand that their remedies aren't going to work in this case. You have to make them understand that there are treatments more advanced than the ones they know and that they have to accept them. . . . We don't deny their treatments. If they think that an herb is going to cure them, they take it. But they can't forget that they have to submit to an operation, or that they have to go for radiation. We can't oppose their beliefs, because then we make enemies out of them . . . the patient as well as the family. What we try to do is gain their confidence.

Physicians' concern with making patients understand their diagnoses and with establishing professional authority fosters the patterns of frank disclosure discussed above. When the doctors consider how to address patients, their overriding goal is to establish a relationship with patients wherein compliance with treatment regimens is assured. This results in habitual frankness, to the point that there is little effort to screen patients from the details of their cancer. Even when the doctor opts to withhold information, his purpose may be to ensure compliance rather than to protect patients from unpleasant facts. A medical oncologist illustrates this point with the following comments.

[To learn that the prognosis is poor] is a psychological blow for them, and implicates an obstacle and they may not finish treatment, because they now have the idea that they are going to die, and then it doesn't make sense to suffer so much, no? . . . You have to understand which group of patients to tell: "Really, you're prognosis is good." . . . If I give a treatment, I hope the treatment will go with the good percentage, with the better percentage, and I help the patient and the family to think on the positive side. . . . I explain that God wants everything to go well.

The Political Economy of Treatment

The anticancer therapies that Mexican physicians in provincial communities can offer are constrained by the economic resources of patients and of the society at large. Pharmaceuticals for chemotherapies are largely imported from the United States; costs to uninsured patients, as well as to the government's health insurance programs, can be exceedingly high (U.S. $200 per month). In addition, one medical oncologist noted that even among his physician colleagues, many were skeptical of chemotherapies and questioned their efficacy to cure cancer or prolong life. Radiation therapy is available only in a few large metropolitan medical communities, and although treatment costs for some patients may be covered by government insurance, patients must travel to these centers and bear the burden of other expenditures. Radiation technology, like the chemotherapies, is imported from the United States; some equipment is recycled from American hospitals, but again the cost to the Mexican system suggests access will continue to be limited. Surgery, in contrast to chemo- and radiation therapies, is often the first and only option fully available to many patients. Frank and assertive disclosure may well be a response of Mexican oncologists to these economic and market constraints on treatment options; and instilling a sense of urgency may be more critical in getting patients into those treatments that are most available and economically feasible.

A Comparative Perspective

In our introduction, we proposed that a comparative analysis of biomedicine should investigate the cultural foundations of practice, and we suggested that these may have serious consequences for how treatment processes are structured and biomedical interventions availed. The practice of oncology and professional ideologies about disclosure of cancer diagnoses, prognoses, and therapies provide a powerful lens for the comparative analysis of biomedicine as a cultural system. The cost and complexity of anticancer therapies, the uncertainty of treatment outcomes, and the menace of the disease intensify difficulties in clinical communication and sharply delineate the cultural and economic constraints that pattern interaction.

In our analysis of ideologies of disclosure for our three case examples—American, Japanese, and provincial Mexican—we not only find remarkable cultural distinctions about the ethics of disclosure but variations in the physician–patient relationship, in the cultural authority of physicians, and in patient access to and societal investment in anticancer therapies.

The American case highlights the cultural assumption that the appropriate clinical management of information, including staged disclosure, can enhance hope and encourage patients to engage treatments that are often toxic and difficult. Curiously, the American notion of the "biology of hope"—that a patient's psychological status may influence the course and outcome of disease—is also wedded to American faith in biotechnology. Such faith may also rest on the assumption that patients will have access to the latest anticancer therapies. Individual patients' willingness to pay for experimental treatment is evidenced in the extreme in expensive fee-for-service cancer research (Lind 1986; Oldham 1987). The commitment of American society to biotechnology and the creation of new anticancer therapies is exemplified by the vast and only recently questioned investments in the National Cancer Institute and in the medical–pharmaceutical industries. Although American physicians may perceive an assault on their cultural authority as individual practitioners because of the rising costs of care and the reorganization of medical practice, the cultural foundations of American biomedicine continue to provide high societal commitment to medicine's scientific and therapeutic enterprise.

The Japanese ideologies of disclosure are currently in flux and range from the assumption that diagnoses of cancer should be withheld from patients (and at times from family members) to new considerations that certain patients should be informed about their diseases. However, the assumption that the physician owns the knowledge and may manage it as he or she sees fit continues to prevail. Patients, when informed, often learn their diagnoses at the end stage of their diseases, in time "to accept death" and to shape the ends of their lives. The experience of physicians recounted in Scope (1987) suggests that the encouragement of patients' hope for cure is considered a clinical goal and that nondisclosure and ambiguity are considered the most culturally appropriate paths to that goal.

Japanese physicians are regarded as having exceptional cultural authority and high social prestige and status. Like American physicians in an earlier age, the profession is at times accused of "acting like god"

(*Wall Street Journal* 1990). This form of cultural authority and the idealized paternalism of the traditional physician–patient relationship encourages continuation of practices of nondisclosure. Nevertheless, the campaign by academic physicians such as Fukushima, Kondo, and others to reevaluate the ethics of nondisclosure appears linked to changes in anticancer therapies, as well as to reformulations of patients' rights. The critique by Japanese cancer scientists of the production and marketing of chemotherapies that are nontoxic but also without documented efficacy also suggests that the meaning of the diagnosis of cancer may be changing. As patients are offered new and more efficacious but aggressive and toxic therapies, disclosing information about a cancer diagnosis not only may be necessary but may no longer be viewed as taking away hope. A diagnosis of cancer may not be immediately equated with "a death sentence," as some Japanese physicians currently fear.

The Mexican case is particularly intriguing, perhaps because the language used and the process of disclosure appears most extreme, most frank. This contrast may be a product of the type of data, namely, observations of actual practice. In discussing why they are frank, however, physicians speak less about the patient's right to know and the clinical goal of instilling hope and more of how one persuades and directs patients into treatment. Whereas the Japanese appear to acquire treatment compliance without informing patients about their cancer, American and Mexican physicians view disclosure as part of the initial clinical task; gaining patient acceptance of treatments frequently requires explanation. For the rural and urban poor and the uninsured of Mexico, the rationale requires balancing the cost of compliance, which may be prohibitive, against a family's meager resources. (The uninsured American patient may also be barred from the latest anticancer therapies because of economic constraints and inequities in the system of care for the working and indigenous poor.) Highly directive clinical communications and assertive modes of disclosure may be amplified by class differences, as well as by the contested cultural authority physicians have as individual caregivers and by the limited prestige of biomedicine and biotechnology in this context. The restricted availability of anticancer therapies, the costs—at times prohibitive—of care, and the often dubious but always uncertain efficacy of treatments may contribute to the Mexican physicians' experience of the need to be assertive, especially in a society with limited economic and biomedical resources.

This chapter illustrates that the practice of biomedicine occurs in local worlds, and that its "scientific universalism" remains in tension with local cultural and economic constraints. The cultural foundations and historical developments of varieties of biomedical practice not only shape the physician–patient relationship and the ethics of professional communication, as is so clearly demonstrated by these three cases, but also have consequences for choice of treatment and for the research and production of therapeutics. This linkage between the culture of medicine, biotechnology, and the political economy of medicine suggests several directions for future research.

First, the relationship between dominant biotechnical societies, such as the United States and Japan, and less technologically developed and wealthy societies should be analyzed from the perspective of the marketing of biotechnology, bioscience, therapeutics, and standards and ethics of medical practice. Second, as new efforts are mounted in the less wealthy societies to focus societal investment on the treatment of adult diseases, such as cancer and cardiovascular disorders (as exemplified by the Health Transition or Health and Social Change movement, sponsored by the Rockefeller Foundation and the World Bank), the acceleration of expenditures on imported high-technology medicine should be examined and the relative efficacy of new treatments assessed. Medical knowledge as well as standard therapeutic protocols are exported by societies such as the United States, along with biomedical technology and pharmaceutical products. One form this export takes is illustrated by our Mexican data, which suggest a third focus for comparative research: How are the ethics of disclosure in local medical contexts shaped by the political economy of cosmopolitan biomedicine and biotechnology? We have focused largely on the reverse relationship—how local cultural foundations shape investment and use of biotechnology. Our Mexican case, however, suggests the usefulness of this alternative framing of the relationship in the comparative analysis of biomedicine in developing societies. Physicians from less developed countries who have been interviewed express concern over the changes in the availability of biotechnology and over the expanded options to screen for and treat cancer. Some find these changes disturbing at times because of the limited resources of many patients and of their societies at large; in such contexts of scarcity and inequity, the "availability" of expensive anticancer therapies can appear almost obscene. Thus disclosure of information about treatment options takes on a particularly political and moral cast. Should patients be explicitly told the "efficacy" rating of their drugs and anticancer therapies? Should increase in longevity be assessed and conveyed to patients, who may be utilizing scarce family resources not for cure but for palliation and only a brief extension of life? These ethical difficulties are expressed by physicians in the Third World with passionate distress.[14] Our analyses of the relationship between the culture of biomedicine and the political economy of biotechnology and anticancer therapies needs next to address the concerns that fuel that distress.

NOTES

Acknowledgments: Funding for Mary-Jo Good's research was provided in part by Biomedical Research Support grant no. BRSG S07 RR 05381–27; funding for Linda Hunt's research in Mexico was provided in part by the National Science Foundation, under grant no. BNS8916157, and Wenner-Gren grant no. GR5185; Tsunetsugu Munakata was funded in part by the Department of Social Medicine, Harvard Medical School, and the National Institute of Mental Health, Japan, during his Harvard sabbatical in 1989; Yasuki Kobayashi was a Takemi fellow at the Harvard School of Public Health, 1989–90. Appreciation is expressed to the editors, Peter Conrad and Eugene Gallagher; to Byron Good for editorial suggestions; to Leon Eisenberg and Joan Kleinman for references; and to Margaret Lock for discussions on Japan. Special thanks to Anne Alach of the Schering Library, Department of Social Medicine, Harvard Medical School, who has diligently assisted Good with literature searches for this comparative project.

1. Three sources of data are used in this analysis, which is part of a larger collaborative effort by the authors and their colleagues to examine biomedicine form a comparative and cross-cultural perspective. Discussion of American practices is based on published surveys and studies and on Mary-Jo DelVecchio Good's ongoing research on American oncology. This research with oncologists and cancer patients includes in-depth interviews, survey interviews, and some observations of practice at major teaching hospitals in the northeastern United States. The project began in 1987 (see Lind et al. 1989; Good et al. 1990; Good 1990, 1991; and Good, Munakata, and Kobayashi 1991; see also Gordon 1990, on Italy). Data for the Mexican case is drawn from Linda Hunt's dissertation research (1992); she spent 1989–90 conducting observations and interviews with oncologists, patients, and family members in a provincial capital city in Mexico. She has also contributed to analyzing data from the study of American cancer patients. The Japanese data is primarily drawn from the published Japanese literature concerning cancer and disclosure; this literature was translated in collaboration with Tsunetsugu Munakata and Yasuki Kobayashi, while they were visiting scholars at Harvard in 1989–90 and working with Mary-Jo Good.

2. The Indonesian physicians interviewed (six doctors) reported that they were unlikely to tell patients their diagnoses until the patient was close to death and commented that they follow the Japanese custom; but they questioned their own practice and reflected on what an appropriate procedure should be. Physicians and volunteers at the Cancer Society hostel in Jakarta, who provided an exquisitely tranquil space for patients from outside of Jakarta who had to come to the capital city for treatment, noted that their patients certainly knew their diagnoses but were perhaps unclear about the often dire consequences of their diseases until they were quite close to death. See also GIVIO 1986, for Italian approaches to disclosure; and Feldman 1985, for critique of American approaches.

3. "Living with cancer" and "cancer as a chronic disease" are popular as well as professional glosses that seek to shatter the equation of cancer with death. This contrasts with the traditional and still dominant Japanese tendency to equate cancer with death.

4. Thanks are due to Margaret Lock, who first brought Chiba's book to our attention and who helped work out early ideas on the contrast between American and Japanese patterns of disclosure in the practice of oncology. Munakata, who has been working on quality-of-life issues and who has given workshops for health professionals on "telling the truth," brought the book with him during his sabbatical at Harvard and translated it for this essay and for our collaborative work.

5. The Japanese authors note that Japanese physicians have a duty to inform at least one family member when a patient has cancer. Examples of cases of nondisclosure from the medical literature suggest that physicians often inform family members when the cancer appears to be terminal. Additional research is necessary to clarify when information is conveyed to family members. Case examples suggest that disclosure of diagnoses may not occur until the patient is close to death. In such cases, the "diagnosis" appears to be equivalent to an American "prognosis."

6. The taboo on discussing one's experience of cancer with one's physician led a thirty-seven-year-old patient to begin a support group for women afflicted with breast cancer. The network, begun by Takako Watt twelve years ago, now has branches in every prefecture in Japan and 2,700 members (*Wall Street Journal* 1990). The *Wall Street Journal* quoted Watt: "When people call us they are desperate and have already tried many times to talk with their doctors, but the doctors don't tell them how serious it is."

7. *Shinjitu wo tugeru*, or "telling the truth," and *kokuchi*, "revelation" or "notification," are very positive words in Japanese.

8. The South Koreans were most critical of Japanese medical practices regarding disclosure, with 20 percent responding positively to the statement "It is a Japanese weakness that people do not want to face reality." None of the Korean respondents acknowledged it might be prudent not to notify patients of their disease in some cases. This suggests that the survey was valid, as the animosity between Korean and Japanese cultures was captured by the interview schedule.

9. Concern with the psychological and psychosocial aspects of caring for cancer patients and with quality-of-life research led to the formation of the Japanese Psycho-Oncology Society in 1986, with over 150 members from the medical and health professions, including religious clergy. The first issue of the organization's journal was published in July 1989 (*The Journal of the Japanese Psycho-Oncology Society*), with an opening foreword by a noted American leader in psycho-oncology, Jimmie Holland.

10. Patients occasionally demonstrated an uncanny ability to continue to avoid recognizing their diagnosis, in spite of revealing comments and questions. Some people, even postsurgically and throughout intensive chemotherapy, maintained the fiction that tests had been negative and treatment was really only preventive.

11. Since 1936, Mexico has required a period of "social service obligation" in an underserved rural area as a requirement for completion of medical school. All of the oncologists in this study completed one year of rural service. However, the level of involvement of doctors in these settings with the local culture and people has been shown to be extremely limited (cf. Rubel 1990).

12. An increased demand for higher education, the lack of employment opportunities for university-age students, a doubling of the number of medical schools, and an open enrollment policy in Mexican medical education resulted in a sixfold increase in the number of Mexican physicians between 1960 and 1985. The ratio of physicians to patients in Mexico in 1985 reached 153 per 100,000 persons. Since 1979, only two new medical schools have been established and the number of new graduates is declining. Julio Frenk's 1987 study found 29 percent of Mexican physicians to be underemployed or unemployed. Seven percent had no medical employment at all, and another 22 percent were underemployed. Physicians' salaries are not especially high in Mexico, and they frequently hold nonmedical employment in addition to health-related jobs in order to make ends meet. Physicians who work in the public hospitals have the status of any government employee: they account for the use of their time on daily case sheets and even punch clocks.

13. When a patient brings X rays or test results to a physician in private practice, the physician takes notes of the results or photographs images (X ray plates, for example), then returns the originals to the patient. In the public hospitals, the patient often will keep X rays in his or her possession, although blood-test results may be kept by the doctor and taped into the patient's chart.

14. In addition to physicians in the Mexican study, others from Mexico, Indonesia, the Philippines, and Turkey have been interviewed in preliminary investigations. Many are in a quandary about how to assess cancer-screening and the limits on available biotechnology and chemotherapies, as well as about the uncertain efficacy but high expense of such treatments.

REFERENCES

Agatsuma, Hiroshi. 1985. *Is the Diagnosis of Cancer Taboo?* (in Japanese). Tokyo: Bungei Shinju Press.

Aguilar Medina, Jose. 1980. *El hombre y la urbe: La ciudad de Oaxaca.* Mexico City: Instituto Nacional de Antropología y Historia.

Angell, Marcia. 1985. "Disease as a Reflection of the Psyche." *New England Journal of Medicine* 312:1570–72. (See also correspondence in 313:1354–59 [1985].)

Asociación Nacional de Universidades e Institutos de Enseñanza Superior (ANUIES). 1984. *Asociación Nacional de Universidades e Institutos de Enseñanza Superior: Matrícula y personal docente de la carrera de medicina en México.* Mexico City: ANUIES.

Buchholz, W. M. 1990. "A Piece of My Mind: HOPE (Generic)." *Journal of the American Medical Association* 263:2357–58.

Callado-Ardón, Rolando, Lilla Toledo Manzar, and José Garcia Torres. 1976. *Medicos e estructura social.* Mexico City: Fondo de Cultura Economica.

Cassileth, B. R., William Walsh, and E. J. Lusk. 1988. "Psychosocial Correlates of Cancer Survival." *Journal of Clinical Oncology* 6:1753–59.

Cassileth, B. R., E. J. Lusk, D. S. Miller, L. L. Brown, and C. Miller. 1985. "Psychosocial Correlates of Survival in Advanced Malignant Disease?" *New England Journal of Medicine* 312:1551–55.

Chiba, Atsuko. 1986. *Living with Cancer in New York* (in Japanese). Tokyo: Asahi.

Coombs, David. 1981."Middle-Class Residential Mobility in Mexico City: Toward a Cross-cultural Theory." *Human Ecology* 9(2):221–40.

Cousins, Norman. 1985. Unpublished "Letter to the Editor" to *New England Journal of Medicine*, responding to Cassileth et al. 1985 and Angell 1985. July 16. Courtesy of the author.

———. 1989. *Head First: The Biology of Hope.* New York: E. P. Dutton.

Davis, Diane. 1989."Divided over Democracy: The Embeddedness of State and Class Conflicts in Contemporary Mexico." *Politics and Society* 17(3):247–80.

Davis, Stanley M. 1972. "United States versus Latin America." In *Workers and Managers in Latin America,* ed. Stanley Davis and Louis Goodman, 57–62. Lexington, Mass.: D. C. Heath.

Feldman, Eric. 1985. "Medical Ethics the Japanese Way." *Hastings Center Report* 15(5):21–24.

Frenk, Julio. 1987. "Mexico Faces the Challenge." *World Health* (April):20–23.

Frenk, Julio, Javier Alagon, Gustavo Nigenda, Alejandro Munoz-del Rio, Cecilia Robledo, Luis Vaquez-Segovia, and Catalin Ramirez-Cuadra. 1991. "Patterns of Medical Employment: A Survey of Imbalances in Urban Mexico." *American Journal of Public Health* 81(1):23–29.

Fukushima, Masanori. 1989. "The Overdose of Drugs in Japan." *Nature* 342:850–51.

Geertz, Clifford. 1983. *Local Knowledge.* New York: Basic Books.

GIVIO (Interdisciplinary Group for Cancer Care Evaluation, Italy). 1986. "What Doctors Tell Patients with Breast Cancer about Diagnosis and Treatment." *British Journal of Cancer* 54:319–26.

Good, Mary-Jo DelVecchio. 1990. "Oncology and Narrative Time." Paper presented at the American Anthropology Meetings, December, New Orleans.

———. 1991. "The Practice of Biomedicine and the Discourse on Hope: A Preliminary Investigation into the Culture of American Oncology." In *Anthropologies of Medicine: A Colloquium on West European and North American Perspectives,* ed. Beatrix Pfleiderer and Gilles Bibeau. Heidelberg: Vieweg.

Good, Mary-Jo, Byron Good, Cynthia Schaffer, and Stuart E. Lind. 1990. "American

Oncology and the Discourse on Hope." *Culture, Medicine and Psychiatry* 14:59–79.

Good, Mary-Jo DelVecchio, Byron Good, Tsunetsugu Munakata, Yasuki Kobayashi, and Cheryl Mattingly. 1991. "Oncology and Narrative Time in Comparative Perspective: American and Japanese Examples." Unpublished paper.

Gordon, Deborah R. 1990. "Embodying Illness, Embodying Cancer." *Culture, Medicine and Psychiatry* 14:275–97.

Grindle, Merilee. 1977. *Bureaucrats, Politicians and Peasants in Mexico: A Case Study in Public Policy.* Berkeley: University of California Press.

Hattori, Hiroyuki, S. M. Salzburg, W. P. Kiang, Tatsuya Fugimaya, Yutaka Tejima, and Junji Furuno. 1991. "The Patient's Right to Information in Japan—Legal Rules and Doctor's Opinions." *Social Science and Medicine* 32:1007–16.

Holland, Jimmie C. 1989. "Now We Tell—But How Well?" *Journal of Clinical Oncology* 7:557–59.

Holland, J. C., Natalie Geary, Anthony Marchini, and Susan Tross. 1987. "An International Survey of Physician Attitudes and Practice Regarding the Diagnosis of Cancer." *Cancer Investigation* 5:151–54.

Hunt, Linda. 1992. "Living with Cancer in Oaxaca, Mexico: Patient and Physician Perspectives in Cultural Context." Ph.D. diss., Harvard University.

Inbe, Atsuko, and Yumiko Kato. 1988. "A Case of Not Telling the Diagnosis." *Japanese Journal of Clinical Research on Death and Dying* 11:59–60.

The Japanese Ministry of Health and Welfare. 1989a. *Report of the Task Force on Terminal Care* (in Japanese) (March). Tokyo: Ministry of Health and Welfare.

———(with the Japanese Medical Society). 1989b. *Terminal Care: Its Examination and Report* (June). Tokyo: Chuohouki.

The Japanese Psycho-Oncology Society (JPOS). 1989. *Journal of the Japanese Psycho-Oncology Society* 1(1).

Lind, S. E. 1986. "Fee-for-Service Research." *New England Journal of Medicine* 314:312–15.

Lind, S. E., Mary-Jo Good, Steve Seidel, Thomas Csordas, and Byron Good. 1989. "Telling the Diagnosis of Cancer." *Journal of Clinical Oncology* 7:583–89.

Long S. O., and B. D. Long. 1982. "Curable Cancer and Fatal Ulcers: Attitudes towards Cancer in Japan." *Social Science and Medicine* 16:2101–8.

Martuscelli, J. 1986. "Recursos humanos en salud de México." *Educación medica y salud* 20:382–87.

Mattingly, Cheryl. 1989. "Thinking with Stories: Stories and Experience in a Clinical Practice." Ph.D. diss., Massachusetts Institute of Technology.

Munakata, Tsunetsugu. 1986. "Japanese Attitudes toward Mental Illness and Mental Health Care." In *Japanese Culture and Behavior*, ed. T. S. Lebra and W. P. Lebra, 369–78. Honolulu: University of Hawaii Press.

———. 1989. "The Socio-Cultural Significance of the Diagnostic Label 'Neurasthenia' in Japan's Mental Health Care System." *Culture, Medicine and Psychiatry* 13:203–13.

Murphy, Arthur. 1983. "Three Economic Groups and the City as a Whole." In *Somos Tocayos: Anthropology of Urbanism and Poverty*, ed. Michael Higgins, Lanham, Md.: University Press of America.

Murphy, Arthur, and Alex Stepick. n.d. "Adaptation and Inequality in Oaxaca: Political Economy and Cultural Ecology in an Intermediate Mexican City." Unpublished paper.

New York Times. 1985. "Debate Intensifies on Attitude and Health" (in Japan). (October 29):C1, C7.

———. 1989. "A Fear of Cancer Means No Telling." (January 20):A4.

Novack, D. R., Robin Plumer, R. L. Smith, Herbert Ochitill, G. R. Morrow, and J. M. Bennett. 1979. "Changes in Physician Attitudes toward Telling the Cancer Patient." *Journal of the American Medical Association* 241:897–900.

Ochiai, T. 1988. "A Case of Telling the Diagnosis." *Japanese Journal of Clinical Research on Death and Dying* 11:57–58.

Ohnuki-Tierney, Emiko. 1984. *Illness and Culture in Contemporary Japan: An Anthropological View.* Cambridge: Cambridge University Press.

Oken, Donald. 1961. "What to Tell Cancer Patients: A Study of Medical Attitudes." *Journal of the American Medical Association* 175:1120–28.

Oldham, R. K. 1987. "Sounding Board: Patient-funded Cancer Research." *New England Journal of Medicine* 316:46–47.

Patterson, James T. 1987. *The Dread Disease: Cancer and Modern American Culture.* Cambridge: Harvard University Press.

Reynolds, David K. 1989. "Meaningful Life Therapy." *Culture, Medicine and Psychiatry* 13:457–63.

Rubel, Arthur. 1990. "Compulsory Medical Service and Primary Health Care: A Mexican Case Study." In *Anthropology and Primary Health Care,* ed. Jeannine Coreil and J. Dennis Mull, 137–53. Boulder, Colo.: Westview.

Scope. 1987. "Again We Think about the Notification of Cancer" (in Japanese). *Scope* 26(9):10–29.

Selby, Henry, Arthur Murphy, and Stephen Lorenzen. 1990. *The Mexican Urban Household: Organizing for Self-Defense.* Austin: University of Texas Press.

Serrón, Luis. 1980. *Scarcity, Exploitation and Poverty: Malthus and Marx in Mexico.* Norman: University of Oklahoma Press.

Swinbanks, David. 1989a. "Japanese Doctors Keep Quiet." *Nature* 339:409.

———. 1989b. "Cancer Drugs Restrictions Recommended." *Nature* 339:843.

Taylor, Katherine. 1988. "Physicians and the Disclosure of Undesirable Information." *Sociology of Health and Illness* 10:109–32.

Wall Street Journal. 1988. "Japan Appears at a Standstill as Concerns over Hirohito's Death Preoccupy Nation." (September 27):31.

———. 1990. "In Japan, the Patient's Right to Know Runs Up Against the Medical System." (October 1): A11A.

Chapter 10

Constraints on Successful

Public Health Programs:

A View from a Mexican Community

KENYON RAINIER STEBBINS

Of the many difficult problems facing underdeveloped countries in Latin America, health issues are clearly among the most pressing. In recent decades, the disparity in well-being between the rich and the poor in the Americas has become increasingly apparent. Despite numerous programs designed to improve health status, health and nutrition indexes often have failed to improve significantly for those most in need of help, and in some cases these indexes of well-being for the poor have worsened, even during periods when national indicators reflect economic prosperity (Mahler 1988; Grindle 1981).

For a variety of reasons, the health status of the poor majority in Latin America has long been a serious concern of governmental bodies, international health agencies, interested scholars, and (as is sometimes seemingly forgotten) the unhealthy people themselves. In the mid-1970s, in response to increasingly distressing health indicators for millions of people in Latin America and other impoverished regions, the World Health Organization (WHO) announced the ambitious goal of "Health for All by the Year 2000" (Mahler 1975). Of special significance for this chapter, WHO has repeatedly emphasized that public health concerns are especially critical to the well-being of the world's poor.[1]

This chapter examines a recent attempt by the Mexican government to provide "health for all" as part of a substantial rural development program (COPLAMAR)[2] initiated in the late 1970s. The case of Mexico is especially interesting because, far from being a latecomer to the arena of public concern for the well-being of its citizenry, Mexico's avowed commitment to the health of its people dates back to 1917 (Soberón, Frenk, and Sepúlveda 1986, 674). Following seven years of revolutionary turmoil, the 1917 Mexican Constitution (the most progressive constitution in the world at the time) included among its many innovative declarations the provision that health was to be a constitutionally guaranteed right of all Mexicans. This right was reaffirmed in 1983 when President Miguel de la Madrid introduced a constitutional amendment ensuring all Mexicans the right to protect their health (Soberón, Frenk, and Sepúlveda 1986, 675). Despite impressive government programs and proclamations, however, this chapter suggests that there is little evidence that governmental promises of health have significantly improved the well-being of Mexico's poor majority.

Illness and disease are disproportionately experienced by the poorer segments of the population in underdeveloped countries (Lopez Acuña 1980a). Although their health problems may well concern all classes in an underdeveloped country, it is the poorest who actually experience them. Health projects that could improve the health status of the poor often fail to realize their full potential. Constraints upon successful public health programs such as the one discussed here can be considered on two levels: the macro level and the micro level.

At the macro level, this chapter argues that underdeveloped countries such as Mexico, with dependent capitalist political and economic orientations (Cockcroft 1983),[3] are unlikely to implement meaningful programs to improve the health of the poor unless the ruling elite view such efforts as preserving their own privileged position. At the micro level, this chapter demonstrates how village-level sociopolitical constraints may override health concerns and serve to impede further effective delivery of important health-related services at the village level. These constraints will be discussed below, after placing the discussion in a historical context.

Because of the rural orientation of the COPLAMAR development program, this chapter focuses on recent health services for rural Mexicans. This emphasis on the rural sector, however, should not be taken as an indicator that Mexico's urban population does not have serious health problems. To the contrary, urban Mexico unfortunately includes great numbers of unhealthy and undernourished people whose plight lies beyond the focus of this chapter.

The data upon which the findings reported here are based were gathered during anthropological fieldwork in a highland Chinantec village in Mexico's southern state of Oaxaca over seventeen months between 1980 and 1982, when I conducted research concerning how state penetration (Corbett and Whiteford 1983) affects the health status of the villagers with whom I lived (see Stebbins 1984). The bulk of the field data were collected in the village during fifteen months' residence, by means of participant observation; open-ended, informal interviewing; and copying of official documents (especially at the government health clinic). In addition to the time spent in the village, I spent two months in Oaxaca City and Mexico City obtaining information from various health agencies and archival repositories.

This chapter begins with a brief historical overview of Mexico's attempts to provide "health for all." This is followed by an evaluation of the country's most recent program, which claims to be bringing health to millions of Mexico's most marginalized and economically depressed citizens. Macro-level and micro-level constraints on successful public health programs are then discussed.

Historical Context

Prior to the Mexican Revolution of 1910–17, although private medicine was generally available for those who could afford it (i.e., urban elites), medical care and assistance for Mexico's masses were largely neglected by the State and only partially provided by the Catholic church.

> During the Colonial Period (1521–1821), medical care and help to the indigents were carried out mainly by the Catholic Church. . . . The Christian ideology of helping one's neighbor and giving charity to the poor led to the creation of nursing homes, hospitals, and houses for the care of the needy. After the achievement of independence in 1821, the Christian concept of charity was replaced nominally, but never substantially, by the liberal idea of public welfare. (Lopez Acuña 1980b, 83–84)

Without a legislative mandate to provide philanthropic medical care, such services were neglected for the remainder of the nineteenth century. In the first decades following the revolution, despite the promise of health as a right for all Mexicans, the organization and institutions of health and public welfare did not change, and private medicine continued much as it had been.

It was not until the 1930s, during the Lázaro Cárdenas administration, that serious discussion began concerning "health for all" Mexicans (Lopez Acuña 1980b, 84). Two public welfare agencies were created in 1937 to attend to the health needs of the poorest Mexicans. These were merged into the Department of Health and Welfare (Secretaría de Salubridad e Asistencia, or SSA) in the early 1940s and comprised the only government-sponsored health care option for most poor Mexicans, offering curative medical services at little or no cost for those who could reach the facilities. Rural dwellers, who comprised the majority of the

Mexican population at the time, were disadvantaged in terms of access to health facilities. Currently, the SSA continues to be responsible for the health care of two-thirds of all Mexicans (both urban and rural), despite being allotted a disproportionately small share (only about 15 percent) of the public health sector budget (Musselwhite 1981, 181–82).

Social security coverage has been available for a minority of Mexicans since 1943, when the Instituto Mexicano del Seguro Social (IMSS) was created as a result of pressures brought upon the Mexican government by unionized industrial workers. The IMSS remains the single largest social security agency in Mexico, accounting for 75 percent of those Mexicans who are covered by any social security agency (Wilson 1981, 122).[4] While only 33 percent of all Mexicans receive health coverage from social security agencies, this favored minority enjoys a disproportionate 85 percent of the total public health sector resources (Musselwhite 1981, 180).

It is not surprising, given the enormous inequalities in funding, that the health services provided by the social security agencies (IMSS and the others) in Mexico are universally seen as superior to those offered by the welfare agency (SSA) (Kreisler 1981; Musselwhite 1981; Spaulding 1981; Wilson 1981). This disparity in services is a function of the relative political power of the various sectors of the Mexican populace. The largely urban-based organized workers (primarily government workers and employees in the petroleum, electricity, railroad, and defense sectors) comprise a powerful political force, which the Mexican government would rather placate than alienate. The relatively powerless status of most rural Mexicans, in contrast, has left them largely unable to influence federal health policy in their favor, despite the fact that over 40 percent of Mexico's population live in rural communities with fewer than 2,500 people.

Recent Developments in Health Programs for Rural Mexico

It has long been known that a person's health status has much more to do with adequate nutrition and other structural factors than with whether a physician's services are available (Dubos 1959; McKeown 1979). Nevertheless, medical services are highly valued in Mexico, not only for what they actually deliver but also for what they represent—the promise of improved health. Unfortunately, it is estimated that fully one-half of all rural Mexicans have never received any medical care in their lives (Musselwhite 1981, 91), and one-fifth of the Mexican population does not have "easy access to health services" (Soberón 1986, 675). This is not because of a shortage of doctors in Mexico; to the contrary, there are perhaps twenty thousand unemployed physicians in Mexico (Riding 1984, 331). However, there is a severe geographic maldistribution of physicians; over

47 percent of Mexico's *municipios* (the most important unit of local government) lack a single doctor (Lopez Acuña 1980b, 90).

The ironic contrast of thousands of unemployed doctors with millions of Mexicans without physicians' services is a reflection of class relations wherein urban-oriented upper- and middle-class physicians are trained in expensive, technology-centered medicine, which is impractical in most of rural Mexico. Physicians prefer to remain in urban Mexico pursuing a variety of economic strategies (often combining part-time medical employment with other jobs) over practicing "simplified" medicine in what they view as "primitive" settings.

Mexico's rural people generally live in impoverished conditions which adversely affect their health status. Malnutrition is estimated to be twice as prevalent in Mexico's rural areas as in urban settings (Aylward and Jul 1975, 25),[5] and potable water, adequate housing, and proper sewage disposal are relatively scarce in these areas when compared with urban Mexico. Urban–rural distinctions are potentially misleading, however, because there are tremendous differences in health status and well-being among urban dwellers. Lower-class Mexicans, for example, generally suffer from high infant mortality, gastrointestinal and respiratory ailments, and poor nutrition, the classic "diseases of poverty." In contrast, upper- and middle-class Mexicans enjoy good nutrition and low infant mortality, although experiencing "diseases of development" (i.e., those diseases associated with developed countries) such as heart ailments and cancer (Musselwhite 1981, 128).

In an underdeveloped country such as Mexico, it is more useful to discuss health problems in terms of socioeconomic class, because the urban poor have more in common with the rural poor than they do with the urban middle and upper classes. Inasmuch as this paper focuses on rural Mexicans (virtually all of whom are lower-class), however, the urban–rural distinction is less critical here.

Only an insignificant fraction of rural Mexicans enjoy social security health coverage. For the overwhelming majority of rural Mexicans, private medical care is prohibitively expensive, and other treatment strategies are generally pursued instead (Young 1980, 1981).

In the past three decades the Mexican government's posture toward the provision of health care services has reflected a new interest in the rural population. In 1960, Mexico's welfare agency (SSA) began placing health posts in rural areas, and in 1973 the agency was installing health posts in some communities with fewer than 1,500 people. In the late 1970s, Mexico's rural health services were bolstered by the COPLAMAR program, which promised to help the "marginalized people in the depressed zones" of rural Mexico by allowing them to "participate more equitably in the national wealth" (COPLAMAR 1978a, xvii). This chapter suggests that these goals have, at best, been only partially realized.

Created in 1977, the COPLAMAR program sought to encourage rural development in several arenas, including improved agricultural and timber production, industry, communications, and transportation, as well as health, education, and human affairs. The overall thrust of COPLAMAR is that of resource production and extraction, and the COPLAMAR program assumes—naively—that the wealth derived from increased productivity in Mexico's most marginal and impoverished zones will benefit the local population. Instead of "trickling down" to the local population, however, the wealth derived from any production increase is typically concentrated in the hands of the few elites who control the bulk of the productive resources affected by COPLAMAR.

Although the health component of COPLAMAR is relatively small (only 7.4 percent of COPLAMAR's 1978–82 funds for the state of Oaxaca were targeted for health [COPLAMAR 1978b, 121]), the overall size of the COPLAMAR development agency resulted in significant expansion of rural health facilities. Within three years, COPLAMAR constructed 2,105 new rural health clinics throughout the republic, covering twenty thousand communities and over 11 million Mexicans (COPLAMAR 1981, 43; Zschock 1986). The following services are theoretically available free of charge to the rural beneficiaries: general outpatient consultations, pharmaceuticals, mother–infant care and family planning, health education, nutrition information, sanitation promotion, immunizations, and control of communicable diseases. In addition to the clinics, forty-one rural COPLAMAR hospitals were constructed to treat, at no charge, those patients whose health problems are too complex to be treated at the rural clinics, with services and areas including special outpatient consultations, hospitalization, pharmaceuticals, obstetrical and gynecological care, pediatrics, surgery, internal medicine, preventive medicine, and dental services.

Each COPLAMAR clinic is run by a fifth-year medical student (a *pasante* who is required to spend a year in "social service"), who is assisted by a local female auxiliary called a "physician's aide." This combination of personnel serves two very important functions. First, because a large number of the new COPLAMAR clinics are located in areas where indigenous languages are spoken (and because it is extremely rare for a medical student to have learned an indigenous language), the local bilingual aide serves as an interpreter. Second, because most *pasantes* are men, the female auxiliary (who is no stranger to her community) provides an opportunity for female patients to preserve their modesty in certain situations.

This general overview of the COPLAMAR program to deliver health and health services to millions of "marginalized" Mexicans, by means of 2,105 rural clinics, provides contextual background for examining one specific clinic locality in the highland Chinantec *municipio* of Amotepec (a pseudonym) in the southern state of Oaxaca.

As we turn now to the village setting, we shall see that several constraints limit the effectiveness of such clinics to improve the health of the targeted population. First, a clinic by itself, in the absence of other improvements in the environment, cannot guarantee health. Second, medical education ill prepares—or even "dysprepares"—the *pasantes* for effective functioning in rural settings. Third, the clinic is equipped and stocked more for curative than for preventive services.[6] Fourth, the personality of the *pasante* is often problematic.

It should *not* be assumed that another limiting factor is that people fail to use such clinics because they do not "believe" in them or are not accustomed to seeking "Western" medicine. To the contrary, rural Mexicans are keenly interested in the curative powers of the clinics. Even though millions of rural Mexicans have no locally available physician care, it is not at all uncommon for people to travel great distances to seek cosmopolitan medicine in urban settings.

Micro-Level Analysis: The Research Setting

Nearly half of COPLAMAR's 2,105 rural health clinics were built in Mexico's heavily "Indian" states of Chiapas, Oaxaca, Puebla, Tlaxcala, Hidalgo, San Luis Potosí, and Guerrero. The particular COPLAMAR clinic under study in this chapter is one of 239 such clinics built in Oaxaca, Mexico's "poorest" state in terms of many economic indicators (Aspe and Beristain 1984).

The highland Chinantec *municipio* of Amotepec is located roughly seventy-five miles north of the state capital of Oaxaca, with which it is linked by a seven-hour bus ride, road conditions permitting. During the 1970s, many important changes occurred in Amotepec, including the opening of a new school, the village's first road access, "potable" (questionably) water, a federally subsidized food staples store (CONASUPO), electricity, bus service, and, in 1979, a COPLAMAR clinic.

The *municipio* has a semipermanent population of about 2,179 people on 325 square kilometers of land, about seventeen degrees north of the equator. With steeply sloped lands between five thousand and eight thousand feet above sea level, the primary economic livelihood of Amotepecans is below-subsistence plow agriculture. On part of their land, villagers cultivate mainly locally consumed corn, beans, and squash, which are completely dependent upon rainfall for water. The bulk of their land is uncultivated and covered with scrub oaks and pines.

Almost all villagers have some land that they work, but very few families can subsist without supplemental income earned outside the village. Therefore, Amotepec men often work as self-employed traveling salesmen (selling primarily herbs and spices) in the adjacent state of Veracruz, or work in a variety of occupations in Mexico City. Also, many Amotepec women work for varying periods of time as domestic servants in Mexico City. Because of this time spent outside of the village, most men and many women can converse in Spanish, although virtually all village conversations are in Chinantec.

Land feuds have been an integral part of life in Oaxaca for several hundred years (Dennis 1976a). The highland Chinantec villages on which this chapter focuses are no exception (Luna 1980). In fact, land ownership and control are sources of constant concern in Amotepec, where many people believe that "land is life."[7]

Amotepecans have long maintained that their landholdings have been illegally exploited for their timber value by the neighboring Chinantec *municipio* of San Polinar (a pseudonym). Amotepec villagers are quick to recount numerous acts of brutality perpetrated by San Polinar caciques (regional power bosses), including the cold-blooded murder of the Amotepec *municipio* president in 1965. In addition to killings, many other examples of physical, verbal, and psychological abuse were shared with me, and I witnessed several others. Tensions between these two neighboring villages are so strained that photographs of the most feared San Polinar residents are passed around in Amotepec so that their faces will be well known. As is shown below, these intervillage rivalries heavily influence how the COPLAMAR clinic in Amotepec is viewed by the villagers who are included in its coverage.

The Macro Level: COPLAMAR in the Broader Context

Until Amotepec obtained its clinic in 1979, it had been among the largest *municipios* in the region without any government health services. The villagers had been petitioning various state and federal agencies for a health post for years and were relieved when their efforts were finally rewarded (Stebbins 1986b). Their initial gratitude has since been dampened, however, because the clinic has proved ineffective in curing their most fundamental recurring health problems (Stebbins 1987).

The health status of the people of Amotepec does not differ significantly from that which is reported for rural Mexico in general. Gastrointestinal and upper respiratory ailments were the most common health problems seen at the COPLAMAR clinic in Amotepec during its first three years of operation, and there was no reduction in the numbers (or percentages) of patients presenting these ailments during this time (see

Stebbins 1986a).[8] That little has changed during the 1980s is reflected in the most recent report from the Mexican Secretary of Health (Instituto Nacional de Estadistica 1989, 24), which notes that acute respiratory infections, enteritis, and other diarrheal diseases are the most commonly reported health problems for the state of Oaxaca.

Malnutrition is also widespread in Amotepec, affecting over two-thirds of the children under age five (more than 25 percent of whom were second- or third-degree malnourished), and there is no indication that conditions are improving, even though the COPLAMAR program is designed to include "nutrition information" among its services. It is doubtful, however, that "nutrition information" would do much toward helping undernourished rural Mexicans. Most do not have sufficient productive land to meet their households' food needs, and they lack the income to purchase adequate food and other health-sustaining resources.

Adequate nutrition and improved environmental sanitation are critical to improving the health and well-being of people throughout the underdeveloped world, where an impoverished population lacks the wherewithal to address these root causes of their afflictions. "Most health problems [in Mexico] have their origin in the poverty, ignorance and unsanitary environmental conditions existing in the countryside and in urban slums. . . . A large part of the [Mexican] population lives in unhealthy conditions and in a state of undernourishment that make them particularly vulnerable to infectious and parasitic diseases" (Riding 1984, 327).

Discussions of poverty in the Third World often neglect to note that these so-called poor countries in fact have enormous wealth. Mexico, for example, enjoyed enormous economic growth during the 1950s, 1960s, and 1970s. What is too often overlooked is the distribution of a poor country's income and wealth (Navarro 1974). Few countries in the world, for example, have a greater concentration of wealth among a small elite than Mexico (Soberón 1986, 675). Economists report that "in only eight countries in the world were the shares of national household income of the top five percent of households greater, and the share of the poorest 40 percent of households smaller, than in Mexico" (Felix 1977, 111).

The promises of the 1917 revolution have yet to become reality for most Mexicans. Nearly seventy years later, Mexico's social indicators differ little from those for countries in the region that have had no revolution (Riding 1984, 316). Although COPLAMAR explicitly emphasizes the importance of adequate nutrition and improved environmental sanitation, this knowledge has yet to be transferred into action, and the people who have been waiting for seventy years for improved health have not yet received what they have long been promised. That so little has improved is perhaps less surprising (though no less acceptable) when one recalls that COPLAMAR is not a community-based organization and thus lacks popular support among the local population.[9]

Importance of Micro-Level Considerations

The people of Amotepec expressed serious frustrations about their new clinic, for several reasons. For example, many were disillusioned that their new health resource, which had held out the promise of better health, had not really improved their health very much, in their eyes. Moreover, most Amotepecans resented the *pasante*'s absenteeism, his arrogance, and his indifference toward patients.

Officially, the clinic is open from 8 A.M. to I P.M. and 3 to 6 P.M. daily except Sundays, when the *pasante* is expected to be available for emergencies. In reality, the *pasante* would often leave the village for five-day weekends and was often publicly drunk during working hours. Understandably, villagers were skeptical of the *pasante* and his commitment to their health.[10]

On those days when patients would find him in the clinic, the *pasante* frequently spoke to them paternalistically, perhaps insulting them for not washing their hands or bathing regularly or for not wearing shoes. He would often appear to be quite irritated when they would "interrupt" his day by seeking his services. On some occasions he would refuse to leave his living quarters because he was watching television, and would instead have his aide act as intermediary and tell her how to deal with the patient.[11]

Thus the villagers were especially dissatisfied with their *pasante* because of his chronic absenteeism, his authoritarian air of superiority, and his frequent drunkenness. However, this paper demonstrates that much more than a diligent *pasante* is needed to prevent recurrence of the villagers' persistent ailments.

Despite their deep frustrations with the clinic's failure to bring improved health into their daily lives, the marginalized and economically depressed people of Amotepec have compelling reasons for not having filed formal complaints about their situation. These reasons become apparent only when viewed from the perspective of the villagers in question (Stebbins 1986b). At this micro level of analysis, Amotepecans, although concerned about their health status, are far more concerned about being dominated and further exploited as a community by the long-hated neighboring *municipio* of San Polinar.

Amotepec's concern about being dominated by a neighboring *municipio* involves much more than pride. The state government of Oaxaca occasionally suggests consolidating any of the state's 270 *municipios* that do not have a population of at least ten thousand. This would include Amotepec, whose residents do not want to become part of any consolidated *municipio*, especially not one that includes San Polinar.[12]

The long-standing hostilities experienced by Amotepecans at the hands of San Polinar villagers have resulted in Amotepec being continuously preoccupied with remaining legally independent from San Polinar. Fearing to share a *municipio* with rival San Polinar, Amotepecans are extremely concerned about being equal or superior to their rivals in every possible way. Because San Polinar had had a government health post for several years, Amotepec had been seeking a clinic of their own for many years and was very pleased to be awarded a COPLAMAR clinic. Amotepec village officials and influential town elders believe that having such an important and impressive public amenity as the COPLAMAR clinic will help their village withstand any potential consolidation with San Polinar.

Even though the villagers of Amotepec had been petitioning for a clinic for its *health* benefits, they clearly recognized the coincidental *political* advantages that came with the clinic. From this perspective, the widespread shortcomings that Amotepecans consider their clinic to have as a provider of health services may be seen in a different light; they judge the clinic's value by the foregoing *municipio* consolidation criteria. Rather than risk losing the clinic by complaining about it to COPLAMAR officials (and thereby appearing to be ungrateful or too demanding), Amotepecans have chosen to tolerate the health-related shortcomings of their clinic because of more serious intervillage political concerns.

The WHO Mandate for "Health for All by the Year 2000": The Mexican Case

Mexico's recent interest in expanding the coverage of its health services into previously unserved rural areas is philosophically in agreement with the WHO goal of "Health for All by the Year 2000." However, it did not originate in response to the WHO mandate but rather evolved from historical circumstances that were significantly influenced by the enormous petroleum revenues Mexico was enjoying during the 1970s.

Historically, despite the 1917 constitutional guarantee of health for all Mexicans, rural Mexicans were ignored until the late 1930s, when modest health services were extended into some rural areas. Little else was done concerning rural health until 1960, when the SSA extended its health care delivery for the first time to rural areas with populations smaller than 2,500.[13] This extension of health services to the least politically powerful segment of the Mexican population was extraordinary and served as a harbinger of programs that have followed, including the most recent 2,105 COPLAMAR clinics.

In 1973, health services were expanded to include rural health posts for communities with fewer than 1,500 people.[14] The 1973 program was unique in that it was designed to extend health care to rural regions not covered by the SSA or the IMSS. By 1976, 310 rural medical units at this lowest level were in operation (COPLAMAR 1981, 46), and they served as a pilot project for the COPLAMAR clinics that soon followed (COPLAMAR 1981, 95). These services were extended to some of the most remote parts of Mexico and by 1978 were reported to have reached roughly 3.3 million people (Wilson 1981, 133).

The COPLAMAR program discussed here, with its 2,105 recent clinics potentially providing health services to 11 million previously neglected rural Mexicans, represents an enormous financial commitment on the part of the Mexican government (Thalmann 1984, 433), paid for in part by oil revenues that have since declined dramatically. Despite this surge in attention to rural health concerns in the late 1970s and early 1980s, decent health for rural Mexicans is far from guaranteed (Horn 1983).

Summary and Conclusions

While the curative medical services that are now generally available in Amotepec are not without merit, they comprise only part of what is required to improve the villagers' health status. Probably more important is the need for public health programs that would seriously attack the malnutrition and the unsanitary environmental conditions that remain (Behrhorst 1975). Because two-thirds of Amotepec's young children are malnourished, they are potentially more seriously affected by such common ailments as intestinal diseases and respiratory infections. Amotepecans' health problems are compounded by their impoverished living conditions, which typically include barefoot children, domestic farm animals roaming freely in living areas, unheated sleeping quarters, and generally unhygienic food preparation and eating environments. Regrettably, the schools do almost nothing to impart health-related information to the children.

The Amotepec clinic's failure to reduce the prevalence of malnutrition and gastrointestinal and upper respiratory diseases is not surprising, given the COPLAMAR program's emphasis on curative medicine (Stebbins 1986a).[15] Because of the choice to emphasize curative rather than preventive medical services, the conditions that contribute to the onset, persistence, and recurrence of Amotepec's most common diseases are left largely unaffected. "The fact that the principal causes of death in Mexico—pneumonia and enteritis—fall into the category of avoidable diseases underlines the difficulty of separating health questions from broader socioeconomic problems" (Riding 1984, 327). Not surprisingly, similar shortcomings are reported elsewhere in Mexico, despite improved access to medical care (Simonelli 1987).

Even though COPLAMAR's clinics are failing in their attempts to deliver health to all citizens, they are succeeding in other ways that serve to benefit Mexico's ruling elite. By appearing to be improving health, the COPLAMAR clinics comprise a type of "preemptive reform," which serves to reduce the likelihood of political instability (Coleman and Davis 1983). The mere existence of such clinics, regardless of their performance, allows the Mexican government to declare that it is actively delivering on the decades-old constitutional promise of health for all Mexicans, including the most "marginal" ones.

Mexico's development strategy for the 1980s was based on previous high growth rates, which were stifled by the dramatic decline in oil prices. Even if the high growth rates had been realized, it is highly questionable that the poorest sector of the Mexican population would have benefited much (Hardy 1982, 510). The economic austerity programs associated with decreased oil revenues have further jeopardized the well-being of Mexico's poor. For example, a 20 percent increase in Mexico's minimum wage in mid-1984 did little to offset price increases of up to 400 percent during the previous eighteen months, during which time government subsidies on many food staples were removed or decreased (Simonelli 1987, 33).

The fact that avoidable ailments persist in the Mexican countryside should not be blamed solely on the COPLAMAR *pasantes*. The greater responsibility for the poor health indexes among rural Mexicans (including Amotepecans) rests with the health planners and the medical institutions that train physicians to work primarily in highly technical urban settings, with almost no training in public health measures or low-technology, simplified health care delivery in cross-cultural settings. At yet a higher level of responsibility are the successive governments that emphasize political stability over programs that could reduce the social injustice that has been evident since long before the 1917 revolution. At the highest level of responsibility, the formulation and implementation of health-related programs in dependent capitalist economies such as Mexico's are greatly affected by fluctuations in the world economy, over which they have very little control (Chossudovsky 1983; Wallerstein 1974).[16]

This chapter has shown that the delivery of health services to a rural population in an underdeveloped country is an extremely complex problem that involves unanticipated expectations and priorities. Macro-level social, political, and economic forces, when viewed in a historical context, help to explain the disadvantaged health status of the rural Mexican population. Micro-level analysis reveals that, despite undesirable health conditions, rural Mexicans may tolerate unsatisfactory health care delivery for reasons quite unrelated to health.

If Mexico's recent COPLAMAR health program is any indication, the

WHO goal of "Health for All by the Year 2000" is unlikely to be realized. This chapter suggests that improved health status for the poor majority in the Third World does not necessarily follow from showy and expensive health clinics. Significant financial resources and meaningful community participation are necessary but not sufficient conditions for providing health for all. What is also needed is the political desire on the part of the ruling elite to see that both preventive and curative health services (including adequate food, water, housing, sanitation, and education) are not only called for but also effectively delivered. Socialist nations such as Cuba, Tanzania, and, more recently, Nicaragua provide examples of such an orientation (Aldereguia Valdes-Brito and Aldereguia Henriquez 1983; Donahue 1986; Gish 1973, 1976; Heggenhougen 1984). Unfortunately for the impoverished masses in dependent capitalist countries such as Mexico, the ruling elite generally lack the political will to prioritize such actions, and the likelihood of a truly healthy world remains remote.

NOTES

Acknowledgments: An earlier version of this paper was presented at the 1987 meetings of the American Anthropological Association in Chicago. I would like to thank Lynn Morgan and Gene Gallagher for their helpful suggestions.
   1. For a critique of the ideological and political assumptions of the "Health for All by the Year 2000" declaration, see Vicente Navarro (1984).
   2. COPLAMAR stands for Coordinación General del Plan Nacional de Zonas Deprimidas y Grupos Marginados, or the General Coordinating Board for the National Plan [to aid economically] Depressed and Marginalized Groups. Created by President José Lopez Portillo, COPLAMAR was subsequently dismantled by his successor (Miguel de la Madrid), and its functions were reassigned to eight different ministries (Riding 1984, 321).
   3. "Dependent capitalist economic and political orientations" refers to the nature of political and economic linkages between developed and underdeveloped countries, resulting in much of the resources of the poor countries being siphoned into the wealthy countries. For elaboration, see Fernando Henrique Cardoso and Enzo Faletto (1979), Ronald H. Chilcote (1981), and Andre Gunder Frank (1969).
   4. In addition to the IMSS, other social security agencies cover employees of the government (the Instituto de Seguridad y Servicios Sociales de los Trabajadores del Estado [ISSSTE], the petroleum industry, the federal electricity commission, the national railroads, and the defense ministry and the navy (Riding 1984, 330).
   5. A 1975 study by Mexico's National Nutrition Institute revealed that 65 percent of all Mexicans (and over 90 percent of the rural population) had inadequate diets (COPLAMAR 1982, cited in Spaulding 1985, 1250).
   6. Rural peasants often express much greater interest in curative services than in preventive services, despite the importance of both.
   7. For an interesting discussion from Oaxaca on how the state benefits from a divided peasant population, see Philip Dennis (1976b).
   8. In September and October of 1979 (when the COPLAMAR clinic in Amotepec had first opened), fully 50 percent of all diagnoses made at the clinic were for gastrointestinal (GI) problems (26.6 percent) and upper respiratory (UR) ailments (23.4 percent). For the same two months in 1980, these same problems accounted for 60.3 percent

(34.6 percent GI and 25.7 percent UR) of all clinic diagnoses, and for the same months in 1981 they accounted for 53.6 percent (39.7 percent GI and 23.9 percent UR) of all clinic diagnoses (Stebbins 1984, 147).

9. The federal elementary school in Amotepec similarly reflects the shortcomings of externally imposed "improvements."

10. *Pasantes* are allowed four days vacation each month, plus three days per month to attend a required meeting in the state capital. In addition, there are fourteen annual vacation days. Thus a *pasante* should be in the village about 265 days per year. However, one *pasante* in Amotepec was observed to have been in the village only 153 days, an absentee rate more that twice that officially allowed.

11. Although similar reports are not uncommon in Mexico and elsewhere, it should be emphasized that not all *pasantes* neglect their duties. In fact, many *pasantes* are extremely dedicated, even to the point of losing their lives while trying to reach their remote posts.

12. Although census figures show San Polinar to be slightly smaller than Amotepec, San Polinar has demonstrated an ability to influence state officials (possibly through bribery) far beyond that of Amotepec. Therefore Amotepecans fear that in a consolidated *municipio* they would quite possibly be dominated by San Polinar.

13. Over 40 percent of Mexico's population live in some 97,615 rural communities of fewer than 2,500 people (COPLAMAR 1981, 39).

14. Most of the 4 million rural Mexicans "eligible" for these new health services "were no more than potential or at best sporadic users of these very rudimentary, primitive, and inexpensive services" (Kreisler 1981, 228).

15. For a revealing discussion of macro-level obstacles impeding a Mexican government program to reduce malnutrition by restoring self-sufficiency in food staples production, see Rose J. Spaulding (1985). For a more recent report on the COPLAMAR program, see Margaret Sherrard Sherraden (1991).

16. The powerful impact of the world economy on life in Mexico is most recently reflected in the dramatic decline in the price of oil in the 1980s, as noted above. For an anthropological critique of dependency theory in the political economy of health, see Lynn M. Morgan (1987).

REFERENCES

Aldereguia Valdes-Brito, Jorge, and Jorge Aldereguia Henriquez. 1983. "Health Status of the Cuban Population." *International Journal of Health Services* 13(3):479–86.

Aspe, Pedro, and Javier Beristain. 1984. "Distribution of Education and Health Opportunities and Services." In *The Political Economy of Income Distribution in Mexico*, ed. Pedro Aspe and Paul E. Sigmund, 265–326. New York: Holmes & Meier.

Aylward, Francis, and Mogens Jul. 1975. "Nutrition in Pregnancy in Central America and Panama." *American Journal of Disease and Children* 129:427–30.

Behrhorst, Carroll. 1975. "The Chimaltenango Development Project in Guatemala." In *Health by the People*, ed. Kenneth Newell, 30–52. Geneva: World Health Organization.

Cardoso, Fernando Henrique, and Enzo Faletto. 1979. *Dependency and Development in Latin America*. Berkeley: University of California Press.

Chilcote, Ronald H. 1981. "Issues of Theory in Dependency and Marxism." *Latin American Perspectives* 8(3 and 4):3–16.

Chossudovsky, Michel. 1983. "Underdevelopment and the Political Economy of Malnutrition and Ill Health." *International Journal of Health Services* 13(1):69–83.

Cockcroft, James D. 1983. *Mexico: Class Formation, Capital Accumulation, and the State*. New York: Monthly Review.

Coleman, Kenneth M., and Charles L. Davis. 1983. "Preemptive Reform and the Mexican Working Class." *Latin American Research Review* 18(1):3–31.

COPLAMAR. 1978a. *Programas integrados*. Vol. 22: *Region Mixteca de Oaxaca*. Mexico City: Presidencia de la Republica.

———. 1978b. *Programas integrados, Zona Mixteca, Resumen*. Mexico City: Presidencia de la Republica.

———. 1981. *Primera reunión anual de análisis del desarrollo del programa IMSS–COPLAMAR: Unidades Médicas Rurales*. Mexico City: Instituto Mexicano del Seguro Social.

———. 1982. *Necesidades esenciales en México*. Vol. 1: *Alimentación*. Mexico City: Siglo XXI.

Corbett, Jack, and Scott Whiteford. 1983. "State Penetration and Development in Mesoamerica, 1950–1980." In *Heritage of Conquest: Thirty Years Later*, ed. Carl Kendall, John Hawkins, and Laurell Bossen, 9–33. Albuquerque: University of New Mexico Press.

Dennis, Philip. 1976a. *Conflictos por tierras en el Valle de Oaxaca*. Mexico City: Instituto Nacional Indigenista.

———. 1976b. "The Uses of Inter-Village Feuding." *Anthropological Quarterly* 49 (3):174–84.

Donahue, John M. 1986. *The Nicaraguan Revolution in Health: From Somoza to the Sandinistas*. South Hadley, Mass.: Bergin & Garvey.

Dubos, Rene. 1959. *Mirage of Health*. New York: Harper & Row.

Felix, David. 1977. "Income Inequality in Mexico." *Current History* 72(425):111–14, 136.

Frank, Andre Gunder. 1969. *Capitalism and Underdevelopment in Latin America*. New York: Modern Reader.

Gish, Oscar. 1973. "Resource Allocation, Equality of Access, and Health." *International Journal of Health Services* 3(3):399–412.

———. 1976. "Alternative Approaches to Health Planning." *Carnets de l'enfance* 33: 32–51.

Grindle, Merilee S. 1981. *Official Interpretations of Rural Underdevelopment: Mexico in the 1970s*. Working Papers in U.S.–Mexican Studies, no. 20. La Jolla, Calif.: University of California at San Diego.

Hardy, Chandra. 1982. "Mexico's Development Strategy for the 1980s." *World Development* 10(6):5501–12.

Heggenhougen, Harald K. 1984. "Will Primary Health Care Efforts Be Allowed to Succeed?" *Social Science and Medicine* 19(3):217–24.

Horn, James J. 1983. "The Mexican Revolution and Health Care, or the Health of the Mexican Revolution." *Latin American Perspectives* 10(4):24–39.

Instituto Nacional de Estadistica. 1989. *Salud y bienestar en Oaxaca*. Secretaría de Salud. Mexico City: Instituto Nacional de Estadistica.

Kreisler, Robert. 1981. "Politics and Health Care in the Republic of Mexico: A Study of the Dynamics of Public Policy." Ph.D. diss., Columbia University, New York.

Lopez Acuña, Daniel. 1980a. *La salud desigual en Mexico*. Mexico City: Siglo XXI.

———. 1980b. "Health Services in Mexico." *Journal of Public Health Policy* 1(1):83–95.

Luna, Jaime Martinez. 1980. "Penetración de capital y reproducción comunitaria en la Sierra Juárez de Oaxaca, México." Unpublished manuscript.

McKeown, Thomas R. 1979. *The Role of Medicine, Dreams, Mirage and Nemesis*. Oxford: Blackwell.

Mahler, Halfdan. 1975. "Health for All by the Year 2000." *World Health Organization Chronicle* 29:457–61.

————. 1988. "Present Status of WHO's Initiative, 'Health for All by the Year 2000.'" *Annual Review of Public Health* 9:71–97.

Morgan, Lynn M. 1987. "Dependency Theory in the Political Economy of Health: An Anthropological Critique." *Medical Anthropology Quarterly* n.s. 1(2):131–54.

Musselwhite, James C. 1981. "Public Policy, Development, and the Poor: Health Policy in Mexico." Ph.D. diss., Johns Hopkins University, Baltimore.

Navarro, Vicente. 1974. "The Underdevelopment of Health or the Health of Underdevelopment: An Analysis of the Distribution of Human Health Resources in Latin America." *International Journal of Health Services* 4(1):5–27.

————. 1984. "A Critique of the Ideological and Political Position of the Brandt Report and the Alma Ata Declaration." *International Journal of Health Services* 14(2):159–72.

Riding, Alan. 1984. *Distant Neighbors: A Portrait of the Mexicans.* New York: Vintage.

Sherraden, Margaret Sherrard. 1991. "Policy Impacts of Community Participation: Health Services in Rural Mexico." *Human Organization* 50(3):256–63.

Simonelli, Jeanne M. 1987. "Defective Modernization and Health in Mexico." *Social Science and Medicine* 24(1):23–36.

Soberón, Guillermo, Julio Frenk, and Jaime Sepúlveda. 1986. "The Health Care Reform in Mexico: Before and After the 1985 Earthquake." *American Journal of Public Health* 76(6):673–80.

Spaulding, Rose J. 1985. "Structural Barriers to Food Programming: An Analysis of the 'Mexican Food System.'" *World Development* 13(12):1249–62.

————. 1981. "State Power and Its Limits: Corporatism in Mexico." *Comparative Political Studies* 14(2):139–61.

Stebbins, Kenyon R. 1984. "Second-Class Mexicans: State Penetration and Its Impact on Health Status and Health Services in a Highland Chinantec Municipio in Oaxaca." Ph.D. diss., Michigan State University, East Lansing.

————. 1986a. "Curative Medicine, Preventive Medicine, and Health Status: The Influence of Politics on Health Status in a Rural Mexican Village." *Social Science and Medicine* 23(2):139–48.

————. 1986b. "Politics, Economics, and Health Services in Rural Oaxaca, Mexico." *Human Organization* 45(2):112–19.

————. 1987. "Does Access to Health Services Guarantee Improved Health Status? The Case of a New Rural Health Clinic in Oaxaca, Mexico." In *Encounters with Biomedicine: Case Studies in Medical Anthropology*, ed. Hans A. Baer, 3–27. New York: Gordon & Breach.

Thalmann, Emilio Lozoya. 1984. "Social Security, Health, and Social Solidarity in Mexico." In *The Political Economy of Income Distribution in Mexico*, 397–437. *See* Aspe and Beristain 1984.

Wallerstein, Immanuel. 1974. "The Rise and Future Demise of the World Capitalist System: Concepts for Comparative Analysis." *Comparative Studies in Society and History* 16(4):387–415.

Wilson, Richard R. 1981. "The Corporatist Welfare State: Social Security and Development in Mexico." Ph.D. diss., Yale University, New Haven.

Young, James C. 1980. "A Model of Illness Treatment Decisions in a Tarascan Town." *American Ethnologist* 7:106–31.

————. 1981. *Medical Choice in a Mexican Village.* New Brunswick: Rutgers University Press.

Zschock, Dieter K. 1986. "Medical Care under Social Insurance in Latin America." *Latin American Research Review* 21(1):99–122.

Chapter 11

Implementing Health for All in Nigeria: Problems and Constraints

S. OGOH ALUBO

In pursuit of the goal of the World Health Organization's (WHO's) Alma Ata Declaration of "Health for All by the Year 2000" (HFA/2000), most underdeveloped countries have begun to implement strategies consistent with the declaration. Primary health care (PHC), defined as basic care that is scientifically sound, socially acceptable, and economically afford-able by individuals, is the chosen strategy for the achievement of this ambitious, tough, desirable goal.

Prior to the commitment to the Alma Ata Declaration, a high pre-mium was traditionally placed on health in Nigeria, as expressed in "health is wealth," "a healthy nation is a wealthy nation," and similar aphorisms. This importance of health and health care is underscored by the reasons offered for the 1983 military coup. Prominent among these explanations were the persistent shortages of drugs and other essentials (Abacha 1985a). The ongoing austerity programs that have followed in the wake of the coup, such as the removal of subsidies, are rationalized as painful but necessary measures, which, among other putative benefits, would stabilize the drug supply in hospitals. To be sure, the relationship between health and the overall economy now seems to be recognized in government policy documents (FGN 1986a), at least as an explanation for the crippling shortages in public hospitals. Hence it is now acknowledged in these documents that the shortages can be resolved only when the economic situation improves. The relationship between health, health care, and the economy, however, goes beyond explanations for shortages;

more significantly, the economy adversely affects the health and health indexes for the population.

This chapter examines Nigeria's implementation of strategies to reach the HFA/2000 goal. I first discuss the political–economic context within which this goal is being pursued; thereafter, the implementation program itself is discussed; and in the final section, I turn attention to the problems and constraints of HFA/2000.

Nigeria: A Sketch of Its Political Economy

It is appropriate to outline briefly the worldview that informs this discussion of Nigeria's political economy. The point of departure is the conception of the world economy as a single system, a perspective variously identified as dependency theory, world-system theory, or Marxist political economy of development (Frank 1967, 1973; Wallerstein 1974, 1979; Marx and Engels 1948, 12.[1] This viewpoint identifies two structural locations: the core, also called "metropole"; and the periphery, also known as "satellite."

Put simply, the core countries (of Europe, North America, and Japan) have, through centuries of relationships, extended economic activities to the periphery (Africa, Latin America, Southeast Asia) and incorporated the latter regions into world economy as appendages. Through this intricate process, which began as mercantilism and colonialism, economic activities in the periphery have been structured to reflect the needs of the core, a process Andre Gunder Frank has aptly referred to as the "development of underdevelopment" (Frank 1973).

This conception of development is both a critique of and an alternative to a modernization theory that views problems of development as basically endogenous to individual countries (Rostow 1960). Unlike theories of modernization, the paradigm used in this chapter suggests that the world economy is one system that, depending on the structural locations of countries as well as of individuals within these countries, produces poverty for some and affluence for others (Frank 1973; Wallerstein 1979).

With specific reference to Africa, Walter Rodney has argued that:

Africa helped to develop Western Europe in the same proportion as Western Europe helped to underdevelop Africa. . . .

. . . the operation of the imperialist system bears major responsibility for African economic retardation by draining African wealth and by making it impossible to develop more rapidly the resources of the continent.

. . . one has to deal with those who manipulate the system and those who are either agents or unwitting accomplices. (Rodney 1972, 37; see also Onimode 1988; Ntalaja 1989)

This system is sustained by an intricate web that firmly links external interests with those of the internal dominant classes—the so-called nationalist bourgeoisie and political elites. The internal bourgeoisie is dependent on the metropole for technology, spare parts, and "expertise," without which it cannot sustain production. Similarly, the political elites utilize their position—through vast opportunities for contracts, foreign-exchange regulations, and so forth—as an avenue for accumulation (Ohiorhenuan 1989; Barnet 1990). In this way, the interests of the domestic bourgeoisie and elites are fused with those of multinational corporations, the modern-day representatives of imperialism and foreign domination.

The overall underdevelopment of satellite countries (and classes) is reflected in health services development through the process of modernization. Development in this area has concentrated on (1) the construction of hospitals and other centers for curative therapy; (2) elitist labor-force development, with emphasis on physicians and nurses rather than health assistants or aides; and (3) importation of drugs and equipment (Sanders 1985). In this pursuit of modernization, Third World countries have characteristically equated health problems with medical problems, even though the major causes of morbidity and mortality lie in deprivation. This conception reinforces as well as legitimizes the existing political–economic system. It reinforces through dependency on "Western" countries for drugs, equipment, and sometimes personnel necessary for providing medical care, and legitimizes by equating health care with medical care, thereby sustaining the belief that conditions that result from deprivation can be resolved by biomedical intervention (Navarro 1978).

Nigeria gained political independence from British imperial power in 1960. Since independence, the country has experienced frequent, sometimes violent, changes of government in an alternating democracy–military government scenario. Thus the first democratic government, which took over from the British, was ousted in 1966, after which military rule continued until 1979. Between 1979 and December 1983 there was a second democratic government, which was again overthrown by the military (Falola and Ihonvbere 1984; Othman 1984; Adamolekun 1984). Military dictatorship has continued thereafter, although there is currently a phased program of transition to democracy by January 1993 (FGN 1987; Alubo 1989).

Until the 1970s, the Nigerian economy shared the characteristic features of underdeveloped countries that were incorporated into international capitalism as appendages to the West—that is, it served for the most part as a market and source of raw materials (Frank 1981). Accordingly, Nigeria exported ground (pea)nuts, cocoa, cotton, and palm produce in exchange for manufactured goods (Onimode 1983; Abba et al. 1985).

The demand for and, in consequence, the prices of these primary products are determined from outside by the metropolitan countries.

This economic situation was dramatically altered by the exploitation of oil reserves, which replaced cash crops—as primary agricultural produce were called—as the major source of foreign exchange. The oil boom, as this period (1973–82) came to be known, was characterized by ambitious—some of them white elephant—projects and general expansion, particularly of the public sector (Alubo 1990a). With specific reference to medical services, the number of government hospitals, including medical schools, doubled (FGN 1981). As Ogoh Alubo (1985a) has illustrated, the rallying cry during the oil boom period was that Nigeria was rich, and the only problem was how to spend its fortunes.

In spite of the oil wealth, the majority of the people remained poor. Moreover, the normal indexes of health (infant mortality rates, child death rates, and general morbidity and mortality rates), all of which are good measures of material well-being, continued to reflect poverty. A government document during the oil boom expressed this condition of widespread poverty amidst plenty—and its health consequences: "Twelve preventable and communicable diseases have been identified as currently accounting for 95 percent of all ill health and death in the country. The prevalent ones are malaria, tetanus, measles, tuberculosis, and meningitis" (FGN 1975, 262; see also FGN 1981, 289; FGN 1986a). The three problems of poverty, illiteracy, and disease, which early on constituted the major agenda for an independent Nigeria, continued to afflict the majority of the people. Thus, irrespective of the oil wealth—worth $25 billion annually from 1973–80 (Parfitt and Riley 1989, 3)—diseases of poverty continued to be the major causes of morbidity and mortality. During this boom period, per capita annual income rose sharply from about $350 in 1973 to $1,010 in 1980. Nigeria was then classified in World Bank documents as a *middle-income* economy (World Bank 1984).

The oil boom (which did not alter the dependent nature of the economy) was, however, short-lived, and the economy began to face a major crisis. This crisis, which was related to the unchanging external control of the economy (Onimode 1983; Abba et al. 1985), was manifest in high and rising unemployment, factory closures and low capacity utilization, high inflation, increasing foreign debt, and severe shortages of commodities, particularly food and medical supplies (Alubo 1985a; Bangura 1987). By 1990, Nigeria's per capita annual income has fallen to $290 and the country's status to low-income economy (World Bank 1990).

This unabating crisis was considered by the military as justification for the 1983 coup d'état. According to General Sani Abacha, who announced the coup, intervention was necessary to rescue Nigeria from a "grave economic predicament" and "harsh intolerable conditions" (Abacha 1985a, 4). This same rhetoric, part of the overall military messianism, was repeated as justification for the 1985 palace coup d'état (Babangida 1985; Abacha 1985a).

Despite the promise of deliverance, the harsh and intolerable conditions that the military ostensibly intervened to resolve have been aggravated by the new government's policies. The thrust of the military government's response to the crisis was monetary austerity prescribed by the International Monetary Fund (IMF) and the World Bank. Translated, this policy has entailed retrenchments in the public service and the reintroduction of *haraji* (poll tax) and *jangali* (cattle tax) as well as hospital fees, all of which were abolished during the oil boom. Other aspects of the Structural Adjustment Program (SAP), as monetarism is called in Nigeria, include removal of subsidies, wage-restraint measures, privatization, and commercialization (FGN 1986b).

These austerity programs have had a devastating impact on the population. Apart from the growing unemployment and the physical decay of social infrastructures such as schools, roads, and hospitals, hunger and starvation have reached catastrophic proportions (Bangura 1987; Thomas-Emeagwali 1988; see also Toyo 1986). Consequently, the scavenging of garbage in search for food (a situation once considered impossible by politicians) is commonplace, and nutrition-related conditions now account for over 50 percent of pediatric admissions in Nigerian hospitals. Succinctly, "the pattern of nutritional diseases now manifest in the country was last experienced in the war zones during the Nigerian civil war. As a matter of fact, diseases like kwashiorkor, previously limited to the urban poor and rural population has now begun to be recorded among *senior staff* children—a relatively privileged category" (Alubo 1990a, 1078). This situation also applies to the adult population, many of whom are changing their dietary compositions from tuber-based carbohydrates to grains (cereals). Others, however, go without one or more meals a day, and suffer all that this near-starvation implies for health.[2]

These nutritional problems are superimposed on existing parasitic and infectious conditions. Further, there is a general increase in morbidity rates as the immune system is compromised by hunger and malnutrition. Frequent outbreaks of various epidemics—among them meningitis, cholera, typhoid, and tuberculosis—have been seen, as has a recurrence of yellow fever, which was presumably eradicated during the oil boom (Alubo and Ogbe, in press).[3]

This increase in epidemics and the general deterioration of health are directly related to the debt crisis and attendant austerity programs. As experiences of other underdeveloped countries have shown, declining quality of life and increased morbidity rates are recognized consequences of austerity programs (Davis and Saunders 1987; Green and Singer 1984; Anyinam 1989; Musgrave 1987).

What has been the impact of austerity on medical services? The perennial shortages of drugs, equipment, and other essentials have escalated to crisis proportions. Across Nigeria, hospitalized patients are required to have a relative on hand to buy drugs, surgical dressings, and whatever else might be prescribed (Alubo 1985b). These shortages are on a larger scale related to the overall structure of underdevelopment and attendant dependency on external sources of drugs and equipment (Stock 1985; Alubo 1985b).

Nigeria's military government has addressed the medical aspect of the crisis through a process of rationalization and the commercialization of services in public hospitals. As part of this process, itself integral to the overall austerity programs, user fees have been reintroduced and free meals for patients on admission have been discontinued (Alubo 1990b). The more intricate component of the adjustments is the Drug Revolving Fund (DRF) scheme, whereby public pharmacies are run as businesses (Cross et al. 1986; Kanji 1989) in accordance with the World Bank prescriptions on health care financing (World Bank 1987). The program was based on the hope that "after an initial capital investment, drug supplies are replenished using monies collected from the sale of drugs to the consumer" (Kanji 1989, 115).

On the surface, DRF appears to be a rational response to the shortages of drugs. However, the DRF scheme does not address the structural origins of the shortages, and without such attention a lasting solution to the shortages will be elusive. Consequently, under DRF profits from the sale of drugs cannot in themselves translate into more drugs, which must compete with other commodities for foreign-exchange allocation. Furthermore, by requiring payment before service, as the operation of DRF does, the poor are effectively excluded. As Denis Ityavyar (1988) has shown, services are either denied outright or discontinued. In this way, not only do the austerity programs create health problems, they also constrain responses to such problems.

It is within this political–economic background of oil boom-and-bust and the post-boom austerity programs that HFA/2000 is being implemented in Nigeria.

The Implementation of HFA/2000 in Nigeria

The implementation of the WHO's "Health for All in Nigeria" program (WHO 1978), which is pursued through the PHC strategy, has a checkered history. After its inauguration during the Third Development Plan (1975–80) and subsequent demise, the PHC program was relaunched in August 1987 (FGN 1975; FGN 1986a). Because of this decline, I discuss both attempts here in some detail.

The Basic Health Services Scheme (BHSS)

PHC through the BHSS was designed to correct the persistent problems of the Nigerian health care system, namely, curative bias and the skewed distribution of facilities in favor of urban areas. The ultimate goal of the scheme was to achieve comprehensive health coverage of the population by the year 2000.

As outlined in the Third National Development Plan, BHSS entailed:

1. the provision of adequate and effective primary health care for the entire population through a gradual process—from 35 percent coverage in 1975 to 80 percent in 1985 and 100 percent by the year 2000;
2. the correction of the curative bias by incorporating preventive programs, such as immunization, health education, maternal and child health, family planning, environmental health services, and nutrition, into the health care process;
3. the use of local government authorities as the basic implementation units, and the Federal Ministry of Health as the central coordinating agency. (FGN 1981; Alubo 1983, 162)

BHSS was, by conception, grass roots-oriented; the local government areas—most of which are rural—were its fulcrum. Each local government area was designated basic health unit (BHU), comprising a comprehensive health center with a bed capacity of ninety for every 50,000 persons; four primary health centers, with fourteen beds for every 10,000 persons, twenty health clinics, with two to four beds for every 2,000 persons; and five mobile clinics for each primary health center. The scheme was designed to lead to community participation, to complement other aspects of rural development, and to lead ultimately to self-reliance. As part of this goal of participation, each community was directed to select two of its members for training as village medical helpers, after which they would return and work in the community.

On paper, BHSS seemed practical and workable. Its implementation, however, belies this apparent practicality. In spite of rhetoric about correcting curative imbalance, the major thrust of the scheme was ironically on medical care rather than health care. Aspects such as food, nutrition, water supply, and community participation were hardly included in the implementation. BHSS's implementation therefore reflects the reduction of health problems to medical problems. Further, many of its projects were not completed; consequently, no single BHU had the full complements of health centers and clinics. Whole states, comprising fifteen to twenty BHUs, had three health centers or fewer. Moreover, the mobile clinics—"Clinomobiles"—initially imported to facilitate PHC in rural areas were soon out of service, due to lack of spare parts. A study of

Benue State, for example, has shown that only three comprehensive health centers were built instead of the sixteen planned, and that none was linked systemically to any other facility. Similarly, the few imported Clinomobiles for the state had long since broken down and had been discarded (Alubo 1983).

These problems relate both to the ambitious nature of the scheme and to the structure of Nigeria's underdevelopment. Inspired no doubt by the oil boom, the scheme planned to build and operate over three hundred BHUs, complete with health centers, clinics, and village helpers, in ten years. Moreover, the high, almost total, import component of the scheme—drugs, equipment, Clinomobiles, even syringes—seems similarly misguided by the notion of affluence prevalent at the time. From the beginning, the entire scheme was founded on the precarious assumption of a continuing oil boom.

Further, in addition to its obvious predeliction for modernization, the scheme did not articulate any coherent worldview or ideology. Development programs, including health care development, both are informed by and reflect the dominant ideology. In Nigeria, the government denies that programs are ideologically motivated; yet it sought to transplant the concept of village medical helper, which originated out of some collectivist ideology (as in China or Tanzania), to Nigeria. The dismal outcome of the BHSS is in this sense typical of many transplanted schemes.[4]

An investigative federal government panel found that BHSS had several major problems, particularly of access and deployment of personnel. Regarding access, the scheme made no allowance for rapid increases in the population; consequently, a shrinking percentage of the population had access to medical care. Concerning deployment, the government evaluation panel found that "because the local government and the communities they were to serve participated very little in their selection, they did not feel any obligation to work in rural areas." Further, concerning the personnel, "their predominantly curative skills they acquired in the schools of health technology were inappropriate for the provision of primary health care services. . . . many were [therefore] posted to general hospitals where they were utilized to carry out 'menial jobs'" (quoted in Kuti 1988, 8).

Clearly, in spite of passing commitments to health care—including social and environmental health—the scheme was effectively expunged of these nonmedical components, of which the problem of deployment is a reflection. Hence, rather than work at the grass-roots level, as was originally envisaged, community health workers ended up in curative centers.

The overall implementation of the BHSS is summed up by the government panel as "haphazard and ineffective" (cited in Kuti 1988, 6). Its impact on morbidity and mortality are negligible. This failure suggests a clear disjunction between the BHSS plan and its execution.

The New HFA/2000 Program

The current program is spelled out in the document titled *The National Health Policy and Strategy to Achieve Health for All Nigerians* (FGN 1986a). Through the PHC strategy, the new program is, like its predecessor, grass roots-oriented.

The new program involves:

1. the division of the country into six zones, such that neighboring states are in the same zone;
2. phased implementation of PHC, beginning with 52 local governments in 1986, 80 in 1987, 100 by 1988, and the entire country (over 560 local governments) by 2000;
3. involvement of local governments and communities in data collection on health problems and available resources, as well as in workshops on how to resolve these problems;
4. the involvement of villages in the selection of its members to be trained as village health workers (VHW) and community health extension workers (CHEW). (FGN 1986a)

Through this program, the ultimate objective is to integrate primary, secondary, and tertiary care in such a way that the emergent health care system would be "promotive, protective, preventive, restorative, and rehabilitative to every citizen" (FGN 1986a, 9). As part of the new initiative, there is an intensified immunization drive against measles, tetanus, whooping cough, and diphtheria. Similarly, oral rehydration therapy (ORT) has the objective of teaching mothers how to combat child dehydration, which often accompanies gastroenteritis, with simple salt-and-water solution. Indeed, immunization shots and ORT packages now take precedence over other aspects of HFA/2000. ORT and intensified immunization are part of the United Nations Children's Fund's (UNICEF's) selective implementation of PHC, known as GOBI-FFF: Growth monitoring, Oral rehydration therapy, Breast-feeding, Immunization, Family spacing, Food supplements, and Female education (Kanji 1989; Banerji 1988, 1990).

Already, participating local governments have all the components of the new programs. Moreover, first-aid kits and bicycles have been provided to facilitate mobility of VHMs and CHEWs in rural communities. Regular visits by health teams to remote villages are central to the new program.

The program seems to recognize the social, nonclinical aspects of health—safe water, sanitation, and food and nutrition (FGN 1986a, 9). The document has called for multisectoral cooperation between various government and nongovernmental agencies to achieve implementation. True, both unsafe water and a lack of food, not to discount environmental problems, now constitute major health problems in Nigeria. Less than 35 percent of the population has access to safe water, and the food situation is also critical (NISER 1988).

These problems have been addressed both as part of overall development (FGN 1975, 1981) and on an ad hoc basis. Since Nigeria attained independence four development plans have been implemented, and various programs such as Operation Feed the Nation (1976), agricultural development programs (1974–1980), and Green Revolution (1981) were inaugurated to boost food production. But as Olufemi Adelakun (1984) has shown, these programs were drawn up by visionary but impractical national elites at the behest of foreign agencies and experts and were imposed on the rural producers. Consequently, the programs have led to more dependency for fertilizers and other agricultural supplies, instead of self-reliance in food supply (Gunilla and Beckman 1985; William 1988).

In 1987, the military government created the Directorate of Food, Roads, and Rural Infrastructure (DFRRI), an agency whose objective is the provision of safe water, rural roads, and a sufficient food supply (Koinyam 1987, 1989). DFRRI claims to have sunk boreholes and constructed rural roads across the country. Critics charge, however, that most of DFRRI's claims are false (Analyst Collective 1987).

Besides the failure of programs to provide adequately for the social components of health care, many existing social infrastructures such as roads, water supply lines, and rural electricity services are out of service because of a lack of spare parts and general decay. As Ali Mazrui (1986) and others (Green and Singer 1984; Anyinam 1989; World Bank 1989) have illustrated, the debt crisis is fast eroding existing social infrastructures throughout Africa, including those in Nigeria.

Thus it may be seen that the implementation of HFA/2000 in Nigeria is confronted by serious problems (Achime 1989), not least of which is the fact that the implementation process invariably exacerbates overall dependency in the supply of vaccines, drugs, and equipment. This widening gap between the HFA/2000 goal and the economic base for its achievement is related to the overall political–economic context. In addition to the problems already noted, the material base for sustaining HFA/2000 is being eroded by the economic crisis.

HFA/2000 in Nigeria: Problems and Constraints

So far, we have discussed HFA/2000 in Nigeria and the political–economic tapestry of its implementation. The HFA/2000 program is presented as the apolitical largess of the benevolent state. It appears to offer "health" as a self-sufficient entity, detached from prevailing patterns of class exploitation, poverty, and oppression.

The reality of Nigeria's political economy, however, belies this apolitical ("let's join hands and work for the common good") orientation. As was earlier observed, class antagonisms are now heightened as international capital, backed by a military dictatorship and other representatives of the bourgeoisie, is pitted against the welfare of the underclasses. These escalating class struggles have led to frequent labor strikes and two popular revolts (Alubo 1989).

It must be said that every aspect of all development, including health development, is political and ideological (Frank 1973; Roxborough 1979). Ideological commitments determine whether and how development programs, in this case HFA/2000, will be achieved. But as is common for all ideological motivations, Nigeria's various postcolonial governments have been reluctant to make any overt pronouncements. Aside from the constitutional acknowledgment of a mixed economy (supposedly, elements of socialism and capitalism), the best official statement sets forth these general "national objectives":

· a free and democratic society
· a just and egalitarian society
· a united, strong, and self-reliant nation
· a great and dynamic economy
· a land of bright and full opportunities for all citizens. (FGN 1986a, 7)

In spite of official denials, Nigeria is thoroughly capitalist—not mixed capitalist–socialist—as historical and current political economic trends show. Historically, communal and other indigenous modes of production became subordinate to the market economy as Nigeria became annexed into world capitalism (Nnoli 1981; Shenton 1986; Onimode 1983). This subordinate (periphery) status is particularly reflected in the patterns of ownership and control over key sectors of the economy— manufacturing, oil, banking, commerce, and so forth—which are privately owned and dominated by multinational corporations, the present-day symbols of imperialism (Abba et al. 1985; Onimode et al. 1983).

The ongoing economic crisis and attendant austerity measures have, through the SAP, strengthened Western control over the economy. Consequently, initial gains in indigenization programs are now being reversed through debt–equity swaps, in which debts owed Western creditors are converted to equity shares in publicly owned corporations, and through other policies of the Western-dominated IMF and the World Bank (Parfitt and Riley 1989; Ake 1988; Onimode 1988).

But even as the SAP is regularly monitored by both the IMF and the World Bank, Nigeria's military government insists that the program was homegrown and that it is "the only alternative we have" (Babangida

1989, 8). The political significance of this conception is that the official program is presented, for legitimation purposes, as not only natural but as the only one possible (Navarro 1986). The Nigerian government insists that there is no alternative to the SAP. Accordingly, class contradictions, particularly as manifest in exploitation and increasing morbidity rates, are glossed over. In spite of widening poverty, government assessments of the SAP have concentrated on its supposed gains (FGN 1989).[5] The gross national product (GNP) in Nigeria fell by over 25 percent between 1987–89 (World Bank 1989), and the cost of living doubled between 1986–87 (NISER 1988). The underclasses bear the brunt of this precipitous decline, as is indicated by exponential increases in nutritionally related diseases and the exclusion of the poor from available social services (such as schools and hospitals) through the imposition of higher user fees (Alubo 1990a).

We note here in passing that even if the SAP were yielding gains in terms of GNP and similar indicators, such gains do not in themselves translate to individual consumption. The supposed "economic miracle" of Brazil, for example, coexisted with poverty and deprivation (Horn 1985; Frank 1981, 7; Macedo 1984). Brazil's former president Ernesto Gisel expressed this contradiction thus: The economy is doing well, but the people are not.

The current pursuit of HFA/2000 thus depoliticizes disease by diverting attention from the material conditions in which the people live. The emphasis is on immunization shots and ORT, as if these in themselves can resolve the problems of deprivation, which accounts for most ill health in Nigeria. It is clear that the implementation of HFA/2000 has neglected health care and concentrated on medical care. As Vicente Navarro (1986) has shown, the program was inaugurated during a time of escalating world hunger and general economic decline. As a result, the impression has been created that these problems would be resolved by the HFA/2000 program. The primary objective of the WHO's HFA/2000 is therefore one of legitimation.

This pursuit of legitimation, however, cannot obfuscate many of the contradictions of the HFA/2000 program, primary among which is the economic contradiction. As earlier discussed, the Nigerian economy is in a major crisis that is eroding the material base necessary for the implementation of HFA/2000. For instance, how is the pursuit of health for all compatible with the hunger now exacerbated by the austerity programs, or with the removal of subsidies and continuing retrenchment? Not only does retrenchment swell the already high unemployment, but it also jeopardizes the livelihood of workers' immediate and extended families; and the removal of subsidies has led to higher inflation.

By overlooking these structural issues while emphasizing medical care, the implementation of HFA/2000 depoliticizes disease. Not surprisingly, it has reduced the treatment of children's diseases—mostly nutritional and therefore political—to vaccines and sugar–salt solutions. The significance of immunizations and oral rehydration cannot be denied, but nutritional disorders cannot be resolved by medication alone (Zaidi 1988; Navarro 1986; McKinlay 1990). Yet the Nigerian government equates immunization statistics with the "number of children saved" (Alubo 1985a), regardless of what problems of nutrition, water supply, and disease they face. As Najmi Kanji has pointed out, GOBI-FFF and similar aspects of the selective implementation of PHC imply that

> selective interventions can improve health, without the improvement in people's economic, social, and political environments. The strategy depoliticizes health and . . . naturalizes poverty.
> . . . It can divert attention from the real causes of ill health. It raises false hopes about improving health standards and transforms local organizations into instruments for the delivery of its package. (Kanji 1989), 113)

The present thrust of HFA/2000 seems to contradict the Alma Ata document, which envisaged a shift from the biomedicine that typically, in the Third World situation, only deepens dependency. Some analysts have linked this change to the World Bank who, acting through UNICEF, has found it politically more expedient to divest HFA/2000 of its participatory as well as class content (Kanji 1989; Banerji 1988, 1990; Sanders et al., forthcoming). Debabar Banerji's comment on the role of UNICEF in all this is instructive:

> UNICEF, which was a co-sponsor of the Alma Ata conference on primary health care, started talking of selective primary health care in the form of GOBI. . . . When female literacy was included, it became GOBI-FFF. It is noteworthy that UNICEF did not consider it necessary to test this selective approach in the field before staking all its prestige and power behind it and pushing this approach on Third World countries.
> . . . With considerable support from many powerful agencies, UNICEF has launched a still more ambitious program—the Universal Child Immunization to all by 1990 (UCI–90). It may be noted that this powerful move to promote technocentric programs in Third World countries has been sustained in spite of very categorical disapproval of this approach by an international meeting of public health administrators representing every region of WHO. (Banerji 1988, 297)

Clearly, the class factors that determine who gets sick and from what conditions are ignored by this pursuit of HFA/2000. As Navarro has rightly observed, depoliticization of health problems may be traced to the

Alma Ata Declaration, itself based on the false premise that not only can the interests of all classes coexist but, more importantly, such interests can be realized in peace and harmony in a supposed new economic order. This strategy is characteristic of multilateral agencies like the WHO, the World Bank, and other organizations that Graham Hancock (1989) has called, in the title of his book, the *Lords of Poverty*, exposing as pretensions their claims to be harbingers of development and affluence.

The implementation of HFA/2000 in Nigeria has other problems. When the program is reduced to medical care, several contradictions still remain, not least of which is the reintroduction of user fees in public hospitals (Ityavyar 1988; Achime 1989). Even if such charges have become "inevitable," there are no provisions for protecting the most vulnerable segments of the population. As earlier noted, the poor are either denied service outright or services are discontinued when patients cannot afford the payments. In this way, not only has the economic crisis escalated health problems, particularly of the poor, but it has also constrained opportunities for treatment. Similarly, the now-enfeebled economy cannot sustain the demand for drugs and equipment necessary for the provision of medical care. In consequence, HFA/2000 rests on a shaky financial base.

Conclusion

This chapter has argued that most diseases in Nigeria, as indeed in many other underdeveloped countries, have political–economic origins, and that the implementation of the HFA/2000 program has generally ignored the political nature of disease. I have shown that the implementation of HFA/2000 in Nigeria has many obstacles that derive from two interrelated sources—externally imposed conditions by the World Bank and other agents of international capital, and the internal power structure that enforces as well as sustains this domination. Outside this broader agenda, community participation, appropriate technology, and other aspects the HFA/2000 program would continue to have marginal impact on morbidity and mortality. The crucial issue is that health care, before or after the year 2000, is a political issue, firmly rooted in the economic structure within which individuals live and the material conditions that impinge on their living.

Therefore the struggle for health is organically linked with that for a more humane and egalitarian society where health care will be determined by individual needs and a collective philosophy to meet such needs, rather than by assumptions of the supposed "common good," austerity programs, and other aspects of the oppressive political–economic structure. Indeed, it has been amply documented that economic imperialism is antithetical to health (Navarro 1986; Cornia, Jolly, and Steward 1987; UNICEF 1989).

The conclusion seems inevitable that the HFA/2000 program is politically deceptive, and that the material base needed to achieve even its narrow medical conception is being eroded by the same forces (international capital, the World Bank, and, to some extent, UNICEF) that foisted the program on the Third World, including Nigeria, in the first place. Moreover, "since the causes of disease are so embedded in the socio-economic structure of a country and the world, approaches like HFA/2000 and PHC will not be able to significantly affect the health status of the poor for so long as they remain within the vicious circle that causes their poverty" (Zaidi 1988, 119). In contrast to its purported goal, the implementation of HFA/2000 in Nigeria might provide medical care to some while denying health care to most.

NOTES

Acknowledgments: The author is grateful to Andrew Twaddle, Stanley Ingman, and Musa Ilu for intellectual inspiration, and to Patti Baldwin who kindly provided secretarial services. Needless to say, the author is solely responsible for the content of the paper.

1. We are aware that dependency theory, world-system theory, and Marxist political economy differ in some respects, although they share the same general worldview.

2. The food crisis has compelled most people—particularly the underclasses—to adjust and "improvise," sometimes with fatal consequences. A newspaper article once related how three members of a family died after an "improvised" meal (see Adelakun and Alubo 1989). Going without one or more meals is articulated in the popular parlance in terms of a daily formula: 0-1-0, 1-0-1, and so forth, where 0 means no meal (Thomas-Emeagwali 1988).

3. In the past four years, yellow fever epidemics have ravaged Benue State (1986), Sokoto State (1988), and Oyo State (1988).

4. The use of village health workers and similar "barefoot doctors" derives from the experiences of China and Tanzania. According to Nigeria's health minister, Olikoye Ransome-Kuti, his ministry "understudied" in many countries, including Tanzania, China, and Zimbabwe.

5. Across Nigeria, billboards proclaim the SAP as the solution to the economic crisis. The supposed gains of SAP are periodically advertised in the media by the Ministry of Information, as well as in propaganda literature (see, e.g., FGN 1989).

REFERENCES

Abacha, Sarji. 1985a. Speech announcing the December 1983 coup. In *Return to Military Rule*, ed. Eddie Iroha, 3–4. Lagos: Daily Times.
———. 1985b. Speech during the August 1985 coup. *Newswatch* (September 9):4.
Abba, Alkasum, Yahaya Abdullahi, Muhammed Sanusi Abubakar, Mike Kwanashie, Abubakar Siddique Mohammad, Okello Oculi, Kyari Tijani, and Yusuf Bola Usman. 1985. *The Nigerian Economic Crisis*. Zaria: Academic Staff Union of Universities.

Achime, Nwabueze. 1989. "Health Sector in a Developing Country: An Analysis of Primary Health Care in Nigeria." *Scandinavian Journal of Development Alternatives* 8(4):159–84.

Adamolekun, Lekan. 1984. *The Fall of the Second Republic*. Ibadan: Spectrum.

Adelakun, Femi, and Ogoh Alubo. 1989. "SAP: The Pains of the 'Gains.'" *National Concord* (February 22):3.

Adelakun, Olufemi. 1984. "Social Structure and Rural Development in Nigeria." Ph.D. diss., Cardiff: University of Wales.

Ake, Claude. 1985. "The Political Economy of Development." *International Social Science Journal* 118:485–97.

Alubo, Ogoh. 1983. "The Political Economy of Health and Medical Care in Nigeria." Ph.D. diss., University of Missouri, Columbia.

———. 1985a. "Underdevelopment and Health Care Crisis in Nigeria." *Medical Anthropology* 9(4):319–35.

———. 1985b. "Drugging the People: Pills, Profits and Underdevelopment in Nigeria." *Studies in Third World Societies* 24:89–113.

———. 1989. "Crisis, Repression and the Prospects for Democracy in Nigeria." *Scandinavian Journal of Development Alternatives* 8(4):107–22.

———. 1990. "State Violence and Health in Nigeria." *Social Science and Medicine* 31(10):1075–84.

———. 1990b. "Doctoring as Business: A Study of Entrepreneurial Medicine in Nigeria." *Medical Anthropology* 12:305–24.

Alubo, Ogoh, and Michael Ogbe. "The 1986 Yellow Fever Epidemic in Nigeria." *Nigerian Journal of Social Studies* (in press).

Analyst Collective. 1987. "DFRRI: N 3 Billion Bonanza for Big Fish." *Analyst* 2 (April):7–13.

Anyinam, Charles. 1989. "The Social Cost of the International Monetary Funds Adjustment Programs: The Case of Health Development in Ghana." *International Journal of Health Services* 19(3):531–47.

Babangida, Ibrahim. 1985. Maiden speech as Nigeria's president. *Newswatch* (September 9):18–19.

———. 1989. *Speech at the Inauguration of Armed Forces Consultative Assembly*. Lagos: Government Printer.

Banerji, Debabar. 1988. "Hidden Menace in the Universal Child Immunization Program." *International Journal of Health Services* 18(2):293–99.

———. 1990. "Crash of the Immunization Program: Consequences of the Totalitarian Approach." *International Journal of Health Services* 20(3):501–10.

Bangura, Yusuf. 1987. "Structural Adjustment and the Political Question." *Review of African Political Economy* 37:24–37.

Barnet, Richard. 1990. "But What about Africa? On the Global Economy's Lost Continent." *Harper* (May):43–51.

Cornia, Andrea, Richard Jolly, and Frances Steward. 1987. *Adjustment with a Human Face*. Oxford: Clarendon.

Cross, Peter, Maggie A. Huff, Jonathan D. Quick, and James A. Bates. 1986. "Revolving Drug Funds: Conducting Business in the Public Sector." *Social Science and Medicine* 22(3):335–42.

Davis, Rob, and David Saunders. 1987. "IMF Stabilisation Policies and the Effect on Child Health in Zimbabwe." *Review of African Political Economy* 38:3–23.

Falola, Toyin, and Julius Ihonbvere. 1984. *The Rise and Fall of Nigeria's Second Republic*. London: Zed.

Federal Government of Nigeria (FGN). 1975. *Third National Development Plan 1975–80*. Lagos: Federal Ministry of Economic Planning.

————. 1981. *Fourth National Development Plan 1981–85.* Lagos: Federal Ministry of National Planning.

————. 1986a. *The National Policy and Strategy to Achieve Health for All in Nigeria.* Lagos: Federal Ministry of Health.

————. 1986b. *Structural Adjustment Program for Nigeria.* Lagos: Government Printer.

————. 1987. *Transition Program for Return to Democracy.* Lagos: Government Printer.

————. 1989. *30 Questions and Answers on SAP.* Lagos: Federal Ministry of Information.

Frank, Andre Gunder. 1967. "Sociology of Development and Underdevelopment in Sociology." *Catalyst* 7:20–73.

————. 1973. "Development of Underdevelopment." In *The Political Economy of Development and Underdevelopment,* ed. C. Wilber, 103–113. New York: Random House.

————. 1981. *Crisis: In the Third World.* New York: Holmes & Meier.

Green, Reginald, and Hans Singer. 1984. "Subsaharan Africa in Depression: The Impact on the Welfare of Children." *World Development* 12(3):283–95.

Gunila, Andrea, and Bjorn Beckman. 1985. *The Wheat Trap: Bread and Underdevelopment in Nigeria.* London: Zed.

Hancock, Graham. 1989. *Lords of Poverty: The Power, Prestige and Corruption of International Aid Business.* New York: Atlantic Monthly.

Horn, James. 1985. "Brazil: The Health Care Model of the Military Modernizers and Technocrats." *International Journal of Health Services* 15(7):49–68.

Ityavyar, Denis. 1988. "Health Services Inequalities in Nigeria." *Social Science and Medicine* 27(11):1223–35.

Kanji, Najmi. 1989. "Charging for Drugs in Africa: UNICEF Is 'Bamako Initiative.'" *Health Policy and Planning* 4(2):110–20.

Koinyam, Larry. 1987. *The Way Forward: Rural Development.* Lagos: Directorate of Food, Roads, and Rural Infrastructure.

————. 1989. *An Urgent Message to All Nigerian Communities.* Lagos: Directorate of Food, Roads, and Rural Infrastructure.

Kuti, Olijoye. 1988. "Speech at the Opening of National Conference on Problems of Rural Dwellers." National Institute for Policy and Strategic Studies, Kuru (January). Mimeograph.

Macedo, Roberto. 1984. "Brazilian Children and Economic Crisis: Evidence from the State of Sao Paulo." *World Development* 12(3):203–11.

McKinlay, John. 1990. "A Case for Refocussing Upstream: The Political Economy of Illness." In *The Sociology of Health and Illness,* ed. Peter Conrad and Rochelle Kern, 502–16. New York: St. Martin's.

Marx, Karl, and Frederich Engels. 1948. *The Communist Manifesto.* New York: International Publishers.

Mazrui, Ali. 1986. *The Africans: A Triple Heritage.* New York: Little Brown.

Musgrave, Philip. 1987. "The Economic Crisis and Its Impact on Health Care in Latin America and the Caribbean." *International Journal of Health Services* 17(3):411–41.

Navarro, Vicente. 1978. *Medicine under Capitalism.* New York: Prodist.

————. 1986. *Crisis, Health and Medicine.* New York: Tavistock.

Nnoli, Okwudiba, ed. 1981. *Path to Nigerian Development.* Dakar: Codsira.

Nigeria Institute of Social and Economic Research (NISER). 1988. *The Social Impact of the Structural Adjustment Program.* Ibadan: NISER.

Ntalaja, Nzongola. 1989. "The African Crisis: The Way Out." *African Studies Review* 32(1):115–28.

Ohiorhenuan, John. 1989. *Capital and the State in Nigeria.* Westport, Conn.: Greenwood.

Onimode, Bade. 1983. *Imperialism and Underdevelopment in Nigeria.* Lagos: Macmillan.

———. 1988. *The Political Economy of the African Debt Crisis.* London: Zed.

Onimode, Bade, John Ohiorhenuan, and Tude Adeniran. 1983. *Multinational Corporations in Nigeria.* Ibadan: Les Shyraden.

Othman, Shehu. 1984. "Classes, Crisis and the Coup: The Demise of Shagari Regime." *African Affairs* 83(33):441–61.

Parfitt, Trevor, and Stephen Riley. 1989. *The African Debt Crisis.* London: Routledge.

Rodney, Walter. 1972. *How Europe Underdeveloped Africa.* Dar es Salaam: Tanzania Publishing House.

Rostow, Walter. 1960. *Stages of Economic Growth.* Cambridge: Cambridge University Press.

Roxborough, Ian. 1979. *Theories of Underdevelopment.* Atlantic Highlands, N.J.: Humanities Press.

Sanders, David. 1985. *The Struggle for Health: Medicine and the Politics of Underdevelopment.* London: Macmillan.

Sanders, David, Fwoze Marij, and Ogoh Alubo. "The Ukunda Declaration on Economic Policy and Health." Forthcoming in *Health Policy and Planning.*

Shenton, Robert. 1986. *The Development of Capitalism in Northern Nigeria.* Toronto: University of Toronto Press.

Stock, Robert. 1985. "Drugs and Underdevelopment: A Study of Kano State, Nigeria." *Studies in Third World Societies* 24:115–40.

Thomas-Emeagwali, Gloria. 1988. "Development Alternatives with Women, Food and Debt Crisis." *Review of African Political Economy* 43:90.

Toyo, Eskor. 1986. "Food and Hunger in a Petroleum Neocolony: A Study of Food Crisis in Nigeria." In *World Recession and the Food Crisis in Africa,* ed. Peter Lawrence, 231–48. Boulder, Colo.: Westview.

United Nations Children's Fund (UNICEF). 1989. *State of the World Children 1989.* Oxford: Oxford University Press.

Wallerstein, Immanuel. 1974. *The Modern World-System.* New York: Academic Press.

———. 1979. *The Capitalist World Economy.* Cambridge: Cambridge University Press.

William, Gavin. 1988. "The World Bank in Rural Nigeria Revisited: A Review of the World Bank's Nigeria Agricultural Sector." *Review of African Political Economy* 43:42–67.

World Bank. 1984. *World Development Report 1984.* Washington, D.C.: World Bank.

———. 1987. *Financing Health Services in Developing Countries: An Agenda for Reform.* Washington, D.C.: World Bank.

———. 1989. *Subsaharan Africa: From Crisis to Sustainable Growth.* Washington, D.C.: World Bank.

———. 1990. *World Development Report 1990.* Washington, D.C.: World Bank.

World Health Organization. 1978. *Primary Care: Report of the International Conference on Primary Health Care, Alma Ata, USSR.* Geneva: WHO.

Zaidi, Akbar. 1988. "Poverty and Disease: Need for Structural Change." *Social Science and Medicine* 27(2):119–27.

Part VI

Applying

Social

Science

Knowledge

in

Health

Settings

Chapter 12

Home and Hospital

Birthing in Oman:

An Observational Study with

Recommendations for

Hospital Practice

CAROL J. PIERCE COLFER *and*
EUGENE B. GALLAGHER

In recent years, the medical profession has begun to accept the importance of such amorphous factors as trust, security, and emotional support in various medical contexts. This acceptance sets the stage for more meaningful incorporation of indigenous knowledge and practice—such as we document here—into medical routine.

Health care consumers in rural areas of developing countries frequently lack the wherewithal to challenge new medical establishments when they are not responsive to people's needs. In such countries, illiteracy is typically widespread, information is hard to gather and disseminate, and governments may have an authoritarian cast not conducive to either political dissent or critical analysis of social institutions such as medicine. Analyses like ours can serve as a bridge for policymakers to help them mold health care institutions in more culturally appropriate directions.

In this chapter, we show how the traditions and procedures of Western medicine can unnecessarily conflict with the values and expectations of consumers. In the end, we distill our findings into recommendations for use by professional personnel.

Focus, Locale, and Methodology of the Study

This study deals with the birthing experience in Oman. First, it describes the perspective that indigenous rural midwives have toward their task of assisting the mother in giving birth at home. Then it compares birthing under medical auspices in a modern rural hospital with home birthing. It describes the beliefs and attitudes that underlie the contrasting midwife and hospital modes.

The Sultanate of Oman lies along the southeastern coast of the Arabian peninsula, covering 82,000 square miles. Although a census has never been done in Oman, estimates of the population range from one to two million. (All statistical population data for Oman are suspect—and changing.) With the exception of an unknown but sizable number of foreign workers, the population is almost completely Muslim. Arabic is the language of the majority, but there are a significant number of other languages spoken by Omanis.

Most Omanis work in agriculture and fishing, though oil supplies over 95 percent of Oman's national income. The World Bank's estimates (World Bank 1990) provide a rough idea of education and health care in Oman: adult life expectancy in years for men is 55, and for women, 58. There is one hospital bed per 331 persons, and one physician per 1,071 persons. The annual rate of population increase is 3.9 percent. In 1989, Saleh Khusaibi (1989) provided a fairly reliable estimate of infant mortality at thirty deaths per one thousand infants.

The nation entered a phase of accelerated development starting in 1970, when the present ruler, Sultan Qaboos bin Said, ousted his conservative father in a palace coup. Under Qaboos there has been a rapid expansion of health facilities, schools, and physical infrastructure for transportation and communication.

Indigenous Midwifery in the Interior: An Interview Study of Six Midwives

One of the authors (Carol J. Pierce Colfer), trained in anthropology and public health, conducted the study of midwives during 1989–90. At that time she held an academic appointment in the Department of Community Health at Sultan Qaboos University's College of Medicine. The other author (Eugene B. Gallagher) is a medical sociologist with research experience in the development of health services in the Middle East and in infant–maternal health.

This study was prompted in part by the desire of health professionals to understand why there were difficulties in dealing with the Omani mothers at the time of delivery. Many mothers came to the hospital too late in the course of labor, according to medical opinion. It was also known that many mothers delivered at home; estimates on home deliveries ranged between 20 percent and 35 percent.

The general policy of the national Ministry of Health (MOH) favors hospital delivery, and in recent years the government has substantially increased its provision for this service. Nevertheless, many women live in rural areas remote from existing hospitals. Others, for reasons to be described below, prefer not to use hospitals for birthing. Their various reasons for reluctance could become sources of difficulty on the occasions—at other births or in cases of illness—when they do come to the hospital.

Many Omani MOH personnel, as in other developing countries, strongly disapprove of midwives or traditional birth attendants. Midwives are widespread throughout the Middle East; social scientists have studied their role and position in the community, as well as the varying stances, predominantly negative, that officials and medical professional have adopted toward them (Newman 1981; Pillsbury 1978).

Whatever the official and professional attitudes toward midwives, it was clear that their influence was significant in the catchment communities of the hospital studied here (Al Jebel Hospital—a pseudonym). Understanding the practices and theories of midwives could help health professionals in the hospital deal with patients in a more culturally appropriate and sensitive fashion.

Colfer spent a total of thirty-four hours interviewing six midwives who lived in the rural area served by Al Jebel Hospital. Each midwife was interviewed in Arabic at least twice. Notes taken during the interviews were shared with physicians and nurses at Sultan Qaboos University, to obtain medical perspectives on the efficacy of, and problems with, the midwives' procedures.

The midwives responded positively to being interviewed; in view of their awareness of official disapproval, it was anticipated that they might be reluctant. However, they were quite willing to convey their knowledge of labor, birth, anatomy, and fertility. Interviews invariably elicited lively discussions among the midwives, as well as among other women who dropped by to visit and observe. It gradually appeared that many older women—not only the identified midwives—help out with births, and that the midwives themselves do not consider midwifery to be a highly specialized activity.

Although official disapproval of midwives focuses on objective health risk factors such as lack of sanitation and sterile procedure, we believe other, more subtle factors may also be at stake. The midwives were modest, even self-deprecating in their conception of their role. They viewed giving birth as a normal part of female life. They saw themselves as concerned, neighborly helpers in a situation that usually turned out well and required no great skill on their part. They did not see themselves as decisive interveners. Though they were quite aware of complications and bad outcomes in delivery, holding in reserve special stratagems for such contingencies, they also had a fatalistic sense about them. These attitudes conflict with the somewhat unrealistic posture of assertive, analytic control and scientific manageability that health professionals and officials often display in their work.

Before turning to specific findings of the midwives' study, we wish to note that among medical consumers in the developed world, the situation of childbirth has evoked strong protest. Evidence showing that pregnancy and childbirth have become unnecessarily medicalized is easy to marshal (Martin 1987). Women in the West, like Omani midwives and mothers, are beginning to emphasize that pregnancy and childbirth are normal, expectable events in the female life cycle.

Many aspects of medical science applied to childbirth have unquestionably spared the lives of many infants and mothers, who would have died in previous times. In the attempt to make pregnancy and childbirth safer, a whole range of hospital procedures have developed that serve to transfer childbirth out of women's control and into the hands of professionals—a transfer many women resist. Yet the fact that normal pregnancy and deliveries far outweigh those with problems lends support to those who wish to normalize pregnancy and reduce medical intervention and control.

This study of Omani midwives was designed to ascertain which aspects of their knowledge and procedures might be adaptable to the hospital setting (deemed safer by most medical personnel). Omani midwives' views are presented first in regard to normal deliveries and then in regard to problem deliveries.

Normal Delivery

Labor

The midwives' stance toward labor can be summed up in one word: waiting. Their expectation is that things will go smoothly and that when the time comes, they will simply cut the umbilical cord. This is in distinct contrast to the hospital's focus on "managing" labor—timing it, monitoring it, remaining ever alert to possible problems. It should be noted, however, that not all doctors share a common stance on labor. A Canadian study found that general practitioners are less prone to interference in the birth process than are obstetricians (Klein 1988).

Position

Views on the best position for delivery vary among the Omani midwives, though there is a preference for a standing position. Every midwife interviewed allowed the woman considerable discretion in determining her own position.

Midwife Maimune (pseudonyms are used to protect their privacy) recommended that the mother sit and lean back against the midwife's stomach or chest, or stand while clinging to a pipe firmly anchored to the ceiling in most homes. Midwife Esme described the woman standing with legs slightly bent and arms clinging to the pipe, while Esme embraced her just below the breasts. Midwife Salame told how the woman pushed forward against a wall, her legs bent, while Salame pressed upon her perineum from behind. Midwives also described mothers kneeling on one leg or two, squatting, or lying down all as legitimate positions.

Opinion in Western medicine is shifting toward the traditional views espoused by the Omani midwives. Brigitte Jordan (1983) summarizes some of the problems now perceived with the lithotomy position (mother on her back) used in most hospitals: negative effects on the mother's blood pressure and breathing and undue stretching of the perineal tissue, leading to more frequent tears. Not surprisingly, this shift in medical opinion has been applauded by Western feminist thinkers who wish to enhance female autonomy in childbirth, as in other spheres of health behavior (Martin 1987).

Apparel

All the midwives insisted that women should give birth with their pants on. Women's pants are typically baggy at the crotch and held up by a drawstring or elastic at the waist. Such apparel seems sensible, particularly for the woman giving birth in a vertical position. It is, however, strikingly different from what women wear in hospitals, and it was severely disparaged by physicians and nurses at Al Jebel Hospital, who made dire predictions of asphyxiation of the baby. Women in the hospital wore hospital gowns that could easily be raised—and regularly were—for visual inspection during labor.

The sentiment behind wearing pants is that of modesty, far from unknown among Western women but no doubt stronger among Omanis. Related to this sentiment is the strong belief that exposing female genitalia is contrary to Koranic teachings. (Educated Omani Muslims say that this is inaccurate; there are many such disputes in Islam, particularly around the status of women, health practices, and norms for dress in public.) Midwives try not to look at the woman's vagina, though they also hint that sometimes it is necessary for them to do so. They consider that exposure of the vagina is a major source of objection to hospital delivery, even though all the hospital personnel in the labor–delivery areas are female. They stress that, in their own practice, the mother is alone with the midwife during the delivery. Female friends and family members wait in an adjoining room, to be called in soon after the birth.

Delivery of the Baby and the Placenta

In normal births, the delivery of the baby "happens." The baby simply comes out. The midwife's main job is to cut the cord. Every midwife said modestly, "I just cut the cord." The interviews all suggested that, if things are seen to be proceeding normally, there is no intervention whatsoever.

Once the baby is born, the woman's pants are removed and the baby is laid on the floor. Esme described the woman as squatting while the cord was cut and then reclining, with her genital area covered by a headscarf draped over her knees, to wait for delivery of the placenta.

Some midwives deliver the placenta before cutting the cord; others, after. Esme has a metal bar around which she wraps the umbilical cord, to help along the delivery of the placenta. Maimune and Salame massage the woman's abdomen for the same purpose. All the midwives are aware of the importance of delivering an intact placenta. They report checking to determine whether the placenta is complete, and reaching inside to get any remaining bits. A retained bit is believed to travel upward to the heart (fu'ad), where it can cause the death of the mother. Although anatomically incorrect, this belief about the probable result—maternal death—of incomplete delivery of the placenta is accurate. Placental delivery is one feature of the birth process in which the midwife is vigilant.

The midwife wraps thread, usually white, tightly around the umbilical cord "the width of two fingers" from the baby's belly. The cord is then cut with a razor blade or with scissors. When asked about the cleanliness of instruments, Maimune stated that she used each side of a double-edged razor only once. Salame said that she washes her scissors with soap and warm water. Indigo (nile) is then dabbed onto the baby's umbilicus.

Placenta and Cord Disposal

The placenta and cord are buried in a hole dug about eighteen inches deep in the courtyard outside the front door of the house. They are covered with ashes and salt to prevent odor. The midwives did not mention any special meanings or rituals connected with the placenta, though such beliefs are common elsewhere (e.g., the superstition in medieval Europe that if a dog or cat should dig up this tissue, the baby would grow up to be a vagrant).

Salame mentioned the practice of saving the stub of the umbilical cord when it drops from the baby's navel. If the baby develops an eye infection during the next several months, a bit of the cord is ground on a stone, mixed with water, and applied to the infected eye with a marwad (a metal stick used to apply kohl, a mascara-like substance applied to the eyes of women and children for beauty and health). The stub can also be tossed into a creek bed (*wadi*) during flood, in the belief that this will help the child walk earlier.

Care after Birth

The midwives reported that immediately after birth they cleaned the mother and the baby. They applied warm water and salt to the mother's vagina. Maimune said she added a little thyme to the solution. The midwives said that tearing of the tissues was unusual, but when it did occur they applied *hal halil*, a hair oil. They do no cutting or suturing. In the past, the midwives also inserted a lump of salt into the vagina, to rid the mother of the birth wastes and to hasten return to her prepregnancy state. They are aware of official disapproval of this practice and all maintained that they no longer did it.

When the birth is complete, Salame reported that she sits facing the mother, putting her heel into the mother's perineum. She and the mother cross arms and pull, increasing the heel pressure on the mother's perineum. Salame says that this reduces back pain. Sheila Cosminsky (1983) reports a similar practice in India, used there, however, to facilitate labor. Other midwives wrapped a cloth tightly around the woman's upper abdomen to prevent back pain and to speed abdominal recovery (cf. the "abdominal binder" used in Central America, noted by Cosminsky [1983]).

Food

The midwives give the new mother a mixture of clarified butter and black pepper soon after the birth. They believe that this helps to reduce pain and to restore the mother to her previous state. This and other ingested substances are linked to indigenous theories of bodily functioning.

Maimune mentioned that she gives the mother *helba* (*Trigonella foenum graecum*) to rid the body of birth wastes. *Helba* is also used in the community and the hospital to increase breast-milk flow.

In addition to breast-feeding, the baby is given a mixture of clarified butter and honey called *henuk*. The baby receives this for seven days to increase its strength. Esme gives it to the mother as well, to decrease postnatal pain.

The Postpartum Period

Women in the community traditionally practiced a kind of "mother-roasting" (*xaamuud*), similar to a Malaysian practice described by Carol Laderman (1987). In this procedure a fire was built on the floor, over which were laid dried leaves of date palm and other trees. A mat was spread over this layer, and the mother lay down with her back on it. The purpose was to relieve pain. Esme said that this procedure was repeated for an hour or so daily for three days. Following that, the mother was free to resume her normal life, except for sexual intercourse. Maimune, in contrast, thought that the woman should rest for fifteen days, during which time her mother, mother-in-law, or husband should carry out her responsibilities.

In many Islamic countries, sexual intercourse is prohibited for forty days after delivery. The restriction is lifted once the woman has taken a ritual cleansing bath, similar to that taken following her menstrual periods.

Problem Deliveries

The midwives differ considerably in their responses when labor does not proceed normally. Maimune's first response is to insert her hand into the mother's vagina and massage her cervix, pulling downward forcefully. Internal massage by midwives runs the risk of introducing infection. A potential benefit of such massage, however, is the release of oxytocin, a hormone that increases the number and strength of contractions. (Synthetic oxytocin was regularly administered intravenously in the hospital when contractions slowed down during prolonged labor.)

Nafadh is a technique used by all the midwives for prolonged labor. It consists of turning the woman upside down, holding her by her legs, and shaking her. Although this procedure typically elicits laughter (even among Sultan Qaboos Hospital's Omani medical students), there may be some beneficial effect (Simkin 1987).

Esme described another technique she uses. She sits with one knee up, placing the woman on her knee, facing away. Esme then presses her knee into the back of the woman's perineum. Sometimes, she reported, the baby then slides out easily.

Esme maintained that this is her entire repertoire of special techniques; beyond this, the lives of the baby and mother are entirely in Allah's hands.

Maimune described two additional techniques that she uses: *xabaan* and *wasm*. Both of these are used for other purposes in Omani traditional healing.

Xabaan is similar to the technique of cupping or moxibustion, familiar in Chinese traditional medicine. It requires a broad, cloth wick and a wide-mouthed pottery jar. The burning wick is placed on the lower abdomen and immediately covered with the inverted jar. The jar is pushed downward with a twisting pressure. The fire generates a strong vacuum in the jar before it goes out. The resulting suction on the abdomen feels like a birth contraction to the woman. The procedure is repeated, moving up the mother's abdomen. It is sometimes applied on the woman's back as well. Medical personnel view this treatment as ineffective.

Wasm is a form of branding that is widespread on the Arabian peninsula (Moloney 1982). Maimune had three branding devices. One was the head of a large nail embedded in a wooden handle. The second was a thick wire, bent to about an inch in length at the branding end. The third was a large needle. Whichever instrument is used, it is heated and then placed on the woman's skin on the right side of her pelvis and on the lower back.

The other midwives did not use *wasm*. They considered it unsuitable for use in birthing and of potential harm to the baby.

Most medical personnel deplore the practice of *wasm*, not only in birthing but in all its other applications. Many hospital doctors in Oman have seen patients with *wasm* burn wounds that subsequently became infected. Nevertheless, most Omanis—including those who are well educated and generally comfortable with Western medicine—see it as an effective treatment for many problems, including infertility.

Midwives rely heavily upon storytelling about their difficult cases as a way of teaching their techniques to others; narrative skill is part of their traditional oral culture (Jordan 1983). Thus, for example, Maimune launched into a lengthy description of a difficult breech presentation that she managed to an ultimately successful outcome. In her account, the baby's foot came out first. Maimune then inserted her hand into the uterus and rubbed downward on it for a long time. She tried to align the baby's legs side by side. Then she got hold of the baby's hands and held them firmly against its stomach. In this way she was able to extricate the baby's feet first. When the placenta was delivered, she slapped and patted it, pushing the blood back into the baby. She spanked the baby on its bottom until it cried.

Despite this ordeal, the baby suffered no bad consequences. At the end of her tale, Maimune proudly pointed nearby to the "baby," now a healthy, bright-eyed girl of nine.

The Midwives' Work Orientation

Many health experts and planners concerned with health in developing societies would prefer an eventual phaseout of the "granny midwives" such as those studied here (Mangay-Maglacas 1990). They anticipate the building of new cadres of educated midwives, linked to the modern health care system and supervised within it (Jordan 1989). Still, in many countries the community-based, traditional midwives will remain important as birth attendants in rural areas during the next twenty to thirty years. We believe that this will be the case in Oman. Despite rapid development of the formal health sector, Oman still has a widely dispersed population and many remote rural areas that must depend on traditional midwives for years to come.

The Omani midwives interviewed here resembled the general pattern set forth by Cosminsky in her 1983 study of Third World midwives. They were middle-aged or older, presently or previously married, mothers, illiterate, part-time practitioners, and trained in an apprenticeship mode in the local community. Although they were not formally organized in an occupational sense, they knew about each other as community members. They had a cooperative rather than competitive approach toward attending births. Some mentioned instances where they had received help from or provided it to another midwife. Although they obviously preferred home delivery for routine cases, they appreciated their fairly new access to hospitals and doctors as a resort for difficult cases. They functioned without collecting set fees; rather, people gave them gifts according to their economic resources. The community expected the midwife not to be unduly interested in recompense.

Two further points are important about their practice. First, although they all lived within the same area, in some instances only a mile apart, they did things somewhat differently. They preferred different birthing positions (although they did not force their preferences on their clients). They varied to some extent even in normal deliveries where their role was relatively slight; more so in problem deliveries. Second, they all shared the sense of being there to help—but also the sense that many things that might happen were beyond their own skill and ultimately up to Allah.

The midwife's outlook is responsive, we believe, to the interest that delivering mothers have in controlling the birth process. This is, in a protean sense, the "consumer interest" that we spoke of above: the desire of the person who receives health services to make those services effective, convenient, familiar—that is, serviceable—and to prevent the service providers from obtaining an exclusive control. Within the relatively simple social and physical structure of the mother's family and home as the scene of delivery, her wishes and expectations can easily retain a dominant place in birthing. The midwife enters as a familiar community figure, prepared to assist rather than dominate the birth process. In sharp contrast, the hospital is filled with foreign professionals of ambiguous status (Colfer 1989), impersonal and seemingly arbitrary routines, and powerful but unfamiliar medical techniques. Much of the stress that the Omani women experience in the hospital can be traced to this basic circumstance, as will become clear from our analysis of birthing in Al Jebel Hospital.

Al Jebel Hospital

Birth Territoriality in Al Jebel Hospital

Births in Al Jebel Hospital are obviously not in the woman's home territory. She has traded—with encouragement from the Ministry of Health—the emotional security of familiar surroundings for the safety and expertise afforded by the hospital setting.

Al Jebel's delivery ward has four labor areas where the mother waits, largely alone, to deliver. An orderly, who is Arabic-speaking and Omani, drops by occasionally to ask her about contractions and pain. If the mother fails to deliver within a certain period of time, the process will be more frequently monitored by inspection of cervical dilation and listening to the baby's heartbeat. An intravenous oxytocin drip to stimulate contractions may be inserted.

In contrast to the home situation, the mother in the hospital is subject to frequent assaults on her modesty (even though all staff in delivery areas are women). The drab hospital gown is both less modest and less colorful than Omani women's usual attire. It may also be stained with blood from previous users. Blood is a more potent symbolic threat among Omanis than in the West.

One of the most alienating aspects of the hospital setting is the fact that all medical personnel (except orderlies) are foreign, and most speak very little Arabic. Omani women come to give birth in a setting where the people with power (nurses and doctors) have different cultural expectations about birth and cannot communicate well with the birthing mother.

As noted above, Omani women typically prefer to walk during labor. Ironically, hospital procedure prohibits walking in the early stages of labor, when the mothers want to walk, but requires it when delivery is imminent. The layout of the labor and delivery room requires that the mother get up, walk to the delivery room, and climb onto a high bed, just when she would prefer to assume her birthing position.

As soon as the baby is born it is removed from the mother to be cleaned, weighed, and observed for scoring on the Apgar developmental scale. The baby is not returned until the mother is moved to the maternity ward. The mothers object to being separated from their babies in this fashion—of course, this does not happen in home deliveries.

The Definition of Childbirth

Territoriality, bodily exposure, mode of dress—these are external features of birthing that can undergird or undercut the mother's sense of security. She also must deal with the different meanings, stimuli, expectations, and symbols that surround her in the hospital.

In these terms, how childbirth is defined becomes a powerful symbolic force. Modern medicine has over the past century formulated a strong conception of childbirth as a medical event. This conception has come to dominate the thinking of both physicians and pregnant women in many industrialized countries. The definition of childbirth in Great Britain and the United States involves healthy pregnant women coming to the hospital to be dealt with as if they were ill. Robert Hahn (1987) documents one influential source for this view: the medical textbook *Williams Obstetrics*, in its successive editions between 1903 and 1985. The medical definition of childbirth is no doubt best suited to the management of critical emergencies that occur in complicated deliveries. In normal deliveries, it offers the physician a full measure of convenient control, but at the price of infringing upon the mother's ability to make her own decisions about important features of the birth process.

Not surprisingly, the medical staff in Al Jebel were the primary sponsors of the medical definition of childbirth. Despite their general primacy in decision-making, however, their authority was not so all-encompassing as to exclude competing definitions from playing an important part in the web of influences that enveloped the mothers. The hospital was an enclave of cosmopolitan medicine located in an outlying area of a thoroughly Arab–Muslim nation. The introduction of Western medicine has made it necessary to recruit staff from many nations, most of them not Arab and not Muslim. Thus all of the dramas of intercultural communication and tension were played out in the hospital.

Nurses and doctors typically came from Kerala State in India and from the Philippines, with smaller numbers from Egypt and Pakistan. The orderlies, in contrast, were all Omani, just like the birthing mothers with whom they had direct contact. Orderlies, who deal most closely with the mothers on the delivery wards, come to the hospital completely unaware of the medical definition of childbirth. Nurses, also in frequent contact with birthing mothers, bring their own cultural traditions from their home countries, spiced with varying degrees of acceptance of medical definitions learned in nursing school. Doctors, rarely seen by birthing mothers (but having the greatest authority in the hospital setting), represent the fullest acceptance of the notion that childbirth is a medical event.

Omani women—including orderlies and birthing mothers—see childbirth as a painful but natural, normal, and happy process. They also see it as exclusively a women's affair, which affords an occasion for the birthing mother to demonstrate her dignity and courage to herself and an audience of supportive peers. Christine Eickelman (1984) found this conception to be a basic element in the Omani picture of motherhood.

In Al Jebel Hospital, the presence of the orderlies ensures some sense of the woman's involvement and accomplishment in birthing. In a typical American hospital, for instance, the woman would likely be *instructed* to push or not to push, depending on the dilation of her cervix, in Al Jebel, orderlies ask women if they *feel* like pushing.

Omani women are probably less compliant than American women partly because the medical model of pregnancy, and of patienthood more generally, has been more intensively disseminated in the United States by the media and the school system. Omani women in the hospital are usually not medicated, so they do retain their critical faculties during labor.

In many cases there is no medically justified reason for the routine hospital procedures. In the case of posture, for instance, the nurses consistently urge women to grip their thighs during contractions. Omani women are used to clinging to something above their heads, so tend to grab for the convenient pipe at the head of the hospital bed. When birth attendants insist women follow this arbitrary hospital policy, many wait for the attendant to leave the room and resume their preferred stance.

Pain Relief

When, in the hospital, Colfer expressed sympathy with the mother's pain or fatigue, the orderlies (sometimes the mothers themselves) responded with remarks such as "Why of course she's tired" and "Naturally! Childbirth is painful!" Most of the mothers deal stoically with the pain of childbirth. They grit their teeth, grimace, and cling to the headboard, but they rarely cry out. (Medical staff with extensive experience confirm this observation.)

A woman's mother often accompanies her to the hospital. Although the mother is not allowed in the labor or delivery rooms, she may see her daughter briefly while retrieving a bundle of clothing or jewelry. She too shows a stoic attitude if she witnesses her daughter's pain.

Women who become noisy or hysterical because of pain are criticized by other Omanis. One woman who was on the point of screaming was slapped sharply by the orderly, to distract her. Another woman, the mother of seven, was ridiculed by the nurses and orderlies as "acting like a primi" (a first-time mother) when she started to moan and writhe. This woman's mother later had to endure listening to a vivid account of her daughter's "misconduct," given by an orderly to one of the groups of coffee-drinking women that characterize Omani hospital settings.

The norm of courage and self-sufficiency may account for a common complaint that Omani women make about their deliveries, namely, receiving episiotomies. Episiotomies are given to the majority of women in their first birth. 1987 data from the hospital show that 12 percent of the total births were first births, and that 10 percent of all the births included an episiotomy.

The Omani mothers react far more negatively to the pain of episiotomy-related suturing than to the pain of childbirth. The research literature on pain experience (Gallagher and Wrobel 1982) suggests that a person's reaction to objectively painful stimuli is greatly affected by his or her interpretation of the source, meaning, and context of the pain. The interpretive scheme of Omani women recommends fortitude during labor and a sense of accomplishment for delivering a baby, but it does not incorporate any response to episiotomies and the other interventions that modern medicine introduces into the birthing situation.

The intended purpose of episiotomy is to forestall uncontrolled tearing of the mother's perineal tissue, should her vagina fail to stretch sufficiently to accommodate the baby. Fear of episiotomy is reported both by medical staff and by Omani women to be a major reason why many women choose not to come to the hospital for delivery. Health care researchers and medical experts in the West (Kitzinger and Simkin 1983; Sleep and Grant 1983) are beginning to question the value of the episiotomy procedure on the wide scale on which it is currently employed. Though few health care researchers question the value of the procedure in certain circumstances, they argue that it has become too routine—that the decision to perform it should be justified in each case, with a bias against performing it in doubtful cases.

In Western hospitals, the woman undergoing episiotomy is routinely given a local anesthetic, if she has not already been centrally anesthetized; but in Al Jebel Hospital, the episiotomized woman is not given any anesthetic. If episiotomies are to continue in Al Jebel on a regular basis, then the mother should be given the option of having a local anesthetic that could be quickly administered by the birth attendant, without routine need for the doctor's direct involvement.

Ideally, expectant mothers—most of whom are illiterate—would be given anticipatory education about episiotomies and anesthetics, in Arabic, as part of antenatal care. Most birthing mothers are fully capable of absorbing and responding intelligently to relevant information presented orally in a nontechnical fashion. As noted above, however, the hospital setting contains significant linguistic and cultural barriers to communication with patients.

Issues of Timing and Control

One of the most common complaints by mothers about the hospital is that the birth process is speeded up to suit medical personnel. The preference of mothers, of course, is to let nature take its course—to allow birthing to proceed at its own, often unpredictable pace. Some admit that they delay coming to the hospital until the very last moment; they fear that if they arrive too soon and labor is not fast enough to suit the doctor, a cesarean section will be performed.

Hospital records support their statements. Of the 365 mothers who came to the hospital for delivery in 1987, 9 percent delivered before reaching it. Of the 299 in-hospital births for which labor time was recorded, 45 percent delivered within fifteen minutes of arrival and another 44 percent delivered within the next forty-five minutes; thus 89 percent delivered within one hour of arrival. Although these figures are somewhat less significant than they would be in the West (due to the fact that only 12 percent were primiparous—the category of birthing mother with the longest labor), they contain the strong hint of delay in coming to the hospital.

The actual rate of cesarean deliveries at Al Jebel was unusually low (about 2 percent for 1987 and the first half of 1988), due to the proximity of better-equipped hospitals in Oman's capital city, only ninety miles away. But whether undergoing a cesarean section at Al Jebel or in the city, these women returned to their communities with stories of their experience.

The mothers' complaints about medical impatience and labor speed-up (by oxytocin drip) embody a latent issue that may be epitomized as "Whose baby is this, anyway?" Hahn's study (1987) shows that, in American hospitals, the birthing mother has virtually no part in decision-making; her sense of accomplishment is diminished by the attending physician, who is credited with "delivering the woman." If the delivery is by cesarean section, on the rise in the United States, then it is still more difficult for the mother to feel that she had anything to do with the birth.

In Al Jebel Hospital, women on the whole retain a greater sense of involvement and accomplishment than in Hahn's picture of American hospitals. Nevertheless, there are many reasons for them to feel uninvolved and powerless. The hospital environment is far from homelike; the patient is continuously exposed to routines, personnel, and environmental stimuli that she must accept but which she does not understand.

Patients' sense of alienation has been documented in various studies of hospitals in the West; how much more extreme it must be in Oman, where the existence of hospitals is so new, and where all the staff are foreign. The orderlies (representing the lowest rung of the hospital hierarchy) are the only personnel a birthing mother encounters who speak and understand her language and share her culture. Mother and orderly comprise a small, relatively powerless pocket of Omani values in the hospital, which otherwise is animated by the intention of and the supporting technology for meeting her potential medical, rather than her personal, needs. Seen in this light, the contrast between giving birth in the hospital and giving birth at home is a great one.

Conclusions: What Can the Hospital Do?

At the beginning of this chapter, we described a consumer-driven perspective in medical care. A good mesh between patient—consumer on the one hand and professional—provider on the other is rare. There are signs in Al Jebel Hospital that the birthing situation is drifting toward stronger, rather than diminished, medical control and intervention in the birthing process. Nevertheless, we are encouraged by the interest, at high levels in Omani medical circles, in making Oman's hospitals more responsive to the wishes of the citizenry.

The Oman MOH (1989) has recently promulgated a manual of recommendations for perinatal and postnatal care that may lead to changes in birthing practices at Al Jebel Hospital. The manual recommends a reduction in episiotomies, returning the baby to the mother quite soon after birth, and greater flexibility in policies regarding continuous family support for the woman during labor and following the birth.

In the spirit of the MOH manual, we have additionally formulated the following recommendations, drawn from our analyses of home and hospital births.

First, *review existing procedures for their cultural compatibility.* Unless medical safety is compromised, drop those that are inconsistent with Omani culture and instead "do it the Omani way." This recommendation would probably lead to changes such as: (1) allowing the woman to wear her baggy pants during delivery, thus respecting her modesty; (2) allowing the woman to select her own position during labor and delivery (it would almost certainly not be the lithotomy position!); (3) explaining episiotomy and giving her a choice on it, along with pain relief if she desires it; (4) allowing her to have one or two companions, if desired, and giving her baby to her immediately after birth. The goal here is to allow the mother as much decision-making responsibility as possible during normal labor and delivery.

We advance second and third recommendations, broader in scope, that deal with the cultural heterogeneity of the hospital.

Second, *give the birth attendants and orderlies additional training and status as patient advocates and delivery-room support personnel.* The orderlies already serve important support roles for birthing mothers and perform critical communication functions between mothers and medical personnel (nurses and doctors). The ability of medical staff to communicate with patients is largely dependent on the cooperation of the orderlies. This function is essential in patient care and should be accorded greater recognition and legitimacy.

Third, *train medical (including nursing) personnel in cross-cultural communication and Omani culture.* Medical personnel could interact more effectively with patients if they were more systematically attuned to Omani traditions and preferences. Such traditions and preferences, as long as they do not endanger health in the labor and delivery situation, can be merged with hospital practices. Some medical obstetric practices are in their own way "traditions," and, insofar as they conflict with Omani preferences, may contribute little toward a positive approach to labor as a normal, healthy, and joyful experience.

REFERENCES

Colfer, C.J.P. "Nursing in Oman—An Intercultural Experience." Keynote address at Workshop on Psychosocial Aspects of Care: The Neglected Role of the Nurse, Muscat, Oman, May 15, 1989.

Cosminsky, Sheila. 1983. "Traditional Midwifery and Contraception." In *Traditional Medicine and Health Care Coverage: A Reader for Health Administrators and Practitioners*, ed. Robert H. Bannerman, John Burton, and Ch'en Wen-Chien, 142–62. Geneva: World Health Organization.

Eickelman, Christine. 1984. *Woman and Community in Oman*. New York: New York University Press.

Gallagher, Eugene B., and Sylvia Wrobel. 1982. "The Sick Role and Chronic Pain." In *Chronic Pain: Psychosocial Factors in Rehabilitation*, ed. Ranjan Roy and Eldon Tunks, 36–52. Baltimore: Williams and Wilkins.

Hahn, Robert A. 1987. "Division of Labor: Obstetrician, Woman, and Society in Williams Obstetrics 1903–1985." *Medical Anthropology Quarterly* 1(3):256–82.

Jordan, Brigitte. 1983. *Birth in Four Cultures*. London: Eden Press.

———. 1989. "Cosmopolitical Obstetrics: Some Insights from the Training of Traditional Midwives." *Social Science and Medicine* 28(9):925–43.

Khusaibi, Saleh. "The Neonatal Problem." Paper presented at the National Woman and Child Care Plan Meeting, Institute of Health Sciences, Muscat, Oman, June 1, 1989.

Kitzinger, Sheila, and Penny Simkin, eds. 1983. *Episiotomy and the Second Stage of Labor*. Seattle: Penny Press.

Klein, Michael. 1988. "Do Family Physicians 'Prevent' Caesarean Sections? A Canadian Exploration." *Family Medicine* 20(6):431–36.

Laderman, Carol. 1987. *Wives and Midwives: Childbirth and Nutrition in Rural Malaysia*. Berkeley: University of California Press.

Mangay-Maglacas, Amelia. 1990. "Traditional Birth Attendants." In *Health Care of Women and Children in Developing Countries*, ed. Helen Wallace and Kanti Giri, 229–41. Oakland, Calif.: Third Party Publishing Company.

Martin, Emily. 1987. *The Woman in the Body—A Cultural Analysis of Reproduction*. Boston: Beacon.

Ministry of Health, Sultanate of Oman, and World Health Organization (WHO). 1989. *Peri-natal and Post-natal Care*. Muscat, Oman: Department of Obstetrics, Department of Pediatrics, and National Health Program.

Moloney, George E. 1982. "Local Healers of Qasim." In *Community Health in Saudi Arabia*, ed. Zohair A. Sebai, 87–98. Monograph 1. Riyadh: Saudi Medical Journal.

Newman, Lucile F. 1981. "Midwives and Modernization." *Medical Anthropology* 5:1–12.

Pillsbury, Barbara L. K. 1978. *Traditional Health Care in the Middle East*. Contract Report no. AID/NE-C-1395. Washington, D.C.: U.S. Agency for International Development.

Simkin, Penny. 1987. *Turning a Breech Baby to Vertex*. Information sheet. Seattle: Penny Press.

Sleep, Jennifer, and Adrian Grant. 1983. "West Berkshire Perineal Management Trial: Three Year Follow Up." *British Medical Journal* 286:749–51.

World Bank. 1990. *World Development Report—1990*. New York: Oxford University Press.

Chapter 13

Strategies for Connecting

Social Science Research to

Actions for Better Health

SALLY E. FINDLEY

Until the 1980s, it was a fairly safe assumption that any given less-developed nation would also have low life expectancy and high mortality. During the late 1960s and 1970s, however, the correlation between economic development and mortality weakened (Preston 1975). Some less-developed nations attained a life expectation at birth of sixty-five years or more, whereas in others, mortality remained excessively high. Though different provision of effective preventive and curative medical services contributes to the variation in the pace of mortality decline, some attribute the differentials in the pace of mortality decline to differences in social, economic, and political factors, such as level of women's education and autonomy, nutritional adequacy, and political priorities for health (see Caldwell 1976; Dunn 1984; Halstead, Walsh, and Warren 1985). It is becoming increasingly evident that further major reductions in the mortality level will involve greater complementarity between social changes and direct health service inputs.

Immunizations against major childhood diseases are a case in point. Through a major worldwide effort to vaccinate all children against polio and other childhood diseases, about one-half of the developing world's children have been completely vaccinated (UNICEF 1989). To reach the other one-half, however, social breakthroughs will be needed. Insufficient personnel and resources do slow down the pace of reaching children, but the low coverage rate cannot be attributed only to these factors. High dropout rates between the first and third vaccinations are a social behavior that limit the effectiveness of the vaccination campaign. Attention must be paid to the social forces behind the low compliance or participation rates in programs such as these.

These social factors might cover a broad range of attitudinal, cognitive, or relational factors. In the example above, the reasons for lack of follow-through on immunizations for children might include misperceptions about the disease processes and the manner in which vaccinations protect children, misunderstandings about coming back for follow-up doses, or fears of additional health threats from the vaccinations themselves. In addition, access may be further constrained by community or structural forces such as poor transport, limited financial resources to pay for the immunizations or related visits, inadequate publicity by the vaccination team, and malfunctioning of the refrigeration or cold-chain system.

Much is now known about the social factors inhibiting more effective health behaviors or consistent use of health services. Among these factors are a lack of awareness of services and their benefits; insufficient money to pay for clinic visits; poor health of the mother, which limits her ability to care for children properly; and little sense of control over health or welfare. Even with clear results, however, social science research often fails to guide social policy as the researchers had hoped (Nathan 1988; Rule 1978).

This chapter outlines some of the factors limiting the application of social science results. The first section briefly reviews the social science research niche within the health research agenda and some of the current problems limiting the application of findings. The second section presents some suggestions for ways to structure the research process to increase the application of the research findings by potential users, whether they are health planners or program managers, community development agents, or others whose activities touch on the pertinent mechanisms of change.

Social Science in the Health Research Agenda

Many now agree that health gains in developing countries over the next decade will depend on changes in individual and household behavior (Bhatia, Saadah, and Mosley 1989; Caldwell 1990; Myntti 1991; Mosley 1992; Simons 1989). Whereas much of the past mortality decline was due to community-wide interventions such as immunization campaigns, vector control programs, and provision of clean water and sanitation, now leading causes of death in developing countries are diseases associated with poverty, malnutrition, and life-style. Reducing the incidence of these diseases will require changes in individual and household behavior (Birdsall 1989).

Because individual choice and behavior are expected to play such a large role in future mortality declines in developing countries, social science research will play a major role in identifying the constraints on such behavioral changes (Adjei 1991; Berman, Sisler, and Habicht 1989; Birdsall 1992; Elder 1987; Kroeger 1983; Mosley 1992). Although much social science research will continue to focus on the provider–patient role and other operational aspects of improving the effectiveness and utilization of health services, increasingly our research focuses on the social and developmental factors influencing health-related behaviors and decisions.

This calls for not only multidisciplinary research but also multisectoral perspectives on the intersection of health and development. A review of recent social science studies yields the following general questions concerning this intersection:

1. What are the social contexts of high versus low mortality risk? In what ways do social and cultural attitudes, roles, and behaviors affect either use of health care services or adoption of preventive health behaviors?

2. How does socioeconomic development generate social contexts contributing to good health behavior? In what ways is it counterproductive?

3. How does ill health hinder development efforts?

4. How can social and economic development programs be modified to achieve a better reinforcement of the underlying good health behaviors, or to work against detrimental health behaviors or risk conditions?

5. When programs—intentionally or unintentionally—have a positive health effect, what project components (process or inputs) were involved? If programs that "should" affect health do not have that effect, why don't they?

6. Given the wider social context of people's daily lives, can the changes necessary to achieve the missing health impact of programs (or the desired utilization rates) be achieved through simple and acceptable techniques, built into their regular interactions with the health or developmental systems?

7. How can these recommended steps be incorporated into the daily life of the community so that they become self-sustaining patterns?

Across the health research community, there is recognition of the need to answer these questions (Adjei 1991; Black et al. 1989; CHRD 1990; Foster 1984; Hammad and Mulholland 1991; Mosley 1992; Vuthipongse 1989). Already there is a growing body of research that describes improvements in health that resulted from programmatic changes inspired by sociological or anthropological research. In Peru, for example, anthropologists demonstrated that high levels of infantile diarrhea were correlated with the use of improperly prepared weaning foods, as well as incorrect assumptions about feeding during severe diarrheal incidents (Black et al. 1989). As a consequence, the Peruvian national nutrition institute now works with mothers' clubs to train them in the preparation and use of improved weaning foods (Lopez de Romana and Lanata 1992). From Bangladesh (Bhuiya, Streatfield, and Meyer 1990; Foster and Weisfeld 1991; Green 1986; Phillips 1990; Stanton et al. 1987), Brazil (Nations and Rebhun 1988), India (Banerji 1986; Gupta 1989), Indonesia (Berman et al. 1989), Kenya (Kaseje 1990), Sierra Leone (Edwards and Lyons 1983), Uganda (Malison et al. 1987), and Venezuela (Briceno-Leon 1991) come reports of improvements in health programs resulting from collaborations between medical and social scientists.

Contrasted with this encouraging evidence, we also find accounts of social science research that failed to make its mark. Too often the research reports languish, and the social scientist finds no changes implemented as a consequence of the research. In India, for example, one observer finds that three decades of social science research failed to lead to any significant improvement in the effectiveness of health programs (Banerji 1986). In his review of behavioral research funded by the World Health Organization (WHO), George Foster (1987) finds that much of the research is of poor quality. When not of poor quality, the research is overly quantitative and too elegant for application. The research does not give the kind of information needed to guide application of the results.

For research to be applied, it is not enough to have appropriate conceptual frameworks. Consideration also must be given to the research process. This means paying more attention to the likely outcomes of health research. Daniel Fox (1992) concludes that potential policy outcomes using social science research depend on how policymakers view disease and, in particular, on how they view public versus private responsibilities for dealing with disease. These views shape how policymakers use research to make program decisions.

To frame research to address these demand issues properly, W. Henry Mosley (1992) argues that the entire research process needs to be integrated with planning and administration. The challenge is to undertake research that connects with people and programs so that the action implications of the research are clearly identified and debated, enhancing the chance that the ultimate research clients (governments, programs, and people) incorporate the findings into their activities.

Application of the Research Findings

Assuming that multidisciplinary, multisectoral research does succeed in addressing the mechanisms of social change with respect to health, how can we make the connections between this evidence and programs? What does it take to apply social science knowledge so that programs actually stimulate these changes?

This section of the chapter identifies a number of research-design issues that appear critical to successful application of research findings: differences between classical and implementation research, identification of the demand for social science research, local ownership of the research process, identifying potential levels of action, involving the community in evaluation and monitoring, and communicating the results.

Differences between Classical and Implementation Research

When we design research, generally we are more preoccupied with identifying the nature of social problems than with applying that understanding to the development of alternative solutions to those problems. Although as researchers our credibility rests on solid scientific results, policymakers or administrators may need additional interpretive information, to clarify the mechanisms by which the effects emerge in real-life situations.

Although application to the real world is a prime motivation for social scientists, for many reasons social science research often is not designed with a view to implementation. Like our natural science colleagues, most of us rely on quantitative procedures to test hypotheses about social structures (Nathan 1988). This may have value for the development of social science theories, but without further translation findings may not be accessible to the general population or to policymakers (Foster 1987; Mosley 1992). Ironically, such research may not succeed in serving the ultimate social science objective of helping society to solve the most pressing problems of the day. For social science research to be relevant, the researcher must carefully consider how and whom his research will benefit, and then ensure that the research allows the proper translation of results for these clients (Rule 1978).

Although purists among us may feel that getting involved with implementation issues can bias or dilute the scientific rigor of our research, classical and implementation-oriented research need not be separate, incompatible activities. According to Milton Hakel and his colleagues:

> Doing research entails considering a large set of issues—selecting and conceptualizing the problem, designing and executing the data collection, analyzing and interpreting the results, extending the design to follow interesting leads, and so on. Doing implementation entails another large set of issues—identifying and diagnosing the problem, gaining sponsorship and resources, setting goals and developing procedures, handling interpersonal "politics," producing results, and the like. (1982, 15)

To increase the chance of implementing social science research findings, we need research that both tests hypotheses and sets the stage for implementation of the findings. Because of the orientation toward producing action, this form of research is referred to as "action" research.

Unlike classical social science research, action research is focused on problem solution rather than on theory development. Whereas in standard scientific research the researcher starts with hypothesis formulation, in applied, action research the researcher starts by outlining a concrete problem, then uses his or her knowledge of the social processes to formulate a trial solution. As in experimental laboratory research, these trial solutions are the research hypotheses. The outcome of the research is not the elaboration of theory but decisions about how the solution works in particular settings (Boehm 1982).

This blending of classical and implementation research styles is not easy to achieve, but there are examples of researchers who have accomplished this marriage. In his search for a more effective means to control Chagas' disease in rural Venezuela, Roberto Briceno-Leon (1991) recast the classical vector control model to an enlarged control model that included community-member participation and control over their lives, not just over disease vectors. He and his colleagues recommended a self-help housing improvement scheme, which proved much more effective in reducing the population of the Chagas' disease vector than had the previous systems of spraying or providing loans for prebuilt homes. Another example comes from Bombay, India, where social scientists considered both individual and administrative or political constraints that contributed to differential mortality and morbidity levels (Crook, Ramasubban, and Singh 1991).

Additional examples may be found in family-planning research. When the original supply-side family-planning programs failed to attract a high level of usage, social scientists began focusing on factors affecting the demand for contraception. Through careful study of pilot projects, much was learned about the process variables that influence contraceptive acceptance. As a result, family-planning programs were modified and acceptance rates began to rise dramatically (Bhatia, Saadah, and Mosley 1989).

The Demand for Research

Focusing on the probable implementation options stemming from a research project requires us to consider the research client and how that client is likely to use research (Fox 1992). Each researcher is likely to have his or her own vision of the proper "client" for research, depending on assumptions the social scientist makes about the likely effect of his or her findings on the client or research user (Rule 1978). In the extreme case, the social scientist can undertake research for which it is assumed there are no net effects and no specific users. The research is for science and the advancement of knowledge. Most social scientists, however, have deep personal commitments to "be relevant" and to make a contribution to society, by translating daily experiences into the "big picture" and then explaining that big picture to people so that they can better understand their world (Berger and Kellner 1981; Mills 1959; Nathan 1988).

The alternative models posit that concrete actions will be recommended based on the research, but different assumptions are made about who will be instrumental in applying the results. Some assume that results will "speak for themselves," and that people will spontaneously understand and incorporate the results into their lives. Close to the classical research model, it is assumed that as soon as we know a better way to live, we will adopt it. This assumption underpins much social science health research, which is aimed at informing the general public about good health practices.

Many are skeptical, however, that simply announcing scientific findings will result in their assimilation. These skeptics prefer to focus their research on particular groups, seen as more likely to use the results to produce change. Some focus on a particular class (e.g., trade unionists, community leaders) who can and will use the results in deciding how to change society. Others aim only at the disenfranchised or the very poorest, who "most need" the social scientists' insights to exercise their voice. Still others concentrate on government actors, who use the information on behalf of the population to design better programs.

Whichever audience is selected—and a case can be made for each audience—the researcher should understand the criteria that expected research clients will use when judging the research. Rather than waiting to see if the findings constitute valid evidence to decision-makers, Fox (1992) argues for a research strategy that, much like defensive driving, anticipates the criteria policymakers use to accept scientific results and the role that evidence plays in their own decisions.

We also must consider what decision-makers want to know. Research should address the problems about which they must make decisions but for which they do not know the answers (Nathan 1988). However, there should not be such urgency for this information that the program planners can't wait for the research to be completed.

Willingness to use results may depend on the political commitment to doing something about a health problem. In Bombay, for example, researchers found that intraurban health differentials were related more strongly to political commitment to clean up the water and neighborhoods than to health care accessibility (Crook, Ramasubban, and Singh 1991). Therefore, they chose to work only with selected communities and nongovernmental organizations committed to developing alternative strategies to reduce the prevalence and risk of leprosy. Similarly, Moni Nag (1990) showed that the commitment of the government of Kerala to actions to improve popular welfare contributed to relatively rapid mortality declines not shared by other Indian states.

Some demand for research findings is likely to be latent, unarticulated, and invisible. Particularly when implementation of research findings may require the participation of mid-level technocrats or others not directly determining policy, it is important for researchers to be sensitive to their questions and research issues (CHRD 1990). Efforts to stimulate demand for research have often been focused on the general public, and the community-participation literature contains numerous examples of the advantages of doing research so that it helps people identify their own problems, making them eager to consider alternatives proposed as a result of the research (for examples, see Banerji 1986; Edwards and Lyons 1983; Hardiman 1986; Kaseje 1990; Morley, Rohde, and Williams 1983). Some of these techniques could be adapted to work with other potential clients such as nonhealth ministry officials, who would not normally participate in the discussions of health research.

Local Ownership of Research

Much health research is funded by international agencies or donors who promote their particular research agendas. Although this standardization may succeed in achieving "comparable" results, many question the validity of those findings or the merit of forcing program designs into a standardized mold (Banerji 1986; Justice 1986; Muhondwa 1989; Vuthipongse 1989). Every country or region has its own unique health and development situation, with different health problems and perceptions of those problems, and global prescriptions may not fit a country's specific situation.

Given the international and internal differences in health problems, many now stress local ownership as the *sine qua non* for credibility and strong linkages to policy-making and action organizations. If local policy-makers or program managers are to influence people's attitudes and behaviors, research findings should consider the local sociocultural and ecological setting. The Commission on Health Research for Development (CHRD) (1990) advocates local ownership of health research as "essential national health research," conducted by local researchers on local priorities in local settings, so that planners have country-specific findings upon which to base their planning.

What does local ownership of the research process really entail? To a certain extent, local ownership of research is the researcher's version of community participation in program implementation. Community participation includes helping the community to resolve conflicts and its members to work together to overcome problems and gain more control over their health and their lives (Hardiman 1986; Midgley 1986; Rifkin 1986; Walt 1990; Werner and Bower 1982).

Local ownership starts with joint discussions about local health research priorities and strategies between researchers and communities and their health and development workers. Recommendations from Colombia (Sevilla-Casas 1989), India (Banerji 1986), Kenya (Kaseje 1990), Liberia (Berney 1990), Nepal (Justice 1986), Nigeria (Yoder 1989), Tanzania (Nangawe et al. 1985), Togo (Eng, Glik, and Parker 1990), and Venezuela (Briceno-Leon 1991) all stress starting with the people, listening to the people, and using these collaborative discussions to discuss problems and perceptions about possible solutions. In Dhaka, Bangladesh, for example, researchers involved twenty-five communities in setting goals for reducing diarrhea. With their input and participation, the health education program was unusually successful in changing personal hygiene practices and bringing down diarrhea rates (Stanton et al 1987).

In these discussions, the researcher can serve as a catalyst to help the community articulate its own understanding of the world, identify priority problems, and recognize its potential to tackle these problems (Chambers 1983). Richard Manoff (1990) calls this communication "feedforward communication" and considers it essential to developing program designs that work with, rather than against, local priorities and potentials for change.

Successful involvement of the community in setting the research agenda requires researchers to go beyond observation to synthesis of issues (Banerji 1986). For example, discussion of priority health problems can help people understand their current health status, but the discussions also should help community residents envision the health they might achieve and identify concrete problems blocking that future (Berney 1990). Essentially, researchers serve as active sounding boards for the community, providing epidemiological and systemic perspectives on the felt needs. We are challenged to do this in ways that facilitate two-way communications, so that learning and information-sharing are built into the process without overwhelming participants and pushing them to revert to the easier role of the "ignorant" poor, alienated and ignored by the experts.

Communities are by no means homogeneous, so researchers should anticipate conflict and be prepared to help communities identify and deal with conflicts of interest and attitudes (Werner and Bower 1982; Midgley 1986). Researchers often prefer to work with the "opinion leaders," but sometimes these are the elites who may use this opportunity to rubber-stamp their own priorities or proposals (Justice 1986). Reliance on their inputs may give a biased perspective which excludes other groups. At a minimum, researchers should acknowledge this bias (Hardiman 1986).

FIGURE 13-1. Potential Levels of Research Clients

Levels of Action	Potential Research Clients
Global or international:	International scientific community Donors International organizations
National:	Ministry of Health Other ministries (e.g. education, social and women's affairs, public works) National development planning body National research institute Nongovernmental organizations promoting health and development Political parties Religious organizations Trade unions, cooperatives, women's groups
Regional:	Regional sections of national organizations District health and development offices Regional government or planning bodies Local nongovernmental organizations (NGOs)
Community or neighborhood:	Local health program managers or workers Local healers, traditional birth attendants (TBAs), pharmacists Local health committee Community development groups Local NGOs Local clubs, women's groups Extension agents or development workers Religious organizations Schools, literacy programs, teachers Transportation and communication services Refuse disposal and sanitation programs
Family or household:	Clan leadership Family elder(s) Informal social networks Shopkeepers and vendors Family enterprises Student groups
Individuals:	Wives, mothers, and mothers-in-law Fathers or husbands Children or siblings Other relatives (aunts, uncles)

Alternatively, procedures could be developed to provide a forum for different community groups, whether that means working with local political parties, health committees, or community advisory panels.

Identifying Potential Levels of Action

Health systems research has been constrained by weak linkages between the researchers of different disciplinary or institutional backgrounds and between the researchers and the other actors in the health system, such as health program managers, nongovernmental organizations, ministry-level planners, and the community itself (Chambers 1983; CHRD 1990; Mosley 1992). When these other actors are not consulted about their priorities, the research may not address their programmatic or information needs. It may turn out that these questions are just as important to resolving program problems as the "big issues" identified by upper-echelon health officials.

As shown in Figure 13-1, the potential actors affecting health behaviors and outcomes range from individuals in local communities to international leaders. Each level of potential action corresponds to a potential user of research results.

Ideally, research would be designed to address information needs of the various clients at different levels and across sectors. In practice, any given research cannot meet the information needs of all potential users, and choices will have to be made.

As more participants are added to the discussions, particularly those drawn from different sectors or levels, the potential for conflict and misunderstanding rises. Even bringing local health program managers into the discussion may be problematic, because health program managers may be outsiders, either ethnically or professionally, members of a foreign "medical" culture (Berney 1990; Werner and Bower 1982). Further, neither the medical staff nor the community may want to bridge the cultural gap. In northeast Brazil, for example, the medical establishment considered information about oral rehydration therapy (ORT) to be a symbol of social prestige, and they had little interest in putting this information in the hands of the poor (Nations and Rebhun 1988). Experiments in Togo (Eng, Glik, and Parker 1990) and Nigeria (Yoder 1989) outline the ways in which the initial communication barriers have been resolved in focus-group and information-exchange discussions, but more consideration is needed of ways to engage different levels of program managers in productive discussions of health research priorities.

Involving the Community in Evaluations and Monitoring

Strong community participation in the research process strengthens the demand for and understanding of research. When people have been involved in data collection, findings will be "real" and not suffer from the usual problems of being foreign or inaccessible (Chambers 1983; Kaseje 1990; Satia 1990). For example, in the Mbale district, Uganda, health workers and the community collaborated in a survey of 2,700 households near thirty-six rural clinics, and they were surprised to find that even in the area near clinics vaccination coverage was much lower and infant mortality was much higher than expected (Malison et al. 1987). Due to this collaborative participation, it was much easier for the clinics and communities to work together to find better ways to encourage clinic use.

When community residents participate in evaluations or monitoring, discussion of results is meaningful and can facilitate a greater commitment to the proposed actions or changes stemming from the research. In Sembura, Sierra Leone, for example, before conducting a survey of hospital usage and health, schoolchildren were enlisted in a campaign to make sure their parents knew of the importance of the survey. As a result, there was great interest and discussion of the results. The researchers helped residents understand the results with an interactive, question-and-answer style of presentation (Edwards and Lyons 1983). Another example of the positive contribution of popular participation in program monitoring comes from the smallpox eradication campaign, where the high level of local popular participation in disease surveillance is considered to have been a major factor in the success of the campaign (Kitron 1989). By observing their own behavior and health events, it is easier for people to make connections between their own acts and the community health situation (Elder 1987; Kaseje 1990; Manoff 1990; Nangawe et al. 1985; Werner and Bower 1982).

How can researchers involve community residents and local program officers in the data-collection and analysis phases of the project without compromising data reliability? One approach is to incorporate the wider social science research program into a management information system. As proposed by J. K. Satia (1990), an appropriate system includes much more than health-worker records. It is a built-in monitoring system that documents the program process and inputs; evaluates program impacts, especially discrete behaviors of participants; and collects complementary community-level data to permit analysis of nonprogram factors potentially influencing the participants' behavior or health (Satia 1990). In Ghana's Danfa project, for example, simply finding out where patients lived prompted managers to propose more satellite services (Adjei 1991). Monitoring service delivery and health status of the community also was helpful in Nepal for that country's evaluation of the primary health care system (Justice 1986). The challenge is to design a monitoring system that neither is unwieldy nor involves such long delays between observing and reporting that community participants have difficulty grasping the connections between the outcomes they have observed and the program interventions.

A disadvantage of reliance on an expanded management information system, however, is the absence of controls or nonparticipants. Based on a study of several behavior modification programs that were focused on improving nutritional behaviors, family-planning practices, and participation in well-baby clinics, John Elder (1987) recommends observation of both adopters and nonadopters, so that people can make the connections between health outcomes with and without the behavior in question.

Process-documentation research is another strategy for involving the community in the collection of information about their own behavior changes relative to ongoing participation in a health or development program. In Bangladesh, for example, observation of individual and maternal behaviors along with health outcomes gave new insights into ways by which to reduce measles mortality (Bhuiya, Streatfield, and Meyer 1990). Other studies that monitored behavior changes gave important clues to how education works to protect health (Lindenbaum, Chakraborty, and Elias 1989; Stanton et al. 1987).

Process-documentation research can be used to document both the planned and unplanned outcomes of the program (Mosley 1992; Bhatia, Saadah, and Mosley 1989). In Nepal, for example, process-documentation research showed that the peons (local messengers and custodians) in the system were actually the most effective village health workers (Justice 1986). Because process documentation includes information about program and nonprogram communities, process-documentation research has great potential to document the actual way in which structural or resource changes affect behavior.

In process-documentation research, the researcher serves as an information conduit between the community and program managers (Veneracion 1988). Rapid sharing of information from the system with program managers and the community increases the chance that all can learn from their experience and quickly incorporate procedures that "work" and modify those that do not, as shown by researchers working in Serabu, Sierra Leone (Edwards and Lyons 1983).

Process-documentation research also generates the details needed to identify requisite operational changes when demonstration or pilot projects conducted by nongovernmental organizations or district programs are to be expanded to regional or national coverage (Abed and Chowdhury 1989; McGinn, Adjei, and Dupar 1990; Phillips 1990; Yeon 1989). If new programs or approaches are to be grafted onto existing practices, process-oriented research will play a key role in matching up the key operational mechanisms of the pilot study with the existing health culture and system. Debabar Banerji (1986) attributes the success of India's National Tuberculosis Institute's program to the ability of local social scientists to use their research to identify the ways to blend the new with existing systems of care.

Communicating the Results

It seems obvious that a key factor in connecting research to action is the communication of research results to policymakers and program managers. Nonetheless, this aspect of the research process is often overlooked. Several commentators find that social science research reports are not prepared quickly enough, are not communicated to the people who can actually use the information to make programmatic decisions, or are not communicated so that the findings can be understood by the relevant audiences (Banerji 1986; Justice 1986; Manoff 1990; Nathan 1988; Yoder 1982, 1989).

Experience suggests that communication of results works well with a two-way exchange, with researchers simultaneously soliciting ideas about what to do about the findings (Manoff 1990; Berney 1990; Korten 1980). This two-way exchange is obviously most pertinent if it is conducted prior to final interpretation of results. In addition, the research should be reported in nonscientific terms, to make it easier for non-researchers to feel competent in discussing the results.

When the results suggest the need for a public education campaign, researchers can work with local communities to identify the most appropriate communication channels. Just as it has been proposed that implementation strategies build on traditional customs or existing programs, the communication of findings could also make use of traditional communication methods such as plays, ceremonial songs, and so forth. (Werner and Bower 1982; Manoff 1990).

Another possibility is to adapt local educators' or healers' work so that they convey the new information. In northeast Brazil, for example, the formal medical system was not doing a very good job of motivating the use of ORT. Anthropologists showed that local healers promoted the use of special teas for the treatment of diarrhea, so they helped the healers adapt their teas to incorporate the requisite amounts of sugar and salt. These teas were promoted in traditional healing ceremonies, and the healers established "healing rooms" where severely dehydrated children could be left for rest and rehydration while their mothers worked. After one year of working with the traditional healers, there were significant increases in the numbers of mothers who knew about ORT and who knew to continue breast-feeding children throughout a diarrheal episode (Nations and Rebhun 1988).

Concluding Perspectives

Focusing on how we expect the research to affect program and behavioral decisions will help us shape our research so that it has a greater chance of generating concrete steps toward better health. We need to be more specific in our assumptions about the ways research findings might be used to guide policy or program decisions. Discussions prior to conducting the research can help the researcher identify the types of information that program managers and decision-makers are likely to use, what amounts of change in these data are sufficient to prompt action by the managers, and what complementary information they need in order to choose among options and chart a new program direction.

In addition, the case studies cited in this chapter suggest that we have a better chance of connecting research with action if the research corresponds to issues high on the list of problems or issues with which program managers and decision-makers are concerned. Their participation in setting the research agenda will enhance the relevance of the research to real-world problems while stimulating interest in the findings, which further increases the chance that findings will be considered seriously and incorporated into program or daily decisions.

For the research to yield the richest set of suggestions for effective programmatic or behavioral options, our conceptual frameworks need to incorporate more process variables that reflect how factors such as education actually lead to better health. Much ingenuity will be needed to design research that measures both outcome and behavioral process, whether in or out of a formal health care delivery system.

The challenge of connecting research to action is further magnified by the underfunding of health research and especially of social science perspectives on health. The study by the CHRD (1990) showed that over two-thirds (68 percent) of research funded through overseas development assistance was allocated to agriculture, compared to only 14 percent for health, population, and education studies. Globally, a total of $1.6 billion (or only $0.43 per capita) was spent on research into developing-country health problems. About one-half of this was spent for research conducted in industrialized countries, mostly for biomedical research. The level of expenditure in developing countries was low, at $0.08 to $0.65 per capita, with a median of $0.29 per capita in 1986 in the nine countries examined by the commission.

Of the funds allocated to health research, the majority have gone to biomedical research. Though there are no comprehensive figures on the social science share of the $0.29 per capita, figures for Thailand, the Philippines, and Mexico give some indication that the upper limit for the social science share is 40 percent of the health research figure, or $0.11 per capita per year (CHRD 1990).

Ideally, if politicians, program officials, and people incorporate the recommendations from research in their decisions or behaviors and begin to see the positive health consequences derived from these changes, they will demand an increase in funding of social science research. In this time of massive cutbacks in research funding, even strong research success stories are unlikely to result in major increases in funding levels. Given the likely continuation of low funding levels for social science research on health problems, it is essential to employ research strategies that get the most out of these scarce investments. We must explore the ways in which the broader sweep of developmental studies can yield more information pertinent to health problems. At the same time, we can explore ways in which ongoing program activities, such as management information systems or regular program evaluations, might be designed to answer some of the questions regarding the demand for health care services or improved health behaviors.

For this type of integration to occur, researchers outside the health sector need to address the often overlooked health dimensions of their research problem. Similarly, those concerned with the more narrow monitoring of health services need to expand their perspective to include the collection of data measuring selected social variables likely to affect the use of those services. We all need to consider each other's questions posed by health social scientists, so that mutual areas of concern can be identified and appropriate measurements included.

REFERENCES

Abed, F. H., and A.M.R. Chowdhury. 1989. "The Role of NGO's in International Health Development." In *International Cooperation for Health: Problems, Prospects and Priorities*, ed. Michael R. Reich and Eiji Marui, 76–90. Dover, Mass.: Auburn House.

Adjei, Sam. 1991. "Ways in Which Design and Delivery of Health Services May Influence Uptake: Methods of Enquiry." In *The Health Transition: Methods and Measures*, ed. John Cleland and Allan Hill, 217–26. Canberra: Australian National University Press.

Banerji, Debabar. 1986. *Social Sciences and Health Service Development in India*. New Delhi: Lok Paksh.

Berger, Peter L., and Hansfried Kellner. 1981. *Sociology Reinterpreted: An Essay on Method and Vocation*. New York: Anchor Books.

Berman, Peter, Daniel G. Sisler, and Jean-Pierre Habicht. 1989. "Equity in Public-Sector Primary Health Care: The Role of Service Organisations in Indonesia." *Economic Development and Cultural Change* 4:771–803.

Berney, Karen Tomkins. 1990. "Training for Transformation: A Handbook for Community Workers." Christian Health Associates of Liberia. *R & D Feedback*, International Health Programs Office, Centers for Disease Control, Atlanta (January 16).

Bhatia, Shushama, Fadia Saadah, and W. Henry Mosley. 1989. "Analytical Review of the Development of Family Planning Program Strategies, Operations, and Research as a Model for Primary Health Care Programs." Paper prepared for the International Commission on Health Research for Development, Harvard University, January.

Bhuiya, Abbas, Kim Streatfield, and Paul Meyer. 1990. "Mothers' Hygienic Awareness, Behaviour, and Knowledge of Major Childhood Diseases in Matlab, Bangladesh." In *What We Know about the Health Transition: The Proceedings of an International Workshop, Canberra, May 1989*, ed. John Caldwell, Sally Findley, Pat Caldwell, Daphne Broers-Freeman, and Wendy Cosford, 462–77. Canberra: Australian National University Press.

Birdsall, Nancy. 1989. "Thoughts on Good Health and Good Government." *Daedalus* 118(1):89–117.

———. 1992. "Understanding Health and Development: Does Research Matter?" In *Advancing Health in Developing Countries: The Contributions of Social Science*

Research, ed. Lincoln Chen, Arthur Kleinman, and Norman Ware, 159–86. Westport, Conn.: Auburn House.

Black, Robert, Guillermo Lopez de Romana, Kenneth Brown, Nora Bravo, Oscar Bazalar, and Hilary Kanashiro. 1989. "Incidence and Etiology of Infantile Diarrhea and Major Routes of Transmission in Huascar, Peru." *American Journal of Epidemiology* 129(4):785–99.

Boehm, Virginia R. 1982. "Research in the 'Real World': A Conceptual Model." In *Making It Happen,* 27–38. See Hakel et al. 1982.

Briceno-Leon, Roberto. 1991. "The Four Dimensions of Chaga's Disease." In *The Health Transition: Methods and Measures,* 321–28. See Adjei 1991.

Caldwell, John C. 1976. "Routes to Low Mortality in Poor Countries." *Population and Development Review* 12(2):171–220.

————. 1990. "Introductory Thoughts on Health Transition." *What We Know about the Health Transition,* xi–xiii. See Bhuiya, Streatfield, and Meyer 1990.

Caldwell, John C., Indra Gajanayake, Pat Caldwell, and Indrani Peiris. 1989. "Sensitization to Illness and the Risk of Death: An Explanation for Sri Lanka's Approach to Good Health for All." *Social Science and Medicine* 28(4):365–79.

Chambers, Robert. 1983. *Rural Development: Putting the Last First.* London: Longman.

Commission on Health Research for Development (CHRD). 1990. *Health Research: Essential Link to Equity in Development.* Oxford: Oxford University Press.

Corbett, Janet. 1989. "Poverty and Sickness: The High Costs of Ill-Health." Institute of Development Studies, Sussex. *IDS Bulletin* 20(2):9–15.

Crook, Nigel, Radhika Ramasubban, and Bhanwar Singh. 1991. "A Multi-dimensional Approach to the Social Analysis of the Health Transition in Bombay." In *The Health Transition: Methods and Measures,* 303–20. See Adjei 1991.

Dunn, Frederick. 1984. "Social Determinants of Tropical Disease." In *Tropical and Geographic Medicine,* ed. K. S. Warren and A.D.F. Mahmond, 1086–96. New York: McGraw-Hill.

Edwards, Nancy, and Mary Lyons. 1983. "Community Assessment: A Tool for Motivation and Evaluation in Primary Health Care in Sierra Leone." In *Practicing Health for All,* 101–13. See Morley, Rohde, and Williams 1983.

Elder, John P. 1987. "Applications of Behavior Modification to Health Promotion in the Developing World." *Social Science and Medicine* 24(4):335–49.

Eng, Eugenia, Deborah Glik, and Kathleen Parker. 1990. "Focus Group Methods: Effects on Village-Agency Collaboration for Child Survival." *Health Policy and Planning* 5(1):67–76.

Foster, George M. 1984. "Anthropological Research and Perspectives on Health Problems in Developing Countries." *Social Science and Medicine* 18(10):847–54.

————. 1987. "WHO Behavioral Science Research: Problems and Prospects." *Social Science and Medicine* 24(9):709–17.

Foster, Stanley O., and Jason S. Weisfeld. 1991. "Epidemiological Methods for Monitoring the Health Transition." In *The Health Transition: Methods and Measures,* 259–68. See Adjei 1991.

Fox, Daniel. 1992. "Using Social Science to Prevent and Control HIV Infection: The Experience of Britain, Sweden and the US." *Advancing Health in Developing Countries,* 85–98. See Birdsall 1992.

Green, Edward C. 1986. "Diarrhea and the Social Marketing of ORS in Bangladesh." *Social Science and Medicine* 23(4):351–66.

Gupta, Prakash C. 1989. "International Cooperation in Dealing with Health Problems Caused by Tobacco." In *International Cooperation for Health,* 209–33. See Abed and Chowdhury 1989.

Hakel, Milton D., Melvin Sorcher, Michael Beer, and Joseph L. Moses, eds. 1982. *Making It Happen: Designing Research with Implementation in Mind.* Studying Organization: Innovations in Methodology 3. Beverly Hills: Sage.

Halstead, S. B., J. A. Walsh, and K. Warren, eds. 1985. *Good Health at Low Cost.* New York: Rockefeller Foundation.

Hammad, Aleya El Bindari, and Catherine Mulholland. 1991. "The Health Status of Vulnerable Groups: A Valuable Indicator for National Development." In *The Health Transition: Methods and Measures,* 165–92. *See* Adjei 1991.

Hardiman, Margaret. 1986. "People's Involvement in Health and Medical Care." In *Community Participation, Social Development and the State,* 45–69. *See* Midgley 1986.

Justice, Judith. 1986. *Policies, Plans and People: Culture and Health Development in Nepal.* Berkeley: University of California Press.

Kaseje, Daniel C. O. 1990. "Community-based Health Care: The Saradidi, Kenya Experience." In *Why Things Work: Case Histories in Development,* ed. Scott B. Halstead and Julia A. Walsh, 69–82. Boston: Adams Publishing Group.

Kitron, Uriel. 1989. "Integrated Disease Management of Tropical Infectious Diseases." In *International Cooperation for Health,* 234–63. *See* Abed and Chowdhury 1989.

Kleinman, Arthur. 1978. "Concepts and a Model for Comparison of Medical Systems as Cultural Systems." *Social Science and Medicine* 12:85–93.

Korten, David C. 1980. "Community Organization and Rural Development: A Learning Process Approach." *Public Administration Review* 40 (September–October): 480–511.

Kroeger, Axel. 1983. "Anthropological and Socio-medical Health Care Research in Developing Countries." *Social Science and Medicine* 17(30):147–61.

Lindenbaum, Shirley, Manesha Chakraborty, and Mohammed Elias. 1989. "The Influence of Maternal Education on Infant and Child Mortality in Bangladesh." In *Selected Readings in the Cultural, Social and Behavioral Determinants of Health,* ed. John C. Caldwell and Gigi Santow, 112–31. Health Transition Series 1. Canberra: Australian National University Press.

Lopez de Romano, Guillermo, and Claudio F. Lanata. 1992. "International Program to Control Diarrheal Disease in Peru." In *Advancing Health in Developing Countries,* 129–40. *See* Birdsall 1992.

McGinn, Therese, Sam Adjei, and Marsha Dupar. 1990. "Expanding the Pilot Project to the Nation: The Case of the Ghana TBA Programme." Paper presented at the Annual Meeting of the American Public Health Association, New York, Sept. 30–Oct. 4.

Malison, M. D., P. Sekeito, P. L. Henderson, R. V. Hawkins, S. I. Okware, and T. S. Jones. 1987. "Estimating Health Service Utilization, Immunization Coverage, and Childhood Mortality: A New Approach in Uganda." *Bulletin of the World Health Organization* 65(3):325–30.

Manoff, Richard K. 1990. "Social Marketing: Why It Makes Things Work." In *Why Things Work,* 167–74. *See* Kaseje 1990.

Midgley, James. 1986. "Community Participation: History, Concepts and Controversies." In *Community Participation, Social Development and the State,* ed. James Midgley, 13–44. London: Methuen.

Mills, C. Wright. 1959. *The Sociological Imagination.* Oxford and New York: Oxford University Press.

Morley, David, Jon E. Rhode, and Glen Williams, eds. 1983. *Practicing Health for All.* Oxford and New York: Oxford University Press.

Mosley, W. Henry. 1992. "Potential for Social Science Research to Inform and Influence the Delivery of Health Care in Less Developed Countries." In *Advancing Health in Developing Countries,* 187–206. *See* Birdsall 1992.

Muhondwa, Eustace P. Y. 1989. "The Role and Impact of Foreign Aid in Tanzania's Health Development." In *International Cooperation for Health*, 173–206. *See* Abed and Chowdhury 1989.

Myntti, Cynthia. 1991. "The Anthropologist as Storyteller: Picking up Where Others Leave Off in Public Health Research." In *The Health Transition: Methods and Measures*, 227–36. *See* Adjei 1991.

Nag, Moni. 1990. "Political Awareness as a Factor in Accessibility of Health Services: A Case Study of Rural Kerala and West Bengal." *What We Know about the Health Transition*, 356–77. *See* Bhuiya, Streatfield, and Meyer 1990.

Nangawe, Elihuruma, Francis Shomot, Erik Rowberg, Therese McGinn, and William VanWie. 1985. "Community Participation in Health Programs: Experiences from the Massai Health Services Project, Tanzania." Working Paper. New York: Columbia University, Center for Population and Family Health.

Nathan, Richard P. 1988. *Social Science in Government: Uses and Misuses*. New York: Basic Books.

Nations, Marilyn, and L. A. Rebhun. 1988. "Mystification of a Simple Solution: ORT in Northeast Brazil." *Social Science and Medicine* 27(1):27–38.

Phillips, James F. 1990. "Translating Pilot Project Success into National Policy Development: The Matlab and MCH-FP Extension Projects in Bangladesh." In *Why Things Work*, 19–38. *See* Kaseje 1990.

Preston, S. H. 1975. "The Changing Relation between Mortality and Level of Economic Development." *Population Studies* 29(2):231–48.

Rifkin, Susan. 1986. "Lessons from Community Participation in Health Programs." *Health Policy and Planning* 1(3):240–49.

Rule, James. 1978. *Insight and Social Betterment: A Preface to Applied Social Science*. Oxford and New York: Oxford University Press.

Satia, J. K. 1990. "Management Information Systems for Health and Population Programs." In *Why Things Work*, 179–82. *See* Kaseje 1990.

Sevilla-Casas, Elias. 1989. "An Anthropological Approach to the Study of Human Circulation and Malaria Risk." *Social Science and Tropical Diseases Network Newsletter* 3(8):3–8.

Simons, John. 1989. "Cultural Dimensions of the Mother's Contribution to Child Survival." In *Selected Readings in the Cultural, Social and Behavioral Determinants of Health*, 132–46. *See* Lindenbaum, Chakraborty, and Elias 1989.

Stanton, Bonita F., John D. Clemens, Tajkera Khair, Khodeza Khatun, and Dilwara Akhter Jahan. 1987. "An Educational Intervention for Altering Water-Sanitation Behaviours to Reduce Childhood Diarrhoea in Urban Bangladesh: Formulation, Preparation and Delivery of Educational Intervention." *Social Science and Medicine* 24(3):275–83.

United Nations Children's Fund (UNICEF). 1989. *The State of the World's Children 1989*. Oxford: Oxford University Press.

Veneracion, Cynthia C., ed. 1988. "A Decade of Process Documentation Research: Reflections and Synthesis." Paper presented at the Workshop on Process Documentation Research, January 21–24, Tagaylay City, Philippines. Quezon City: Institute of Philippine Culture, Ateneo de Manila University.

Vuthipongse, Prakorn. 1989. "Institutional Capacity to Address Health Problems." In *International Cooperation for Health*, 37–57. *See* Abed and Chowdhury 1989.

Walt, Gill. 1990. "Community Involvement." In *Why Things Work*, 199–206. *See* Kaseje 1990.

Werner, David, and Bill Bower. 1982. *Helping Health Workers Learn*. Palo Alto, Calif.: Hesperian Foundation.

Yeon, Ha Cheong. 1989. "An Approach to Developing Primary Health Care in Korea." In *International Cooperation for Health*, 119–44. *See* Abed and Chowdhury 1989.

Yoder, Stanley P. 1982. "Issues in the Study of Ethnomedical Systems in Africa." In *African Health and Healing Systems: Proceedings of a Symposium*, ed. Stanley Yoder, 1–20. Los Angeles: Crossroads.

———. 1989. "Reporting Research Results as Information Exchange: A View from Niger State, Nigeria." Working Paper no. 105, Center for International Health and Development Communication, University of Pennsylvania, Philadelphia.

Chapter 14

Modernization and Medical Care

EUGENE B. GALLAGHER

Would we consider a society "modern" if its economy were based primarily in industry but it had a backward system of medical care? Imagine, conversely, an agricultural or maritime society with little industry but an advanced system of medical care. Would we consider this second society to be "modern"? The thematic aim of this article is to explore the connection between modernity—the condition, on a societal scale, of being modern—and health care (in this paper, I use the terms "medical care" and "health care" interchangeably). I examine, conceptually and with empirical illustration, the position of health care within the modernization process. The questions stated above evoke this theme.

Though it may seem an unproblematic endeavor to examine the place of health care in the modernization process, it points to a neglected question within the tradition of Western social thought. The Weberian–Parsonian theoretical scheme, taken here as a recognized synthesis of that tradition, reduces human action analytically to ends, means, and conditions of action (Parsons 1949). In this scheme, the health of an individual is regarded, like the physical environment, as a neutral background condition capable of affecting his or her action at the limit but is not in itself a primary focus of attention. There is no concept of "health rationality" comparable to "economic rationality," the latter making up the socially structured motivation that led to major socioeconomic changes in the West. This theoretical scheme does not allow us to regard health as an end state or goal of action; nor does it envisage the emer-

Reprinted from *Sociological Perspectives*, Vol. 31 no. 1 (Jan. 1988):59–87. © 1988 Pacific Sociological Assn.

gence of health as a major societal value that shapes institutional development and stimulates individual consciousness, analogous to the quest for economic profit, for religious salvation, or for scientific knowledge. Although Max Weber and Talcott Parsons were concerned with accounting for social change—"progress" or, with weaker moral conviction, "modernization"—they emphasized phenomena within the sphere of economics and politics, these being the primary and pivotal spheres within which social change occurred. Their scheme did not recognize important facts and trends within contemporary health care that have a significant bearing upon the direction of modern societies. The beginnings of such a recognition can, however, be seen in Parson's well-known analysis (1951) of the professional medical role and in attempts to extend the Weberian concept of patrimonial authority to bases of political legitimation in the contemporary welfare state, which makes explicit provision for the health of citizens.

A second omission, which is significant from the perspective of this article, is that while Weber and Parsons dealt with the political power and socioeconomic transformation within Western societies, their view of the "rest of the world"—the preindustrial part—captured it primarily in colonial status. Their scheme did not envision the new forms of interplay between economic and political forces, the emergence of postcolonial autocracies, and the ambivalent reactivity toward the West seen in many Third World societies today.

Starting in the early 1960s, modernization theory continued the themes of Western social thought. Its perspectives provide ideas for understanding health care in the Third World. It raises the questions, crucial for health care, whether or not the path to Third World development lies simply in the importation of Western technology (value-neutral "technology transfer"), whether Third World societies are also importing Western models of social organization, or whether they will develop their own indigenous equivalents to organizational forms and value complexes such as bureaucracy, the Protestant ethic, and functionally specific professional roles.

A concrete illustration of the implications of this question can be seen when a piece of new medical equipment is imported into a village health center, in the "magical" expectation that it will thereby improve medical care. Yet it may lie there in disuse because no one has been trained in its operation or maintenance. The attitudes of the resident health providers move along an emotional spectrum from the excitement of acquisition to eventual mild embarrassment over its nonuse and desuetude. Such an example is not exceptional. It occurs frequently in Third World settings, to the point that the World Health Organization (WHO) holds seminars and workshops and organizes regional training centers for medical technicians (WHO 1980).[1] Yet to speak of "magical" expectation may be too one-sided. Sheer equipment can of itself be an energizing "icon of modernity" (Berger, Berger, and Kellner 1973). It may be an unrealistic expectation on the part of health planners in the capital city to suppose that local health workers can perform with spirit and dedication in the absence of such technological icons. Such is the situation of health workers in communities too poor to afford new equipment and not fortunate enough to have priority allocation from the central government or international agencies.

This example leads to a brief exposition of modernization theory as a source of concepts for examining medical care in modernizing societies.

Modernization Theory

Modernization theory is characterized more by the questions it raises and the social structures that it investigates than by distinctive propositions or conceptual methods. As propounded by its leading formulators—Peter Berger (1973), Shmuel Eisenstadt (1966), Marion Levy (1966), and Daniel Lerner (1958)—it started from the recognition that a cumulative historical change in the mode of economic production has occurred in the West. It then proceeds to give an analytical description of concomitant changes in institutional forms, in sociocultural values, and in the social psychology of individuals and groups. It searches the sociocultural, political, and economic landscape of the diverse Third World societies to identify their critical developmental processes and to determine whether they are repeating the history of the West or moving along novel paths. (See Goldthorpe 1984, for a recent analysis of theories of Third World development.)

Berger's version of modernization theory provides a convenient account within which to situate a conception of health care. In Berger's view, modernization is a transformation of human consciousness that depends upon two processes: technological production and bureaucratization. Technological production occurs within the real world, in contrast to bureaucracy, which creates and inhabits a symbolic classificatory world. Technological production is accomplished through work, which is carried out in practical terms by the organization of human effort, specialization, cooperation, and coordination, which are subordinated to and driven by the empirical prerequisites for fashioning raw materials in production. Technological production is rooted in empirical fact or principle. In contrast, bureaucracy always has an irreducible social root to it—an idea concerning right, equitable, efficient ways of regulating human relationships that arises within a particular cultural context. Bureaucratic consciousness and bureaucratic institutions find their most refined expression in the political sphere of society.

Technology, in Berger's conception, is goal-oriented and is open to new knowledge, especially scientific knowledge, that will improve the processes of production and lead to new modes of organization of productive effort. Bureaucracy too has its own dynamic, which consists of the refining of its categories for the classification of human actions, the statuses of persons, and the jurisdictional scope of its principles.

Technology and bureaucracy are *primary carriers* of modernity, each of which in its independent fashion exerts a strong force in the formation of modern society. Berger distinguishes these from the so-called *secondary carriers*, "which include a variety of social and cultural processes, most of them *historically* grounded in the primary carriers but now capable of autonomous efficacy" (Berger, Berger, and Kellner 1973, 103). The secondary carriers include urbanization, mass education, the growth of the private sphere of individual life (including the role of individuals as economic and cultural consumers and as "personalities" in social interaction), and the institutions of knowledge and science.

The meaning and salience of the secondary carriers can be illustrated by looking at mass education. As an essential feature of modern society, mass education is linked in various ways with the primary carriers (technology and bureaucracy). Its linkage with technology comes from the fact that it prepares individuals to participate in economic production. To varying degrees, however, contemporary mass education also provides a base of literacy and general knowledge. There is thus some slippage between the demands of technology and the goals of mass education; the latter is more than sheerly "vocational." Further, the character and content of mass education show the historical markings of a given society. Mass education in the United States has been much more affected by the spirit of egalitarianism and the prospect of individual upward mobility, and much less disposed to establish stringent sorting mechanisms that separate the intellectual elite from the mass, than societies such as Great Britain and Japan that have less "room at the top." Similarly, in its bureaucratic dimension mass education prepares its recipients for membership affiliation and participation in social groups, particularly as citizens of the state.

Modernity also has a major impact upon the ways in which individuals conceive of themselves and others. It promotes the awareness of oneself as a person who, whatever one's social identities, memberships, and allegiances, is not exhaustively defined by these categories. The traditional definers of social identity—age, sex, and marital status—become more fluid, less coercive, and less embracing. The modern "individual" has an inner biological uniqueness, the conception of which is a remarkable consequence of contemporary bioscience. The individual has also an external functional style ("personality") that marks him or her as different from other individuals. On these bases, he or she is entitled to recognition and respect apart from any solidaristic affiliations. The value system of universal human rights, which is the moral and legal locus of claims to health care and corporal integrity, has displaced earlier, more invidious systems of status honor and communal protection for socially categorized persons.

Health Care as a Carrier of Modernity

Health care fits into the structure of modernity in a special way. The aims of contemporary health care—to cure, to prevent, to alleviate disease—are not new in human history. The modern, scientifically trained physician is kin to the medieval herbalist and the preliterate shaman in seeking to rid patients of their bodily ills. However, these aims are accomplished in ways profoundly different from premodern health care. The differences between a modern hospital and the practice situation of a traditional bonesetter or midwife are no less in magnitude than the difference between traditional human labor-intensive agriculture and modern agriculture, which is based upon scientific knowledge and the use of mechanical power.

From the standpoint of its provision, modern health care is increasingly the object of calculation and rationalization. Only within the past hundred years have diagnosis and treatment become sharply segregated from magic–religious traditions, forming the content of specialized vocational activities that apply scientific knowledge. From a small, albeit culturally vital feature of the premodern social structure, health care has been transformed into a major productive enterprise in modern societies. The learning of health care skills is not left to the vagaries of informal transmission from one generation to the next, as with traditional healing roles, but is instead carried out systematically through formal education. The practice of health care is generally a full-time livelihood and a lifelong career for those persons trained and authorized to provide it.

The modern notion of health care as a commodity emphasizes its calculability. Health care is not a commodity from the premodern standpoint of the midwife in the village or urban neighborhood where she provides her services. Delivering babies is an activity that, in addition to meeting a human need, validates her worth in an important social role and brings her into sociable contact with clients already known to her (Sukkary 1981). The midwife's work may well provide income in cash or in kind, but it is not a commodity in the sense of consuming calculable resources or constituting a stream of economic value in an ongoing system of production. If the women of the village lowered their rate of pregnancy, the midwife might be less occupied; but would she worry about "the impending midwife surplus"? Her casual economic posture can be contrasted with that of the contemporary obstetrician (or other physician), whose offering has a far more systematic character and tangible monetary value.

In drawing attention to the calculability aspect of modern health care, one need not claim that physicians or other health care providers look upon their patients with venal eyes, that they perform needless procedures for profit, or that they are part of a "medical—industrial complex" (Relman 1980). This is not to deny that these phenomena exist or that they can become widespread within a health care system. I believe, however, that they are an accentuated, rather than an integral, expression of the ways in which modern health care is calculable.

The concept of health care as a calculable resource is an essential feature in its role as a carrier of modernity. It collects and subsumes many interrelated features of modern health care that distinguish it from premodern health care. Among these features are a general presumption that health care is a worthwhile enterprise, whatever its relevance and effectiveness in particular cases; the systematic, specialized application of objective scientific knowledge as "technique"; the transformation of the patient from a socially endowed and identified person into a socially neutral, clinical "case"; and the remuneration of the care provider in money income (whether from insurance disbursement, fees, salary, or capitation payment).

The general presumption that health care is a "good thing" doubtless contributes to whatever tendencies there are toward hasty intervention or overtreatment in the concrete clinical situation. It refers to something more basic, however, namely, a broadly and strongly favorable predisposition toward the creation of a health care system as a major ongoing "establishment" that, though not beyond all need to justify itself in terms of its rationality and effectiveness, nevertheless commands a level of societal respect and support that is not closely tempered to its actual accomplishments, at least not in any immediate cause-and-effect relationship.

This presumption lies behind the rapid diffusion of the technological and organizational structures of modern medicine from the industrialized societies to Third World societies (of course, this does not mean that health delivery structures meanwhile remain static within the industrialized source-societies). A question of significance for social scientists is that of exploring the social, political, economic, and cultural factors that influence this process—those features that impede it and those that impel it.

Much of the health services increase in the Third World consists of bringing, for the first time in a given society or region, health services that are well established in the industrialized societies: the use of pharmaceuticals, prenatal and childbirth service, and, at a higher level of technology and sophistication, surgery and other hospital-based services.

This extension has its counterpart in impoverished, underserved areas of the industrialized societies—their own "Third World enclaves"—when health services become more widely available to persons who previously lacked geographic or economic access, or where they are provided on a more refined, intensive basis, as, for example, when a specialist physician performs a certain procedure that had commonly been performed by non-specialists previously. Health care is introduced into Third World societies within the value context of modernization. This means that it is sought and appreciated not only for the specific tangible benefits it offers but because of its association with, and representation of, the complex of meanings linked with modernity.

Health Value and Endeavor

It is the fact that health care always deals with individuals—with the illnesses and disabilities of individual human beings—that creates the possibility that its techniques can be introduced, almost as a hermetically encapsulated vector of modernity, into social situations that are otherwise marked by cultural isolation and poverty.

Changes in the technological–economic base of a society or in its system of government cannot be effected without concomitant changes in the residential patterns, daily life, and social relationships of people. In contrast, medical care, which can be provided by outside experts, techniques, and equipment, makes no such demands. The patient or recipient need only to present his or her body and to "cooperate with treatment" in the predominantly passive mode of patienthood; he or she need not be able to read or to write or even to speak the same language as the provider. It is logistically possible, for example, to establish transient field stations that provide immunization and elementary medical care for geographically remote nomadic groups, whose culture and technology are otherwise not much touched by modern ways.

The fact that modern medicine asks little of its beneficiary yet offers increasingly effective clinical benefit gives it the status of a greatly desired service in the eyes of individuals and peoples who otherwise are not culturally prepared to embrace modern things. Berger conveys the linkage, in the Third World context, of health care with traditional sentiments and with new expectations: "On the most elementary levels of human experience, modernity is associated with the expectation of being delivered from hunger, disease and early death. Thus modernity has about it a quality of miracle and magic that, in some instances, can link up with old religious expectations of delivery from the sufferings of the human condition" (1973, 139). This implies that medical care, more than most other components and carriers of modernity, has direct appeal for individuals and families. It musters stronger personal concern than the greater, more public works of modernity such as roads, factories, and projects for economic and educational development.

A distinctive characteristic of modernity in the health sphere is the more widespread and penetrating awareness of the value of health and related efforts to preserve it. This focused concept of health as an ongoing state of objective social value, which can be beneficially influenced by individual effort, by a conducive physical environment, and by medical care, stands in sharp contrast to the more passive, often fatalistic attitudes that have prevailed in many traditional cultures. In the modern conception, health is analogous to the notion advanced earlier of health care as a commodity. This conception of health, still formative in industrial societies and only gradually moving into the Third World, converts it from an existential gift into a process-related quasi-commodity that is susceptible to rational calculation and control.

The qualifier "quasi" in "quasi-commodity" indicates that health has an ultimate contingent aspect that eludes full control. The concept of "risk factor" catches this meaning with a thoroughly modern abstractness and ambiguousness. It offers a probabilistic recipe: "If your behavior patterns and your accustomed physical environment expose you to such-and-such, then you have X percent chance of dying or contracting such-and-such disease." The bringing of individual health status—one's somatic destiny—under rational probabilistic purview is an ingredient in its "commodification." But there is an inherent lack of reference in risk factor statements; whatever the actuarial risks, it's not clear what will happen to *me* as someone who smokes cigarettes, consumes high-cholesterol foods and alcohol, and drives recklessly, or who, in the positive direction, walks in that path of health righteousness that eschews all risks. Faced with impersonal statistics, however, many individuals redouble their personal efforts to live on the safe side of risk factors. Government bureaus, schools, and enlightened employers offer incentives to undergird individual efforts. The sum of individual and group sentiments in these directions is, in industrialized societies, a movement buttressing the notion of health as a rationally achievable goal. Both health care and health are regarded as amenable to calculation, control, and—in relation to the political ideal of equity—social distribution.

Within industrialized societies, the public sentiment is growing that the health of individuals is a matter of collective concern that includes, but goes beyond, impairments to their individual productive capacity or their possible danger to others (as through infection). Mark Field articulates this sentiment in these words: "the idea that the welfare of society *as a whole* benefits from a reduction in morbidity and a lengthening of life expectancy" (1980, 401).

As an aspect of modernization, public concern with individual health is incrementally penetrating the health policy and practice of developing societies. One must, of course, distinguish official pronouncements and symbols (such as a showcase hospital in the national capital) from the prevailing reality. In the spirit of the traditional solicitude of the ruler for his subjects who are afflicted, many Third World governments, both autocratic and democratic, have proclaimed lofty health care ideals. Such proclamations may sometimes by the hypocritical gesture of self-serving elites—the substitution of legitimizing rhetoric for actual performance. However, it is also valid to argue that, whatever the shortfall of performance, an accretion of ideals and symbols serves to change popular health values and consciousness, to motivate young health-professional aspirants, and to lay tracks for future genuine accomplishments.

Priorities at the Center and the Periphery

A serious geographic maldistribution of health resources prevails in many Third World societies (the industrialized societies have similar but less extreme problems). Modernization theory provides an analysis of this problem that moves in directions somewhat different from those suggested by many health planners. The conventions of health planning usually prescribe a geographic deployment of resources from the center outward, and a balanced development of medical personnel with a stress upon primary health care, especially maternal and child health (in view of the youthful complexion of Third World societies). Although by no means opposed to rational health planning, modernization theory also recommends that the "mass social psychology" of modernizing populations be taken into account. A certain level of "overconcentration of overspecialized resources" in metropolitan areas may be of symbolic value in the modernization process. It is, of course, difficult to quantify such values and to array them against the maps, labor force statistics, and community health surveys that health planners adduce as objective evidence in favor of a broad geographic deployment. Despite the intangibility of the "modernity" factors, they cannot be ignored. Peter Berger, Brigitte Berger, and Hansfried Kellner write about them as follows:

> In most of the Third World the allure of modernity is strongly linked to city life. . . . Whatever its frustrations and degradations, the city continues to be the place where things are happening, where there is movement and a sense of the future. . . . The governments of newly independent countries of the Third World have often been chastised by Western observers for their lavish expenditures on purely symbolic enterprises. . . . The Western observers in question habitually point out that the governments

cannot afford such expenditures. In purely economic terms this may be true. Men, however, do not live by bread alone—especially not in situations of desperate need and urgent hope. In such situations men at least *also* live on dreams. (1973, 142–44)

An ironic complicating element in the issue of resource deployment is that it is not only the new hospitals and medical schools in the larger cities that bear the allegation of "waste"; precisely the same charge can be directed at many rural health stations in Third World societies. Not infrequently, medical care provided at the periphery is substandard. Pharmaceuticals are improperly stored and prescribed, equipment is poorly maintained, and personnel maintain irregular clinic hours. Nevertheless, it could be held that the very fact that a clinic has been built and staffed—apart from what it delivers—has important symbolic value. That is, the health facility provides local people with a sense of participation in modern things and the assurance that the government is concerned with their community.

The foregoing argument will now be refined by looking at ethnographically based illustrations of low standards in Third World rural health care and by introducing additional modernization concepts that support a centralized bias in deployment, but that do not rest wholly upon the argument about symbolic value.

An example of inadequate service at a rural health clinic comes from a recent field study by Kenyon Stebbins (1986) of a village in Oaxaca, Mexico. Though Stebbins allows that many of the 2,000 clinics recently started by the central government of Mexico may have a better service record, his observations of the clinic he studied are telling. He notes that many of the village residents had major complaints concerning the clinic and states:

Interestingly, many . . . residents are willing to pay cash for certain pharmaceuticals in the cities even though they could obtain the same drugs . . . at the village clinic at no expense. This is because the clinic's pharmaceuticals are widely distrusted and suspected of being outdated. In addition, the clinic medicines are often believed to be of inferior quality, having been rejected by more "educated" wealthy urban elites who . . . had them sent out to rural health posts for "second-class" folks. . . . As for their dissatisfaction with the clinic's services, the *pasante* (doctor) is often absent or drunk, and he is considered to be inexperienced and ineffective regarding the elimination of persistent ailments. (116–17)

The doctor in this clinic was actually a medical student serving as a solo practitioner in this post for one year, which made up the fifth year of his medical education. This is the standard pattern—assignment as part of the "social service" component of medical education. Each doctor–student has the assistance of a village woman who speaks the local Indian language (almost all the Mexican doctor–students are Spanish-speaking men of urban background who are not conversant with the local languages).

A similar picture emerges from the observations of Zohair Sebai (1981), a Saudi public health physician, at a village clinic in the Turabi oasis of Saudi Arabia. Among the clinic failings he noted were lack of physical facilities and equipment (such as thermometer and sphyg-momanometer) for examination of patients, inadequate storage and indiscriminate prescription of drugs (especially antibiotics), lack of adequate record-keeping on patients' diagnosis and treatment, and frequent acquiescence by staff in ill-advised patient expectations and demands (such as the demand for medication by way of injection rather than oral tablet).

The Saudi clinic had a staff of fourteen, including three physicians, two of whom were Pakistani and the other Egyptian. In the Stebbins account of the Mexican clinic, it clearly appeared that the solo physician was derelict in his attention to duty; his low motivation was perhaps in some measure due to the involuntary assignment (as part of the medical curriculum) and his professional isolation. In contrast, at the much larger Saudi clinic the staff were well motivated but overworked; the inadequacies in service were due in considerable measure to poor physical facilities and, with regard to deficiencies in medical treatment, due to the expatriate doctors' reluctance to exercise medical restraint in the face of patient demands for active intervention. Sebai believed that Saudi physicians would have felt more secure in dealing with the patients, who were all Saudi—but it is almost impossible to recruit Saudi physicians to rural outposts, and, unlike the Mexican system, the Saudi medical education system has no semicoercive methods of placing students in the field.

Despite differences, it is possible to discern in both these situations two features that emphasize the characteristic shortcomings of rural health. These features, discussed below, can be regarded analytically as structural mechanisms that express the value tensions and conflicts conceptualized by modernization theory.

First, rural health care frequently juxtaposes an urbanized physician with a rural patient who is attached to local traditions and whose attitudes with regard to health and medical care are an ambivalent blend of admiration for modern medicine, of "show-me" skepticism, and of strong preconceptions about what ails the patient and what he or she needs. The degree of cultural disjunction is greater when the physician is, rather than an urban cosmopolitan of the same country, a "foreigner" who has for the sake of higher pay or better professional and life opportunities elected to leave his or her own country; studies of international medical migration suggest that many immigrant physicians fill positions that physician nationals shun. Although migrating physicians are no doubt highly sophisticated, adaptable professionals, they may be unable to inspire the confidence of their patients, many of whom are deeply rooted in an indigenous culture.

Second, health care outside the metropolitan areas tends to be low in professional opportunity for its providers, low in contact with more experienced professionals who can serve as role models and technical consultants, and low in an ambiance of professional dedication and discipline. These deficiencies are exacerbated in Third World countries by the fact that professional services, including modern medical care and medical education, are still formative. Ideally, no one would engage in clinical practice, particularly in exposed and professionally unsupported outpost areas, until he or she was well trained and until the infrastructural routines of clinic administration, professional relationships, and handling of records, supplies, and equipment were well established. The actual situation is usually far from ideal: the health care delivered may be compromised by the hardships and novelty of the situation, and professional morale may suffer.

The delivery of health care in the Third World must perforce be carried out in the face of many imperfect conditions. Questions abound concerning how to blend ongoing service with education and professional upgrading. Services delivered too far from the "center" tend to start out defectively and then deteriorate. Advocates of primary medical care and the broad geographical distribution of health resources do recognize these problems but believe that social equity in health care is an overriding goal, despite ineffectiveness or poor quality. The international health physician Carl Taylor (1981) recommends that, in implementing the WHO goal of "Health for All by the Year 2000," the accent should fall upon "for all" rather than upon "health." In regard to developing countries, he writes that there should be "some kind" of health care for everybody, with the implication that some care, even if not of high quality, is better than no care. Pressed to the extreme, and in awareness of the deep vacuums in health care resources that exist in many developing societies, this logic might also condone ineffective means of self-care, medical "alternatives" bordering on quackery, and polypharmacy (Van Der Geest 1982).

If, however, first priority goes to the building up of a central base for future delivery of services at a higher level of quality, then the foregoing considerations would urge the accumulation of a strong professionalized core and of exemplary practice leading to orderly but cautious decentralization.

Demodernization Tensions

Progress in the allocation and deployment of health resources reflects the pull between center and periphery, and it depends upon political balances, the power and predilections of health professional groups, expressed population needs, and health values. Many Third World societies, despite strident nationalism vis-à-vis outsiders, are rent by internal ethnic and regional cleavages that retard the sense of national civic welfare. Third World societies also ponder the acceptability of ideas and things that have the cachet "made in the West." Is that cachet a taint?

Attachment to tradition and a related desire to exploit it for future national development have led many Third World societies into a skeptical stance with regard to innovations from the West. Tensions are felt between the dominant trends toward modernization and countertrends toward demodernization.[2]

Demodernization strains are not confined to Third World societies. Modern societies, especially those framed in a democratic pluralism, tolerate strata and subcultures that explicitly cultivate values and traditions at variance with the societal consensus. Youth culture within industrial society is a well-known example. It expresses powerful yearnings for a more integral, communal mode of existence, running counter to the pressures of bureaucracy and technology that are experienced by young people, whether directly or imaginatively, as depersonalizing and false. Through its dress, music, and social relationships, youth culture protests these pressures.

In Third World societies, the demodernizing impulse lacks the stressful divisiveness of protest by an internal age stratum. Instead it is based upon a widespread, unifying desire to assert indigenous traditions against the alleged materialism of the West and against the legacy of colonial domination.

A typical demodernization posture holds that Western technology is acceptable but Western values are not acceptable. A representative statement is the following assertion by Bakr Abdullah Bakr, rector of the King Fahd University of Petroleum and Minerals in Saudi Arabia: "Some countries have sacrificed the soul of their culture in order to acquire the tools of Western technology. We want the tools but not at the price of annihilating our religion (Islam) and cultural values" (Reynolds 1980).

Applied to health care, Bakr's statement raises by implication the question: Is modern health care a set of tools and techniques that embody no value other than the acultural, apolitical, panhuman values of healing and relief from suffering? Or is it a value-skewed program that favors certain value systems over others? By comparison, consider military preparedness as a value that is done in the name of the neutral, internationally recognized right of self-defense. Carried out to an extensive degree, military preparedness is not in fact neutral; it has been historically associated with totalitarian political systems.

Modern health care is a more neutral value than is military preparedness. It finds positive acceptance in Third World societies despite their variable political–economic complexion. Third World governments, though hampered by meager resources and general cultural underdevelopment, have generally committed themselves to the expansion of health care resources and the improvement of health. This commitment occurs in the fields of both public health and clinical medicine. A revealing indication of the clinical commitment can be seen from the fact that Third World nations increased the number of their medical schools between 1955 and 1974 by 124 percent, compared with the figure of 43 percent for the Western industrialized nations (Kindig and Taylor 1985).

This does not mean, however, that modern medicine is exempt from Third World modernization–demodernization tensions. Third World societies and social strata have various bases for objection to modern medicine. For example, modern medicine has a characteristic disregard of indigenous healing traditions and methods. Most physicians instinctively distrust herbal medicines because the effective strength is unknown and therefore cannot be titered, in contrast with manufactured pharmaceuticals. Further, the criticisms of medical care found in industrialized societies (Carlson 1975; Illich 1976; Waitzkin and Waterman 1971) will also come to be found in the Third World. Third World "critics of medicine" would not be, in structural locus, the farming and village peasantry, whose limited exposure to modern medicine occurs mainly in government-sponsored health clinics, but rather urban dwellers, who have greater access to the marketplace for private medical services in the metropolitan areas.

I will give two case examples of criticism of modern medicine that stem from demodernization values. For each case, I will describe the cultural context that produces the demodernization sentiment. Both cases show that, even when modern medical technique is valued, cultural doubts crystallize in relation to the social circumstances of its delivery.

First Case: Amish Attitudes toward High Medical Bills

This example deals with the impact of a particular instance of neonatal intensive medical care among the Old Order Amish in the United States. The Amish are a rural, endogamous, nonproselytizing Christian Anabaptist sect. They coexist with "the world" but largely reject its ways to follow their traditional, "plain" way of life. They use modern medical care, but they also resort to many traditional herbal remedies and to nonmedical practitioners such as chiropractors (Hostetler 1980). Although unmistakably rooted in Western culture, the Amish can be regarded as a highly traditionalized "demodernization pocket" in North America.

The following excerpts (with my explanatory comments in brackets) are taken from *The Diary* (1983 and 1984), a church newsletter circulated in the Old Order society. Published monthly, *The Diary* contains religious materials, genealogies; and listings of births, marriages, deaths, and illnesses among the Amish, as well as news of their farming activities and family migrations to new agricultural areas.

August 1983: *Community Notes from Dunnville, Kentucky.* On Tues. Morning the 26th, John and Marie Detwiler had a little boy weighing only some over 2 lb. The baby was taken to Lexington [the University of Kentucky Medical Center in Lexington, Kentucky] as soon as it could be moved. Marie was in Intensive Care in Somerset Hospital [sixty-five miles from Lexington and twenty miles from the hamlet of Dunnville], Tues. and Wed. Is still in hospital but is gaining. She had to have 12 units of blood.

October 1983. The small son of John and Marie Detwiler is still in Lexington, U.K. Medical Center. He has been named Jake. He now weighs about 3 lb. and can keep his formula down. They are talking of sending him back to Somerset as they need room for sicker babies. Their hospital bill was $33,000 already a week ago. *How can they charge such outrageous prices!*

[Later dispatch in the same issue] The small son of John and Marie Detwiler has been transferred to the Somerset Hospital to make it closer to the parents. They are in the process of bringing him home as soon as the monitor is ready. They are fixing up a monitor with a battery [Amish households, on religious principle, do not use electricity from public utility companies and use battery-generated electricity only exceptionally]. The baby now weighs 4 lb. 14 oz. The bill in Lexington is around $60,000 and they'd appreciate any help that anybody wished to share.

November 1983. Baby Detwiler has made a big improvement and is weighing almost 7 lbs. now but is still on the monitor at home. He had a very bad spell the evening of the 11th when he turned blue and was given artificial respiration and rushed to the hospital after being home.

February 1984. The Detwiler baby spent another 4 days in the Lexington hospital the early part of the month with broncholitis [*sic*] and inner ear infection but is doing good again. He lost quite a bit of weight in that time but is up to over 12 pounds again. They received a nice sum of money on their big hospital bill from different Amish communities that was greatly appreciated and may God Bless each and every one that helped. They are taking him to a chiropractor once a week now and they found a slight back problem that they thought may have happened when he was so tiny. He seems to have more strength and can make himself stiffer.

In March 1984, I interviewed a delegation of four Amish fathers, including the infant's father who had come from Dunnville to the University of Kentucky Medical Center to discuss payment of the bill. It was clear that they had confidence in the medical competence of the Medical Center but that they were greatly perturbed at the size of the bill.

They did not use the words "overcharge" or "greedy," but such thoughts seemed to lie close to the surface of their thinking. In their cultural relationship to medical facilities, the Amish are even more on the "outside" than most patients; being committed to an agricultural way of life and opposed to secondary and higher education (for themselves), no Amish person could ever become a health professional. In the Amish view, doctors, nurses, and hospitals occupied a worthy vocational niche in the plan of life, but something had gone wrong when health professionals could render such huge bills. These Amish men did not seem to have much grasp, I thought, of the cost of materials, services, and overhead in a medical center. Along with much of the American public (of which they are, however, not a representative segment), they perhaps feel that physicians receive inordinately large financial rewards. In cases such as the Detwiler infant, however, even a "leveling out" of physician incomes would still leave very high bills.

In examining this case from the standpoint of demodernization values, I note that the Amish objections focused entirely on money. They were prepared to pay a good deal for the infant's treatment—but in their thinking, about $100 to $150 a day would be the legitimate maximum.

Amish economic values emphasize hard work and self-sufficiency, coupled with a strong pattern of mutual aid to Amish families that experience adversity. The Amish shun "worldly" financial institutions such as insurance companies and U.S. governmental programs of special assistance (despite the fact that they pay taxes and are "entitled"). The Detwiler's attitude is different from that of the average American family that, confronted with a large medical bill, shakes its head in amazement and then proceeds to determine what insurance coverage or governmental entitlements are within its reach. Although distressed, the Amish in this instance were very far from rejecting modern medicine or mounting a call for the reform of its economic organization. Their attitude reflected a traditional set of values, which, juxtaposed to modern medicine, produced a demodernizing critique.[3]

Second Case: Islamic Medicine

The phenomenon of Islamic resurgence, generally familiar through accounts of "return to the veil" on the part of women in Iran and Egypt and the rising political prominence of conservative sects, has a medical dimension that is less well known. Groups of Muslim physicians, all Western-trained or recipients of Western-equivalent training in Middle Eastern medical schools, are attempting to articulate a modality of medical practice—"Islamic medicine"—that reflects the precepts of Islam.

Middle Eastern history provides a provenance for the definition of Islamic medicine. The names and contributions of Arab physicians such as Avicenna (Ibn Sina) and Al-Razi are well known in Western histories of medicine: the work of Arab physicians in starting hospitals in the Middle East, in a period when European civilization was in a low ebb, is also well known (Khairallah 1946). The historical record makes it clear, however, that Arabic medicine, along with broader Arabic culture, burned brightly from the seventh through the twelfth centuries and then quickly spent itself.

If Arabic medicine had maintained its dynamic energy, then there would be no contemporary need to recreate a tradition of Islamic medicine. The purposes and prospects of such a cultural recreation are uncertain. It may be no more successful than Benito Mussolini's invocation of imperial Rome to shore up Italian fascism, or Abdel Nasser's public reminiscing about the glory of pharaonic Egypt. However, the quest for Islamic medicine may have more solid possibilities. Rather than being the fantasy of a single demagogic leader, it is part of a broader cultural movement that is seated in and linked by diverse groups.

The cultural construction of Islamic medicine is a demodernization response because it aims to orient the practice of medicine by the precepts and values of a well-established tradition that predates modern medicine. Although it has varied manifestations and strategies, it has two common features. First, it accepts the technology of modern medicine and, more tacitly, the validity of biomedical knowledge (though doctrinal Islam balks at certain parts of modern science, such as evolutionary biology). Second, Islamic medicine is the project of practicing physicians who are oriented to clinical medicine, rather than of health officials, public health physicians, nonmedical personnel, patients, or the public at large. As a corollary, the only kind of health care with which Islamic medicine concerns itself is that in which the physician is the pivotal figure.

Having stated the common elements, I present three expressions of Islamic medicine that reflect the varied geographic, societal, and medical practice situations of their proponents.

First, there are several thousand Muslim physicians currently practicing in the United States and Canada. Not all have maintained active religious ties; however, the many who have have constituted themselves into the Islamic Medical Association of North America (IMA). Like other professional associations, the IMA publishes a newsletter and a journal and holds conventions.

The IMA physicians offer Islamic critiques and remedies to the problems of contemporary medicine in North America. Consider the following statements in an IMA *Newsletter* editorial by the organization's president, H. F. Nagamia:

> American medicine is undergoing rapid changes . . . the rapid development in technology has enabled medicine to advance at a phenomenal rate. . . . However, American medicine has developed a lot of failures. Most of these are related to the commercial exploitation of medicine. . . . American medicine has become a business and is no longer centered towards the individual physician who had at one time a "one to one" patient-physician relationship. . . .
>
> Are there any answers? . . .
>
> First and foremost the physician needs to gain back the respect of the patient he once enjoyed.
>
> Perhaps very humbly I should point out that the "Muslim physicians" that practiced one thousand years ago had achieved the respect of their patients. . . .
>
> If ever such a practice of Islamic Medicine is restored here in America or in any other nation I think that the physician will regain the confidence of the patient and his respect will be restored. Unfortunately, until that happens we are going to face a decline in medicine for years to come. (1985)

The foregoing statement by Nagamia focuses on the doctor–patient relationship as the redeeming element in health care amid the profuse necessities of technology and the rising importance of nonmedical providers in medical care. His vision of the doctor–patient relationship emphasizes the "whole patient" as against more impersonal organ- or disease-centered models of medical care. However, his vision is strongly "physician-dominated" and shows no awareness of the tendencies toward greater equality and more open communication between patient and doctor than have prevailed in the past (Haug and Lavin 1981; Reeder 1972).

A second manifestation of Islamic medicine occurs in the medical conferences of Islamic medical societies or Islamic nations. These conferences typically have one series of papers presenting clinical and laboratory research in the various medical specialties and a second, Islamic series that seeks to confirm the consistency of Koranic precepts with contemporary biomedical knowledge. Many of the Islamic papers deal with human embryological processes, such as the fertilization of the egg by the sperm and the stages of embryonic genesis; they correlate scientific terminology with texts (sura) from the Koran. Others deal with sexual practices, finding support for Koranic admonitions against promiscuity in current medical knowledge concerning sexually transmitted disease, especially the newer forms such as genital herpes and AIDS.

Representative titles of presented papers from a recent national medical conference in Saudi Arabia (which is a thoroughly Islamic society) include: *Human Sex Development and the Correlation with the Quran and Hadith, The Key of an Embryo's Future*, [and] *The Place of Scientific Aspects of the Holy Quran in the Medical Curriculum (Abstracts* 1983).

A third example of Islamic medicine deals with the use of the Arabic language in medical conferences and medical education. The foregoing Saudi medical conferences started in 1976. They have been conducted in English but increasingly use Arabic as the medium for oral delivery of the Islamic medicine papers and for the publication of written reports and abstracts on all topics. Correspondingly, the four extant Saudi medical schools have relied upon English as the medium of instruction, but they too have recently attempted a greater use of Arabic (greatly hampered, however, by the lack of medical textbooks in Arabic).

The language trend is a critical dimension of Islamic medicine because, among Muslims, Arabic has the status of a hallowed language, even more integral to Islamic religious sensibility and orthodoxy than Latin was to medieval Christianity or German to Lutheranism. Although many educated Muslims speak and read some English or French, to receive education and conference content in Arabic not only is far easier for them but also spares them the cultural discomfort that may come from dependent reliance upon a former colonial language (Gallagher 1985).

None of the foregoing examples of Islamic medicine should be construed to mean that its proponents are intent upon building a non-Western brand of medical practice, or that they want to slow the introduction of modern medical techniques into Islamic societies. Instead, they seek a demodernized, Islamic dimension of medicine that will coexist with and provide a cultural support for modern medicine. Islamic medicine will perhaps be able, in time, to constitute itself as a culturally confirming commentary on modern medicine within a restricted domain, but one doubts that it will ever exert a powerful force, even in Islamic societies.

Comparing the Cases

The foregoing Amish and Islamic case examples, drawn from highly contrasting cultural traditions, illustrate demodernization as a generic cultural process. These cases also show that, like the biological variations that different individuals manifest in response to a common pathogen, demodernization strains vary in a manner that reflects inherent characteristics of the traditional culture that is being challenged by modernization. The basic Amish cultural–historical position—passive endurance of the world's evils—was set in the mold of religious persecution of the Amish in sixteenth- and seventeenth-century Europe. Now safe and respected in their North American refuges, the Amish make a gentle protest against the "persecution" of high medical bills. In contrast, the Islamic tradition has historically been that of social and cultural ascendancy. The efforts to articulate Islamic medicine reflect a desire to envelop modern Western medicine within a cognitive web of Islamic and Arabic legitimation. Whatever actual impact of Islamic medicine, the attempt comes from an ambitious conviction.

The Amish and Islamic examples also refer back to Berger's (1973) categorization of bureaucracy and technology as primary carriers of modernity. The Amish and the Islamic medicine exponents both accept the technology of modern medicine; their reservations focus instead on its bureaucratic or social–organizational context—the ways in which medical bills are generated and borne, and the ways in which medical authority and judgment are eroded in modern medicine. In general, bureaucracy as a primary carrier is more likely than technology to retain residues of traditional values, human relationships, and economic arrangements. Thus demodernization programs tolerate or even embrace technology but strive to conserve social and economic forms that are prebureaucratic.

Summary

This chapter has attempted to bring medical care within the purview of modernization concepts. One of the most characteristic features of modern medicine is its status as a calculable commodity or resource. Premodern systems of health care lack this feature. Traditional cultures react to modern medicine with demodernization strains, which I have illustrated by Amish and Islamic case examples. Further work analyzing the relationships between medical care and modernization will increase conceptual acuity in regard to fruitful concepts in this area and add substantively to the comprehension of modern society.

NOTES

1. Problems in the operation and maintenance of equipment occur in the hospitals and clinics of developed societies, of course (Strauss et al. 1985), but not as frequently as in many Third World societies. Other problematic medical phenomena, such as the geographic maldistribution of resources and demodernization protests, can also be found in developed societies. What characterizes the Third World picture is a consistent difference in degree, not an absolute difference in kind.

2. Parallel with my usage of "modernization," I intend here to use the concept of demodernization in a value-neutral sense, free from the implication that modernization is a wholly benign or progressive process whereas demodernization is a correspondingly regressive or atavistic tendency. The opposite stance is also rejected, namely, that modernization is "bad" (because of depersonalization, loss of personal autonomy, cultural uprooting, or other alleged faults) whereas demodernization is correspondingly "good." It will further be clear that demodernization, as used analytically here, is not concretely tied to Third World events: industrialized societies have their own pockets of demodernization, as revealed in the subsequent discussion of Amish attitudes, within a U.S. setting, toward American medical care.

3. A respected colleague who read this article in draft offered the criticism that the Amish case expresses a questioning of a particular feature of American medical care—namely, the extent to which individual patients must meet their own expenses—more than it expresses a demodernization protest.

This is an instructive criticism, which I nevertheless answer by noting that demodernization is a general concept that subsumes many phenomena and processes. Specific demodernizing tactics and messages always occur within a particular place, time, and social structure. Thus in their raids on the "manufactories" that used the new textile machinery, the Luddites of early nineteenth-century England were attempting to maintain a market demand for their manual skills in the face of technological displacement. Though they were concerned with their immediate economic self-interest and lacked the articulate and morally informed demodernizing ideology of, for example, a Mohandas Gandhi, they were nevertheless authentic demodernizers.

In the Amish example, the Detwiler family confronted a temporally situated social structure—the American medical care system. Two important characteristics of this system are (1) its technological progressiveness, leading to high costs, and (2) its historical lack of comprehensive governmental provision for the organization and financing of medical care.

Though one readily sympathizes with the plight of anyone who is weighed down by medical costs, I believe there is a certain naivete in the Amish objection to their high medical bill. Their traditionalism and otherworldliness keep them innocent of the "facts of life" about medical care. Neonatal care is inherently intense and correspondingly expensive, no matter who pays the bill. The Amish response in this instance is an integral part of their thoroughgoing demodernizing stance in the modern world. One could imagine that a group such as the Amish, who pride themselves on being "old-fashioned," can in perfect character and consistency reject the forms and benefits of virtually everything modern—except modern medical care. Although the Amish do have their own "low-resource" folk remedies, they have no exclusive commitment to these. They thus are peculiarly open to the benefits of modern medicine, but, given their withdrawal from "the world," they do not take a political or ideological interest in shaping medical care delivery to their communal values. Instead, they question its cost that, in the analysis here, counts as a demodernization protest.

REFERENCES

Abstracts of the Eighth Saudi Medical Conference. 1983. Riyadh: Al-Saud National University.

Berger, Peter L., Brigitte Berger, and Hansfried Kellner. 1973. *The Homeless Mind—Modernization and Consciousness.* New York: Random House.

Carlson, Rick J. 1975. *The End of Medicine.* New York: John Wiley.

The Diary. 1983, 1984. Gordonville, Pa.: Pequea Publishers (Monthly Serial).

Eisenstadt, Shmuel N. 1966. *Modernization: Protest and Change.* Englewood Cliffs, N.J.: Prentice-Hall.

Field, Mark G. 1980. "The Health System and the Polity: A Contemporary American Dialectic." *Social Science and Medicine* 4A:397–413.

Gallagher, Eugene B. 1985. "Medical Education in Saudi Arabia: A Sociological Perspective on Modernization and Language." *Journal of Asian and African Studies* 20(1/2):1–12.

Goldthorpe, J. E. 1984. *The Sociology of the Third World.* 2d ed. Cambridge: Cambridge University Press.

Haug, Marie R., and Bebe Lavin. 1981. "Practitioner or Patient—Who's in Charge?" *Journal of Health and Social Behavior* 22:212–29.

Hostetler, John A. 1980. *Amish Society.* 3d ed. Baltimore: Johns Hopkins University Press.

Illich, Ivan. 1976. *Medical Nemesis: The Expropriation of Health.* New York: Pantheon.

Khairallah, Amin. 1946. *Outline of Arabic Contributions to Medicine.* Beirut: American Press.

Kindig, David A., and Charles M. Taylor. 1985. "Growth in the International Physician Supply." *Journal of the American Medical Association* 5:253.

Lerner, Daniel. 1958. *The Passing of Traditional Society: Modernizing the Middle East.* New York: Free Press.

Levy, Marion. 1966. *Modernization and the Structure of Societies.* Princeton, N.J.: Princeton University Press.

Nagamia, H. F. 1985. *Islamic Medical Association Newsletter* 9 (April 1):1–2.

Parsons, Talcott. 1949. *The Structure of Social Action.* 2d ed. Glencoe, Ill.: Free Press.

———. 1951. *The Social System.* Glencoe, Ill.: Free Press.

Reeder, Leo G. 1972. "The Patient-Client as a Consumer: Some Observations on the Changing Professional–Client Relationship." *Journal of Health and Social Behavior* 13:406–12.

Relman, Arnold S. 1980. "The New Medical–Industrial Complex." *New England Journal of Medicine* 303:963–70.

Reynolds, Barry. 1980. "Their Fathers' Sons." *Aramco World Magazine* 31 (January–February):2–11.

Sebai, Zohair A. 1981. *The Health of the Family in a Changing Arabia—A Case Study of Primary Care.* Jeddah, Saudi Arabia: Tihama.

Stebbins, Kenyon R. 1986. "Politics, Economics, and Health Services in Rural Oaxaca, Mexico." *Human Organization* 45 (Summer):112–19.

Strauss, Anselm, Shizuko Fagerhaugh, Barbara Suczek, and Carolyn Wiener. 1985. *Social Organization of Medical Work.* Chicago: University of Chicago Press.

Sukkary, Soheir. 1981. "She Is No Stranger: The Traditional Midwife in Egypt." *Medical Anthropology* 5 (Winter):26–34.

Taylor, Carl E. 1981. "An Interview with Dr. Carl E. Taylor." *International Health News* (August):11.

Van Der Geest, Sjakk. 1982. "The Illegal Distribution of Western Medicines in Developing Countries: Pharmacists, Drug Peddlers, Injection Doctors, and Others. A Bibliographic Exploration." *Medical Anthropology* 6 (Fall):197–219.

Waitzkin, Howard, and Barbara Waterman. 1971. *The Exploitation of Illness in Capitalist Society.* New York: Bobbs-Merrill.

World Health Organization (WHO). 1980. *Annual Report of the Regional Director for the Eastern Mediterranean.* Cairo: WHO.

About the Contributors

Collins O. Airhihenbuwa is associate professor of health education at Pennsylvania State University.

S. Ogoh Alubo is professor of sociology at the University of Jos, Nigeria.

Carol J. Pierce Colfer is a research associate at the East–West Center, University of Hawaii.

Peter Conrad is professor of sociology at Brandeis University.

Sally E. Findley is associated with the Center for Population and Family Health, Columbia University.

Eugene B. Gallagher is professor of sociology in the Department of Behavioral Science, University of Kentucky Medical School.

Rita S. Gallin is director of the Women and International Development Program and professor of sociology at Michigan State University.

Mary-Jo DelVecchio Good is associate professor of sociology in the Department of Social Medicine, Harvard Medical School.

Ira E. Harrison is associate professor of anthropology at the University of Tennessee.

Charles W. Hunt is assistant professor of sociology at the University of Utah.

Linda Hunt is assistant professor of anthropology at the University of North Carolina at Charlotte.

Yasuki Kobayashi is a faculty member at the School of Public Health, Teikyo University, Japan.

Tsunetsugu Munakata is associate professor of health and sports sciences at University Tsukoba, Japan.

Stella R. Quah is professor of sociology at the National University of Singapore.

Joseph W. Schneider is professor of sociology at Drake University.

Kenyon Rainier Stebbins is associate professor of anthropology at West Virginia University.

Janardan Subedi is assistant professor of sociology at Miami University, Ohio.

Sree Subedi is assistant professor of sociology at Miami University, Ohio, at Hamilton.

Index

Migrant labor. *See* AIDS and migrant labor in Africa

Ministering and monitoring as tasks of family care work, 161–62

Modernization, 78, 100–101, 135; alternative to theory of, 229–30; de-modernization tensions, 297–304; family care work and, 174–76; health care and (*see* Health care and modernization); theory, 287–89

Modern medicine: in developing countries, xvii–xix; curative (clinical) versus preventive, xi–xii, 141, 234; history, strength, weaknesses, and contributions of, in Nepal, 112–19; integration of traditional medicine and, 126–29; traditional medicine and, xvi–xvii. *See also* Oncology practice and disclosure

Mortality, causes of, in Singapore, 85

"Mother-roasting" birthing practice, 253–54

Moxibustion technique, 254–55

Muslim Law Act, 83

Muslim medicine. *See* Islamic medicine

Nafadh technique, 254

National health policies and traditional medicine, 129–31

Nepal, 276, 277. *See also* Traditional medicine and modern medicine in Nepal

Nicaragua, 224

Nigeria, traditional health care in, 123–24, 124–25. *See also* Public health programs in Nigeria

Nurses: birthing and, 258; family care work and, 169–74

Oaxaca, Mexico. *See* Public health programs in Mexico

Oil boom in Nigeria, 231

Oman. *See* Birthing practices in Oman

Oncology practice and disclosure, 180–210; comparative perspective on, 202–5; in Japan, 184–93; in Mexico, 193–202; in United States, 181–84

Optimism and American oncology practice, 182–84

Oral rehydration therapy (ORT), 236, 275, 278

Ownership: of social science research, 272–74; of traditional medical knowledge, 127, 128–29

Pain relief during birthing, 259–60

Pakistan, health indicators for, 111

Pasantes in Mexico, 216–17, 220

Patent laws, 128–29

Patients: characteristics of emergency, 63–64; disclosure to (*see* Oncology practice and disclosure); perspectives on medical urgency, 69–70; types of emergency, 66–69

Peiban, Chinese, 156. *See also* Family care work in Chinese hospitals

Periphery-core concept, 8–9, 229–30

Permission form-signing as task of family care work, 162–63, 171

Peru, 267–68

Philippines, development and health indicators, 83–84

Physicians: class relations and Mexican, 215; experiences of disclosure in Japan by, 189–91; family care work and, 169–74; Mexican *pasantes*, 216–17, 220. *See also* Oncology practice and disclosure; Training of physicians

Placenta, delivery and disposal of, 252–53

Politics. *See* Sociopolitics of health

Position during birthing, 250–51

Postpartum period, 253–54

Poverty and distribution of wealth, 219

Preventive medicine, curative medicine versus, xi–xii, 141, 234. *See also* Ethnicity and health behavior in Singapore

Primary care, emergency services as, 72

Process-documentation research, 277

Professional authority of Mexican physicians, 200–202

Prostitution, AIDS and, 12–13, 17, 23, 26–28

Public health programs, xix; clinical versus preventive medicine, xi–xii; in Nepal, 117–18; in Saudi Arabia, 295

Public health programs in Mexico, 211–27, 294–95; historical context, 213–17; Mexican Constitution and, 212; research setting and conclusions, 217–21, 222–24; WHO HFA/2000 program and, 211, 221–22

Public health programs in Nigeria, 228–45; implementations of HFA/2000, 233–37; political economy of Nigeria and, 229–33; problems and constraints of, 237–42

Relationships (*guanxi*), Chinese, 165–69

Religion and health behavior: in Africa, 123–24; Amish attitudes toward high medical bills, 298–300, 303–4; Islam and, 96–97, 99–100, 139, 149;